HEALTHCARE PROFESSIONAL GUIDES

DISEASES

Springhouse Corporation
Springhouse, Pennsylvania

Staff

Senior Publisher
Matthew Cahill

Editorial Director
Patricia Dwyer Schull, RN, MSN

Clinical Manager
Judith Schilling McCann, RN, MSN

Art Director
John Hubbard

Senior Project Editor
Kathy E. Goldberg

Clinical Project Manager
Helene K. Nawrocki, RN, MSN

Clinical Editors
Stanley W. Nawrocki, RN, CEN; Beverly Ann
Tscheschlog, RN; Marybeth Morrell, RN, CCRN,
Collette Bishop Hendler, RN, CCRN

Copy Editors
Cynthia C. Breuninger (manager), Karen C.
Comerford, Stacey A. Follin, Brenna H. Mayer,
Pamela Wingrod

Designers
Arlene Putterman (associate art director),
Elaine Ezrow, Joe Clark, Jacalyn Facciolo, Susan
Hopkins Rodzewich, Jeff Sklarow, Mary Stangl

Illustrators
Jacalyn Facciolo, Jean Gardner, John Gist,
Francis Grobelny, Bob Jackson, BJ Krim, Bob
Neumann, Judy Newhouse, George Retseck,
Phillis Carol Nathans

Typography
Diane Paluba (manager), Joyce Rossi Biletz,
Phyllis Marron, Valerie Rosenberger

Manufacturing
Deborah Meiris (director), Pat Dorshaw
(manager), T.A. Landis, Otto Mezei

Production Coordinator
Margaret A. Rastiello

Editorial Assistants
Beverly Lane, Mary Madden

Indexer
Barbara Hodgson

Printed in the United States of America.
HCPGDIS-021198

 A member of the Reed Elsevier plc group

**Library of Congress Cataloging-in-Publication
Data**
Diseases.
    p. cm. — (Healthcare professional guides)
    Includes bibliographical references and index.
    1. Diseases — Handbooks, manuals, etc.
    2. Nursing — Handbooks, manuals, etc.
    I. Springhouse Corporation. II. Series.
    [DNLM: 1. Diseases — handbooks. 2. Thera-
    peutics — handbooks. QZ 39 D611 1997]
RT65.D49 1997
616 — dc21
DNLM/DLC   97-24667
ISBN 0-87434-913-3   CIP

Contents

Advisory board

Foreword

The patient in room 327 has just been diagnosed with histoplasmosis. What kind of disease is that? You don't remember. What precautions, if any, must you take when caring for this patient?

Where can you get this information immediately? There's no time for a visit to the hospital library. You need the facts now!

Where will you start looking? To find information about a specific disease or condition, you usually need to know at least what type of disease it is before you can locate the information. And you might need to consult several references before you can find exactly what you want.

As a busy health care professional, you don't have that kind of time.

Face it. You can't know everything related to health care, even if you've worked in your profession for many years. What's more, the amount of knowledge in medicine and science keeps growing at a mind-boggling rate.

But now there's help. *Diseases* supplies up-to-the minute information on over 350 diseases and disorders. The book is a real boon for all health professionals involved in patient care — both the experienced practitioner and the student. This valuable reference has close to 400 pages, yet is extremely compact.

What's more, because diseases and conditions are arranged in alphabetical order, you don't need to know the disease type to locate the one you're looking for. You'll also find information presented in a consistent manner and in a concise format. Each entry starts with a brief description of

the disease, then details the causes and characteristic signs and symptoms. Next, you'll learn about appropriate diagnostic tests, standard treatment, and potential complications of the disease. Each entry ends with special considerations, such as tips on preventing the spread of the disease and instructions on dealing with a potential life-threatening crisis.

This valuable book offers more than 50 illustrations as well as numerous charts. Attention-getting graphics highlight four recurrent themes: pathophysiology, urgent interventions, prevention guidelines, and patient teaching.

At the end of the volume, you'll find a critical thinking self-test, a summary chart that provides concise information on dozens of additional disorders, and a list of patient outcomes for selected diseases.

In short, you'll find everything you need for an informed overview — so you can get back to your patient fast. In fact, this little volume contains so much information in such an easy-to-read format that you may find you don't need any other references.

Diseases should become a welcome addition to the book collections of all health care practitioners and an indispensable reference in your daily practice.

Ellen P. Digan, MA, MT (ASCP)
Coordinator, MLT Program
Professor of Biology
Manchester Community-
  Technical College
Manchester, Conn.

Abdominal aneurysm

In an abdominal aneurysm, an abnormal dilation in the arterial wall generally occurs in the aorta, between the renal arteries and iliac branches. Over 50% of all people with untreated abdominal aneurysms die within 2 years of diagnosis, mainly from aneurysmal rupture.

These aneurysms develop slowly. A focal weakness in the muscular layer of the aorta, caused by degenerative changes, allows the inner and outer layers to stretch outward. Blood pressure within the aorta progressively weakens the vessel walls and enlarges the aneurysm.

CAUSES
About 95% of abdominal aortic aneurysms result from arteriosclerosis; the rest, from cystic medial necrosis, trauma, syphilis, and other infections.

SIGNS AND SYMPTOMS
Although abdominal aneurysms usually don't produce symptoms, most are evident (unless the patient is obese) as a pulsating mass in the periumbilical area, accompanied by a systolic bruit over the aorta. A large aneurysm may cause symptoms that mimic renal calculi, lumbar disk disease, or duodenal compression.

Pain, rupture, and hemorrhage
Lumbar pain that radiates to the flank and groin (from pressure on lumbar nerves) may signify aneurysm enlargement and imminent rupture. If the aneurysm ruptures into the peritoneal cavity, it causes severe, persistent abdominal and back pain.

Signs and symptoms of hemorrhage include weakness, sweating, tachycardia, and hypotension. Patients with rupture into the retroperitoneal space may remain stable for hours before shock and death occur; 20% die immediately.

DIAGNOSTIC TESTS
This aneurysm is often detected accidentally on X-ray or during a routine physical examination. Ultrasound can determine its size, shape, and location. Aortography shows the condition of vessels near the aneurysm and the extent of the aneurysm.

TREATMENT
Usually, an abdominal aneurysm must be resected and the damaged aortic section replaced with a Dacron graft. If the aneurysm is small and causes no symptoms, surgery may be delayed. Regular physical examinations and ultrasound checks are necessary to detect enlargement, which may precede a rupture. Large aneurysms or those that produce symptoms pose a significant risk of rupture and require immediate repair.

SPECIAL CONSIDERATIONS
 ACTION STAT: Stay alert for signs of rupture — decreasing blood pressure; increasing pulse and respiratory rates; cool, clammy skin; restlessness; and decreased sensorium.
• The patient is usually helped to walk as soon as possible (generally the 2nd day after surgery).
• Provide psychological support for the patient and family. Appropriate explanations and answers to their questions will help ease their fears about the intensive care unit, the threat of impending aneurysm rupture, and surgery.

Acquired immunodeficiency syndrome

One of the most widely publicized diseases, acquired immunodeficiency syndrome (AIDS) is marked by progressive failure of the immune system, which makes the patient susceptible to opportunistic infections, unusual cancers, and other abnormalities. AIDS is characterized by gradual destruction of cell-mediated (T-cell) immunity. However, the disease also affects humoral immunity and even autoimmunity.

Since AIDS was first described by the Centers for Disease Control and Prevention (CDC) in 1981, the CDC has declared a case surveillance definition for AIDS and modified it several times, most recently in 1993.

CAUSES

AIDS is caused by human immunodeficiency virus (HIV) type I. HIV transmission occurs by contact with infected blood or body fluids. HIV strikes cells bearing the CD4+ antigen. The latter serves as a receptor for the retrovirus and lets it enter the cell. HIV prefers to infect the CD4+ lymphocyte but may also infect other CD4+ antigen-bearing cells.

AIDS begins with infection by the HIV retrovirus and ends with the severely immunocompromised, terminal disease stage. The time elapsed from acute HIV infection to the appearance of symptoms to the diagnosis of AIDS and, eventually, to death varies greatly. Current antiretroviral therapy and prophylaxis and treatment of common opportunistic infections can delay the progression of HIV disease and prolong survival.

The HIV infection process takes three forms:
• immunodeficiency (opportunistic infections and unusual cancers)
• autoimmunity (lymphoid interstitial pneumonitis, arthritis, hypergammaglobulinemia, and production of autoimmune antibodies)
• neurologic dysfunction (AIDS dementia complex, HIV encephalopathy, and peripheral neuropathies).

Transmission

HIV is transmitted by direct inoculation during intimate sexual contact, transfusion of contaminated blood or blood products, sharing of contaminated needles, and transplacental or postpartum transmission from infected mother to fetus (by cervical or blood contact during delivery and in breast milk).

SIGNS AND SYMPTOMS

HIV infection manifests itself in many different ways. After inoculation, the infected person may experience a mononucleosis-like syndrome and then may remain asymptomatic for years. In this latent stage, the only sign of HIV infection is laboratory evidence of seroconversion. When symptoms appear, they may take many forms, including:
• persistent generalized adenopathy
• nonspecific symptoms (weight loss, fatigue, night sweats, fevers)
• neurologic symptoms resulting from HIV encephalopathy
• opportunistic infection or cancer.

DIAGNOSTIC TESTS

Diagnosis is confirmed by the presence of an opportunistic infection with laboratory evidence of HIV infection and a CD4+ T-cell count of less than 200 cells/μl.

Antibody tests indicate HIV infection indirectly by revealing HIV antibodies. Initial screening is done with an enzyme-linked immunosorbent assay (ELISA) test. A positive ELISA test should be repeated and then confirmed by another test — usually the Western blot or an immunofluorescence assay. (Antibody tests are unreliable in neonates because transferred maternal antibodies persist for 6 to 10 months.)

Direct tests can also be performed. These tests include antigen tests (p24 antigen), HIV cultures, nucleic acid probes of peripheral blood lymphocytes, and the polymerase chain reaction.

Current drug treatment for AIDS

Drugs currently used to treat acquired immunodeficiency syndrome (AIDS) include:
- antiretroviral agents, designed to inhibit or inactivate the human immunodeficiency virus (HIV)
- immunomodulatory agents, which boost the weakened immune system
- anti-infective and antineoplastic agents, which combat opportunistic infections and associated cancers; some are used prophylactically to help patients resist opportunistic infections
- protease inhibitors (such as saquinavir [Invirase]), which inhibit the activity of HIV protease, thus preventing cleavage of proteins essential for HIV maturation.

Combination therapy

Most patients receive two or more agents to gain the maximum benefit with the fewest adverse reactions and to help inhibit the production of resistant, mutant HIV strains.

Additional tests are performed to support the diagnosis and help evaluate the severity of immunosuppression.

TREATMENT

No cure has been found for AIDS. However, at least four beneficial forms of treatment are available for HIV disease. (See *Current drug treatment for AIDS.*) Supportive treatments help maintain nutritional status and relieve pain and other distressing symptoms.

Many pathogens in AIDS respond to anti-infective drugs but tend to recur after treatment ends. For this reason, most patients need continuous anti-infective treatment. Zidovudine (AZT) has proved effective in slowing the progression of HIV infection, decreasing opportunistic infections, and prolonging survival. However, it often causes serious adverse reactions and toxicities.

SPECIAL CONSIDERATIONS

- Diligently practicing standard precautions can prevent inadvertent transmission of AIDS.
- Recognize that a diagnosis of AIDS is profoundly distressing because of the disease's social impact and poor

prognosis. The patient may lose his job, financial security, and support of family and friends. Coping with an altered body image, the emotional burden of serious illness, and the threat of death may overwhelm the patient.

Acute respiratory failure in COPD

In patients with chronic obstructive pulmonary disease (COPD), acute respiratory failure may occur if the arterial blood gas (ABG) values and clinical condition deteriorate. (Unlike people with normal lung tissue, those with COPD often have a consistently high partial pressure of arterial carbon dioxide [$PaCO_2$] and a low partial pressure of arterial oxygen [PaO_2].)

CAUSES

Acute respiratory failure may develop in COPD patients from any condition that increases the work of breathing and reduces the respiratory drive. The most common precipitating factor is a respiratory tract infection, such as bronchitis or pneumonia. Other causes include bronchospasm and accu-

Understanding high-frequency ventilation

Used to treat respiratory failure, high-frequency ventilation (HFV) uses high ventilation rates (60 to 3,000 breaths/minute), low tidal volumes, brief inspiratory time, and low peak airway pressures.

HFV has three different delivery forms — high-frequency jet ventilation (HFJV), high-frequency positive-pressure ventilation, and high-frequency oscillation. Here's a brief summary of how HFJV works.

Mechanics of HFJV

A humidified, high-pressure gas jet pulses through the narrow-lumen gas jet valve on inspiration and accelerates as it flows through the port's narrow lumen and into the patient's endotracheal tube.

The pressure and velocity of the jet stream cause a drag effect that entrains low-pressure gases into the patient's airway. These gas flows combine to deliver 100 to 200 breaths/minute to the patient.

The gas stream moves down the airway in a progressively broader wave front of decreasing velocity. Tidal volume is delivered to airways under constant pressure. The gas stream creates turbulence, which causes the gas to vibrate in the airways. Alveolar ventilation increases without raising mean airway pressure or peak inflation pressure.

Benefits of HFJV

- Improved venous return
- Decreased airway pressures and

(possibly) improved pulmonary artery pressure
- Improved arterial gas exchange
- Decreased right ventricular afterload
- Reduced chance of pulmonary barotrauma and decreased cardiac output

Points to remember

- The mechanical setup, parameter alarms, and tubing connections must be checked frequently.
- The patient's respiratory status is assessed regularly.
- If airway secretions are extremely viscous, increased humidification may prevent formation of mucus plugs.

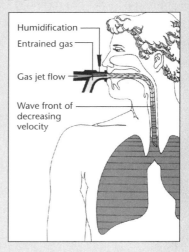

Labels: Humidification — Entrained gas — Gas jet flow — Wave front of decreasing velocity

mulating secretions brought on by cough suppression.

SIGNS AND SYMPTOMS

Increased ventilation-perfusion mismatching and reduced alveolar ventilation cause decreased PaO_2 (hypoxemia) and increased $PaCO_2$ (hypercapnia). The resulting hypoxemia and

acidemia affect all body organs. Specific signs and symptoms include:
- increased, decreased, or normal respiratory rate
- shallow or deep respirations, or alternation between the two
- air hunger, cyanosis, crackles, rhonchi, wheezes, and diminished breath sounds
- restlessness, confusion, irritability,

poor concentration, tremulousness, diminished tendon reflexes, papilledema, and coma
- tachycardia with increased cardiac output and mildly elevated blood pressure
- arrhythmias (with myocardial hypoxia)
- pulmonary hypertension.

DIAGNOSTIC TESTS
Progressive deterioration of ABG levels and pH, when compared to the patient's usual values, strongly suggests acute respiratory failure in COPD. Other findings, such as increased bicarbonate levels and cardiac arrhythmias, support the diagnosis.

TREATMENT
Acute respiratory failure in COPD patients is an emergency that requires cautious oxygen therapy (using nasal prongs or a Venturi mask) to raise the PaO_2. If significant respiratory acidosis persists, mechanical ventilation may be necessary. High-frequency ventilation may be used if the patient doesn't respond to conventional mechanical ventilation. (See *Understanding high-frequency ventilation*.) Treatment routinely includes antibiotics for infection, bronchodilators and, possibly, steroids.

SPECIAL CONSIDERATIONS
- Oxygen is given at concentrations to maintain a PaO_2 of at least 50 to 60 mm Hg. The patient is monitored for improvements in breathing, color, and ABG values.
- If the patient is retaining carbon dioxide, encouraging him to cough and breathe deeply with pursed lips can help maintain a patent airway. If he's alert, urge him to use incentive spirometry. If he's intubated and lethargic, he must be turned every 1 to 2 hours.
- Postural drainage and chest physiotherapy help to clear secretions.
- Monitor the patient closely for signs of respiratory arrest. Keep in mind that changes in breath sounds and ABG values indicate distress.

- The cardiac monitor is closely observed for arrhythmias.
- If the patient requires mechanical ventilation, use of minimal leak technique and a cuffed tube with high residual volume (low-pressure cuff), a foam cuff, or a pressure-regulating valve on the cuff can prevent tracheal erosion caused by artificial airway cuff overinflation.
- To prevent nasal necrosis, the nasotracheal tube should be kept midline within the nostrils and good hygiene should be provided.

Acute tubular necrosis

Acute tubular necrosis (ATN) accounts for about 75% of all cases of acute renal failure. It's the most common cause of acute renal failure in critically ill patients. ATN injures the tubular segment of the nephron, causing renal failure and uremic syndrome. Mortality ranges from 40% to 70%.

CAUSES
ATN results from ischemic or nephrotoxic injury, most commonly in debilitated patients, such as the critically ill and those who have undergone extensive surgery.

In ischemic injury, disruption of blood flow to the kidneys may result from circulatory collapse, severe hypotension, trauma, hemorrhage, dehydration, cardiogenic or septic shock, surgery, anesthetics, or reactions to transfusions. Ischemic ATN can cause lesions in the renal interstitium.

In nephrotoxic injury, damage may follow ingestion of certain chemical agents or result from a hypersensitive reaction of the kidneys. Because nephrotoxic ATN doesn't damage the basement membrane of the nephron, it's potentially reversible.

SIGNS AND SYMPTOMS
ATN can be hard to recognize in early stages because effects of the critically ill patient's primary disease may

mask symptoms. The first obvious effect may be decreased urine output. Generally, hyperkalemia and uremic syndrome soon follow, along with oliguria and confusion, which may progress to uremic coma. Other complications may include congestive heart failure, uremic pericarditis, and pulmonary edema.

DIAGNOSTIC TESTS
ATN is hard to diagnose accurately until the advanced stage. Significant laboratory clues are urinary sediment containing red blood cells (RBCs) and casts, and diluted urine with low specific gravity, low osmolality, and a high sodium level.

Blood studies reveal elevated blood urea nitrogen and serum creatinine levels, anemia, defects in platelet adherence, metabolic acidosis, and hyperkalemia. An electrocardiogram may show arrhythmias and, with hyperkalemia, a widening QRS segment, disappearing P waves, and tall, peaked T waves.

TREATMENT
During the acute phase of ATN, the patient requires vigorous supportive measures until normal kidney function resumes. Initial treatment may include diuretics and infusion of a large volume of fluids. Long-term fluid management requires daily replacement of projected and calculated losses.

Other measures to control complications include packed RBC transfusions for anemia and antibiotics for infection. Hyperkalemia may warrant emergency I.V. administration of 50% glucose, regular insulin, and sodium bicarbonate. Sodium polystyrene sulfonate with sorbitol may be given to reduce extracellular potassium levels. Peritoneal dialysis or hemodialysis may be needed if the patient is catabolic.

SPECIAL CONSIDERATIONS
 ACTION STAT: Report fever and chills (indications of infection) immediately. If the patient has an indwelling urinary catheter in place, flank pain may also indicate infection.

• Because the debilitated patient is vulnerable to infection, aseptic technique must be strictly applied.

• Foods containing sodium and potassium, such as bananas and orange juice, must be restricted. Prescribed medications should be checked for potassium content.

• Providing adequate calories and essential amino acids while restricting protein intake ensures an anabolic state.

 PREVENTION: To help prevent pulmonary complications, encourage the patient to do coughing and deep-breathing exercises.

Adenoviral infections

Adenoviruses cause acute self-limiting febrile infections, with inflammation of the respiratory or ocular mucous membranes, or both.

Adenoviruses have 35 known serotypes. Adenoviral organisms are common and can remain latent for years. They infect almost everyone early in life.

CAUSES
Adenoviruses cause five major infections, all of which occur in epidemics. Adenovirus transmission can occur by direct inoculation into the eye, by the oral-fecal route, or by inhalation of an infected droplet. The incubation period is usually less than 1 week; acute illness lasts less than 5 days and may be followed by prolonged asymptomatic reinfection.

SIGNS AND SYMPTOMS
Clinical features vary. (See *Major adenoviral infections.*)

DIAGNOSTIC TESTS
A definitive diagnosis requires isolation of the virus from respiratory or ocular secretions or fecal smears. During epidemics, typical symptoms alone can confirm the diagnosis.

PATHOPHYSIOLOGY

Major adenoviral infections

DISEASE	AGE-GROUP	CLINICAL FEATURES
Acute febrile respiratory illness	Children	Nonspecific cold-like signs and symptoms, similar to those of other viral respiratory illnesses: fever, pharyngitis, tracheitis, bronchitis, pneumonitis
Acute respiratory disease	Adults (usually military recruits)	Malaise, fever, chills, headache, pharyngitis, hoarseness, and dry cough
Viral pneumonia	Children and adults	Sudden onset of high fever, rapid infection of upper and lower respiratory tracts, skin rash, diarrhea, intestinal intussusception
Acute pharyngoconjunctival fever	Children (particularly after swimming in pools or lakes)	Spiking fever lasting several days, headache, pharyngitis, conjunctivitis, rhinitis, cervical adenitis
Acute follicular conjunctivitis	Adults	Unilateral tearing and mucoid discharge; later, milder signs in other eye
Epidemic keratoconjunctivitis	Adults	Unilateral or bilateral ocular redness and edema, preorbital swelling, local discomfort, superficial opacity of the cornea without ulceration
Hemorrhagic cystitis	Children (boys)	Adenoviruria, hematuria, dysuria, urinary frequency

TREATMENT

Supportive treatment includes bed rest, antipyretics, and analgesics. Ocular infections may require corticosteroids and direct supervision by an ophthalmologist. Hospitalization is required in cases of pneumonia (in infants) to prevent death and in epidemic keratoconjunctivitis (EKC) to prevent blindness.

SPECIAL CONSIDERATIONS

• During the acute stage of the illness, the patient's respiratory status and fluid intake and output are monitored.

• EKC can be prevented through sterilization of ophthalmic instruments, adequate chlorination in swimming pools, and avoidance of swimming pools during EKC epidemics.

 PREVENTION: To help reduce the incidence of adenoviral disease, instruct all patients in proper hand washing to reduce fecal-oral transmission.

Adrenal hypofunction

Adrenal hypofunction is marked by partial or complete failure of adrenocortical function. In primary adrenal hypofunction or insufficiency (Addison's disease), which originates within the adrenal gland, secretion of mineralocorticoids, glucocorticoids, and androgens decreases.

Adrenal hypofunction can also occur secondary to a disorder outside the adrenal gland or when a patient abruptly stops taking long-term exogenous steroids. Secondary hypofunction results in glucocorticoid deficiency.

Adrenal crisis (addisonian crisis) — a critical deficiency of mineralocorticoids and glucocorticoids — generally follows acute stress, sepsis, trauma, surgery, or omission of steroid therapy in patients with chronic adrenal insufficiency. This medical emergency necessitates immediate, vigorous treatment.

CAUSES
Primary adrenal hypofunction occurs when more than 90% of both adrenal glands is destroyed. Such destruction usually results from an autoimmune process. Other causes include tuberculosis, bilateral adrenalectomy, hemorrhage into the adrenal gland, neoplasms, and infections.

Secondary hypofunction can stem from hypopituitarism, abrupt withdrawal of long-term corticosteroids, or removal of a nonendocrine, corticotropin-secreting tumor.

Adrenal crisis may follow trauma or other physiologic stress, exhausting the glucocorticoid stores of a person with adrenal hypofunction.

SIGNS AND SYMPTOMS
Primary adrenal hypofunction typically causes fatigue, weight loss, GI disturbances, bronze skin discoloration, increased mucous membrane pigmentation, orthostatic hypotension, reduced cardiac output, electrolyte abnormalities, and decreased tolerance for even minor stress.

Secondary adrenal hypofunction causes clinical effects similar to those of primary hypofunction, but *without* hyperpigmentation, hypotension, or electrolyte abnormalities.

Adrenal crisis leads to profound weakness, nausea, vomiting, hypotension, and dehydration. If untreated, it can lead to vascular collapse, renal shutdown, coma, and death.

DIAGNOSTIC TESTS
Blood samples confirm adrenal insufficiency. Secondary hypofunction is identified through the metyrapone test. A corticotropin stimulation test may be ordered to evaluate for primary or secondary hypofunction.

TREATMENT
Lifelong corticosteroid replacement is the primary treatment. Some patients with Addison's disease may also receive I.V. desoxycorticosterone or oral fludrocortisone.

Adrenal crisis requires prompt I.V. bolus administration of hydrocortisone, with later doses given I.M. or I.V. until the patient's condition stabilizes. After the crisis, maintenance hydrocortisone doses preserve physiologic stability.

SPECIAL CONSIDERATIONS
• During adrenal crisis, vital signs are monitored carefully for evidence of shock, such as hypotension and volume depletion.
• Until onset of mineralocorticoid effect, fluids are given to replace excessive fluid loss.
• Steroid replacement may necessitate adjustment of insulin dosage in a patient who has diabetes.

TEACHING TIP: If the patient receives maintenance steroid therapy, teach the patient to recognize symptoms of a steroid dosage that's too high or too low, to increase the dosage during times of stress, to always carry a medical identification card that states that he takes a steroid, to keep an emergency kit containing hydrocortisone available for use in times of stress, and to consume foods that help to maintain sodium and potassium balance. Also review the conditions that can trigger adrenal crisis (infection, injury, and profuse sweating in hot weather).

• In a patient receiving steroids, cushingoid signs (such as fluid retention around the eyes and face) must be identified early.

Adult respiratory distress syndrome

Adult respiratory distress syndrome (ARDS) is a form of pulmonary edema that causes acute respiratory failure. Also called shock lung or stiff lung, ARDS results from increased permeability of the alveolar capillary membrane. Fluid accumulates in the lung interstitium, alveolar spaces, and small airways, causing the lung to stiffen. This impairs ventilation, impeding adequate oxygenation of pulmonary capillary blood. Severe ARDS can cause intractable and fatal hypoxemia. However, patients who recover may have little or no permanent lung damage.

CAUSES
ARDS can result from a variety of conditions, such as:
• aspiration of gastric contents
• sepsis
• trauma
• viral, bacterial, or fungal pneumonia or microemboli (fat or air emboli or disseminated intravascular coagulation)
• drug overdose or blood transfusion
• smoke or chemical inhalation
• hydrocarbon or paraquat ingestion
• near-drowning.

SIGNS AND SYMPTOMS
ARDS initially causes rapid, shallow breathing and dyspnea within hours to days of the initial injury (sometimes after the patient's condition appears stable). Other features include intercostal and suprasternal retractions, crackles and rhonchi, restlessness, apprehension, mental sluggishness, motor dysfunction, and tachycardia.

Severe ARDS causes overwhelming hypoxemia which, if uncorrected, results in hypotension, decreased urine output, respiratory and metabolic acidosis and, eventually, ventricular fibrillation or standstill.

DIAGNOSTIC TESTS
Arterial blood gas (ABG) analysis helps detect ARDS. Other tests include pulmonary artery catheterization and chest X-rays.

Tests must rule out other lung disorders. To establish the cause, sputum cultures and blood specimens are collected to detect infections and a toxicology screen is done to identify drug ingestion.

TREATMENT
When possible, treatment aims to correct the underlying cause of ARDS and prevent potentially fatal complications. Supportive care consists of administering humidified oxygen by a tight-fitting mask, which allows for use of continuous positive airway pressure (CPAP). Hypoxemia that doesn't respond adequately to these measures requires ventilatory support with intubation, volume ventilation, and positive end-expiratory pressure (PEEP). Other supportive measures include fluid restriction, diuretics, and correction of electrolyte and acid-base abnormalities.

SPECIAL CONSIDERATIONS

ACTION STAT: Immediately report hypotension, tachycardia, and decreased urine output in a patient who's receiving PEEP.

• The patient's respiratory status is monitored frequently. Retractions on inspiration, dyspnea, use of accessory respiratory muscles, and adventitious or diminished breath sounds are danger signs.

• Ventilator settings must be checked frequently and condensate emptied promptly from tubing to ensure maximum oxygen delivery. ABG studies are monitored and checked for metabolic and respiratory acidosis and changes in the partial pressure of arterial oxygen.

• A patient who has suffered injuries to the lungs is watched closely for respiratory changes — especially for the first 2 to 3 days after injury.

Allergic purpura

A type of nonthrombocytopenic purpura, allergic purpura is an inflammation of the cells that line the blood vessels, accompanied by allergic symptoms. The disorder affects the skin, genitourinary (GU) tract, GI tract, and joints. If allowed to develop fully, allergic purpura is persistent and debilitating and may lead to serious kidney disease. An acute attack can last for several weeks and is potentially fatal (usually from renal failure). Most patients, though, do recover.

When allergic purpura primarily affects the GI tract, with accompanying joint pain, it's called Henoch-Schönlein syndrome or anaphylactoid purpura. However, the term *allergic purpura* applies to purpura associated with many other conditions.

CAUSES
The most common identifiable cause of allergic purpura is an autoimmune reaction directed against vascular walls that's triggered by a bacterial infection. Typically, upper respiratory infection occurs 1 to 3 weeks before symptoms appear. Other possible causes include allergic reactions to some drugs and vaccines, insect bites, and some foods.

SIGNS AND SYMPTOMS
Allergic purpura produces characteristic purple skin lesions that are macular, ecchymotic, and of varying size.

Lesions usually appear in symmetrical patterns on the arms and legs and are accompanied by pruritus and paresthesia. Scattered petechiae may appear on the legs, buttocks, and perineum.

Henoch-Schönlein syndrome commonly produces transient or severe colic, tenesmus and constipation, vomiting, and edema or hemorrhage of the intestinal mucous membranes, resulting in GI bleeding, occult blood in the stools and, possibly, intussusception. Musculoskeletal symptoms, such as rheumatoid pains and periarticular effusions, mostly affect the legs and feet. GU symptoms also may occur. (See *Genitourinary features of allergic purpura.*)

DIAGNOSTIC TESTS
No laboratory test clearly identifies allergic purpura, so diagnosis requires careful clinical observation. Small-bowel X-rays may reveal areas of transient edema; tests for blood in the urine and stools are often positive. Increased blood urea nitrogen and serum creatinine levels may indicate renal involvement. Diagnosis must rule out other forms of nonthrombocytopenic purpura.

TREATMENT
Treatment aims to relieve symptoms. For example, severe allergic purpura may require steroids to relieve edema and analgesics to relieve joint and abdominal pain. Some patients with chronic renal disease may benefit from immunosuppression with azathioprine, along with identification of the provocative allergen. An accurate allergy history is essential.

SPECIAL CONSIDERATIONS
• The patient is urged to maintain an elimination diet to help identify specific allergenic foods.

• The patient is observed carefully for complications, such as GI and GU tract bleeding, edema, nausea, vomiting, hypertension, and abdominal rigidity and tenderness.

Genitourinary features of allergic purpura

In about 25% to 50% of patients, allergic purpura is associated with such genitourinary features as:
- nephritis
- renal hemorrhages that may cause microscopic hematuria and disturb renal function
- bleeding from the mucosal surfaces of the ureters, bladder, or urethra
- glomerulonephritis (occasionally).

Allergic rhinitis

This immune disorder is a reaction to airborne (inhaled) allergens. Depending on the allergen, the resulting rhinitis and conjunctivitis may be seasonal (hay fever) or occur year-round (perennial allergic rhinitis). Allergic rhinitis is the most common atopic allergic reaction, affecting over 20 million Americans.

CAUSES

Hay fever reflects an immunoglobulin E–mediated, type I hypersensitivity response to an environmental antigen (allergen) in a genetically susceptible individual. In most cases, it's induced by wind-borne pollens, such as tree, grass, or weed pollens.

In perennial allergic rhinitis, inhaled allergens provoke antigen responses that produce recurring symptoms year-round. Major perennial allergens and irritants include dust mites, feather pillows, mold, cigarette smoke, upholstery, and animal danders.

SIGNS AND SYMPTOMS

Seasonal allergic rhinitis causes paroxysmal sneezing, profuse watery rhinorrhea, nasal obstruction or congestion, and pruritus of the nose and eyes, usually accompanied by pale, cyanotic, edematous nasal mucosa; red and edematous eyelids and conjunctivae; excessive lacrimation; and headache or sinus pain.

In perennial allergic rhinitis, chronic nasal obstruction is common and often extends to eustachian tube obstruction.

In both types of allergic rhinitis, dark circles may appear under the eyes because of venous congestion in the maxillary sinuses. Some patients have chronic complications, such as sinusitis and nasal polyps.

DIAGNOSTIC TESTS

Microscopic examination of sputum and nasal secretions reveals large numbers of eosinophils. Blood chemistry studies show normal or elevated immunoglobulin E levels. A firm diagnosis rests on the patient's personal and family history of allergies and on physical findings during a symptomatic phase. Skin testing, paired with tested responses to environmental stimuli, can help pinpoint responsible allergens.

TREATMENT

Symptoms are controlled by eliminating the environmental antigen, if possible, and by drug therapy and immunotherapy. Antihistamines block histamine effects. Inhaled intranasal steroids (such as flunisolide) produce local anti-inflammatory effects with minimal systemic adverse effects. However, for acute exacerbations, nasal decongestants and oral antihistamines may be needed.

Long-term management includes immunotherapy or desensitization with injections of extracted allergens administered before or during the allergy season or perennially.

SPECIAL CONSIDERATIONS

- The patient must use intranasal steroids regularly, if prescribed, for optimal effectiveness.

 PREVENTION: Advise patients to reduce environmental exposure to airborne allergens by sleeping with windows closed,

Experimental drugs for Alzheimer's disease

Most drugs currently being used to treat Alzheimer's disease are experimental. These drugs, which may slow the disease process, include:
- choline salts
- lecithin
- physostigmine
- enkephalins
- naloxone.

avoiding the countryside during pollination seasons, using air conditioning to filter allergens, and eliminating dust-collecting items, such as heavy drapes, from the home.

Alzheimer's disease

Alzheimer's disease, a progressive dementia, accounts for over half of all dementias. An estimated 5% of people over age 65 have a severe form of the disease, and 12% suffer from mild to moderate dementia. Alzheimer's disease carries a poor prognosis.

CAUSES

Alzheimer's disease is thought to be related to the following factors:
- neurochemical factors, such as deficiencies in acetylcholine, somatostatin, substance P, and norepinephrine
- environmental factors, such as aluminum and manganese
- viral factors, such as slow-growing central nervous system viruses
- trauma
- genetic immunologic factors.

SIGNS AND SYMPTOMS

Onset is gradual. Initially, the patient experiences subtle changes, such as forgetfulness, recent memory loss, difficulty learning and remembering new information, and inability to concentrate. Gradually, tasks that call for abstract thinking and judgment become more difficult. Progressive and severe deterioration in memory, language, and motor function leads to loss of coordination and inability to write or speak.

Personality changes (restlessness, irritability) are common. Eventually, the patient becomes disoriented and physical and intellectual disability progress. Usually, death results from infection.

DIAGNOSTIC TESTS

Early diagnosis is difficult because early signs and symptoms are subtle. Initial diagnosis relies on information provided by a family member, supported by tests of mental status, neurologic examination, and psychometric testing. Other tests can rule out other disorders. However, definitive diagnosis cannot be confirmed until after death when brain tissue is examined for three hallmark features: neurofibrillary tangles, neuritic plaques, and granulovacuolar degeneration.

TREATMENT

Cerebral vasodilators may be used to enhance brain circulation. Hyperbaric oxygen may be given to increase oxygenation to the brain. Psychostimulative drugs such as methylphenidate may be used to enhance mood. If depression seems to exacerbate the dementia, antidepressants are given. Tacrine, a centrally acting anticholinesterase agent, may be used to treat memory deficits. Some patients may receive other drugs. (See *Experimental drugs for Alzheimer's disease.*)

Another approach to treatment includes avoiding antacids, aluminum cooking utensils, and aluminum-containing deodorants to help decrease aluminum intake.

SPECIAL CONSIDERATIONS

- Overall care focuses on supporting the patient's existing abilities and compensating for lost abilities.
- Take steps to maintain a safe envi-

ronment. Serve food on unbreakable dishes. Move unsafe furniture against the walls.

 TEACHING TIP: Teach the patient's family about the disease. Referrals to social service and community resources for legal and financial advice and support are important.

Amyotrophic lateral sclerosis

Commonly called *Lou Gehrig's disease,* amyotrophic lateral sclerosis (ALS) is the most common of the motor neuron diseases causing muscular atrophy. Onset occurs between ages 40 and 70.

A chronic, progressively debilitating disease, ALS is rapidly fatal. About 5,000 new cases are diagnosed each year.

CAUSES
The exact cause of ALS is unknown, but about 5% to 10% of cases have a genetic component. In these, it is an autosomal dominant trait.

Researchers have focused on the following as possible causes of ALS:
• slow-acting virus
• nutritional deficiency related to disturbed enzyme metabolism
• metabolic interference in nucleic acid production
• certain autoimmune disorders.

SIGNS AND SYMPTOMS
Patients with ALS develop fasciculations, accompanied by atrophy and weakness. Other features include impaired speech and difficulty chewing, swallowing, and breathing. Mental deterioration usually doesn't occur, but patients may become depressed in reaction to the disease.

DIAGNOSTIC TESTS
Electromyography and muscle biopsy help show nerve, rather than muscle, disease. Cerebrospinal fluid protein levels are increased in one-third of affected patients. Diagnosis must rule out multiple sclerosis, spinal cord tumor, polyarteritis, syringomyelia, myasthenia gravis, and progressive muscular dystrophy.

TREATMENT
ALS is untreatable. Management aims to control symptoms and provide emotional, psychological, and physical support.

SPECIAL CONSIDERATIONS
• Rehabilitation programs should be designed to maintain the patient's independence as long as possible.
• The patient and family may require help to obtain equipment, such as a wheelchair, as well as to schedule appointments with visiting nurses and to learn about the illness.
• The patient's muscular capacity determines the amount of assistance needed with bathing, personal hygiene, and transfers from wheelchair to bed. Establishing a regular bowel and bladder routine helps to increase patient well-being and reduce caregiver stress.
• Staying upright while eating and consuming soft, solid foods may make swallowing easier. Gastrostomy and nasogastric tube feedings may be necessary if the patient can no longer swallow.
• To help prevent skin breakdown, good skin care should be provided for a bedridden patient. Frequent turning, good skin hygiene, and use of sheepskins or pressure-relieving devices also help prevent problems.
• Because of the fatal nature of the disease, health care workers should provide emotional support, directing efforts toward preparing the patient and family for his eventual death. Patients with ALS may benefit from a hospice program.

TEACHING TIP: Teaching the patient self-suctioning techniques can help him manage increased accumulation of secretions and dysphagia. A suctioning machine kept handy at home can reduce his fear of choking.

Anal fissure

This condition is a laceration or crack in the lining of the anus that extends to the circular muscle. A posterior fissure, the most common type, is equally prevalent in males and females. An anterior fissure, the rarer type, is 10 times more common in females.

CAUSES

A posterior fissure results from passage of large, hard stools that stretch the lining beyond its limits. An anterior fissure usually results from strain on the perineum during childbirth or, rarely, from scar stenosis. Occasionally, an anal fissure occurs secondary to proctitis, anal tuberculosis, or carcinoma.

SIGNS AND SYMPTOMS

Onset of an acute anal fissure is characterized by tearing, cutting, or burning pain during or immediately after a bowel movement. A few drops of blood may streak toilet paper or underclothes. Painful anal sphincter spasms result from ulceration of a *sentinel pile* (swelling at the lower end of the fissure).

A fissure may heal spontaneously and completely, or it may partially heal and break open again. A chronic fissure produces scar tissue that hampers normal bowel evacuation.

DIAGNOSTIC TESTS

Anoscopy showing a longitudinal tear and typical clinical features help establish the diagnosis. A digital examination that elicits pain and bleeding supports the diagnosis. Gentle traction on perianal skin can create sufficient eversion to visualize the fissure directly.

TREATMENT

For superficial fissures without hemorrhoids, forcible digital dilatation of the anal sphincter under local anesthesia stretches the lower portion of the anal sphincter. For complicated fissures, treatment includes surgical excision of tissue, adjacent skin, and mucosal tags and division of internal sphincter muscle from external.

SPECIAL CONSIDERATIONS

• Hot sitz baths, warm soaks, and local anesthetic ointment are used to relieve pain.
• Diarrhea is controlled with diphenoxylate or other antidiarrheals.

 TEACHING TIP: Inform the patient that a low-residue diet, adequate fluid intake, and stool softeners prevent straining during defecation.

Anaphylaxis

Anaphylaxis is a dramatic, acute reaction marked by the sudden onset of rapidly progressive urticaria and respiratory distress. A severe anaphylactic reaction may trigger vascular collapse, leading to systemic shock and even death.

CAUSES

The cause of anaphylactic reactions is ingestion of, or other systemic exposure to, sensitizing drugs or other substances.

Sensitizing substances

Sensitizing substances include serums, vaccines, allergen extracts, enzymes (such as L-asparaginase), hormones, sulfonamides, local anesthetics, salicylates, polysaccharides, diagnostic chemicals, foods, sulfite-containing food additives, insect venom, and antibiotics. (Penicillin induces anaphylaxis in 1 to 4 of every 10,000 patients who receive it.)

Pathophysiology

An anaphylactic reaction requires previous sensitization or exposure to the specific antigen, which results in production of specific immunoglobulin E (IgE) antibodies by plasma cells. IgE antibodies then bind to membrane receptors on mast cells (found throughout connective tissue) and basophils.

On reexposure, the antigen binds to adjacent IgE antibodies or cross-linked IgE receptors, activating a se-

Teaching patients how to use an anaphylaxis kit

If your patient has been advised to carry an anaphylaxis kit to use in an emergency, explain that the kit contains everything he needs to treat an allergic reaction: a prefilled syringe containing two doses of epinephrine, alcohol swabs, a tourniquet, and antihistamine tablets.

Instruct the patient to notify the doctor at once if anaphylaxis occurs (or to ask someone else to call him) and to use the anaphylaxis kit as follows.

Getting ready
●Take the prefilled syringe from the kit and remove the needle cap. Hold the syringe with the needle pointing up. Expel air from the syringe by pushing in the plunger until it stops.
●Next, clean about 4" (10 cm) of the skin on your arm or thigh with an alcohol swab. (If you're right-handed, clean your left arm or thigh. If you're left-handed, clean your right arm or thigh.)

Injecting the epinephrine
●Rotate the plunger one-quarter turn to the right so that it's aligned with the slot. Insert the entire needle — like a dart — into the skin.
●Push down on the plunger until it stops. It will inject 0.3 ml of the drug for persons over age 12. Withdraw the needle.

Removing the insect's stinger when a sting is the cause
●Quickly remove the insect's stinger if it's visible. Use a dull object, such as a fingernail or tweezers, to pull it straight out. If the stinger can't be removed quickly, stop trying. Go on to the next step.

Applying the tourniquet
●If you were stung on an arm or a leg, apply a tourniquet between the sting site and your heart. Tighten the tourniquet by pulling the string.

Taking the antihistamine tablets
●Chew and swallow the antihistamine tablets.

Following up
●Apply ice packs to the sting site. Avoid exertion, keep warm, and see a doctor or go to a hospital immediately.
●After 10 minutes, release the tourniquet by pulling on the metal ring.
  Important: If you don't notice an improvement within 10 minutes, give yourself a second injection. If the syringe has a preset second dose, don't depress the plunger until you're ready to give the second injection. Proceed as before, following the injection instructions.

Special instructions
●Keep the kit handy for emergency treatment at all times.
●Ask the pharmacist for storage guidelines.
●Periodically check the epinephrine in the preloaded syringe. A pinkish brown solution needs to be replaced.
●Note the kit's expiration date and replace the kit before that date.

ries of reactions that triggers the release of powerful chemical mediators (histamine, ECF-A, PAF) from mast cell stores. IgG or IgM enters into the reaction and activates the release of complement fractions.

At the same time, two other chemical mediators, bradykinin and leukotrienes, induce vascular collapse by causing certain smooth muscles to contract and by increasing vascular permeability. This leads to decreased peripheral resistance and plasma leakage from the circulation to extravascular tissues. Hypotension ensues, leading to hypovolemic shock and cardiac dysfunction.

SIGNS AND SYMPTOMS

An anaphylactic reaction produces sudden physical distress within seconds or minutes after exposure to an allergen (although a delayed or persistent reaction may occur for up to 24 hours). The more rapidly signs and symptoms appear, the more severe the reaction is likely to be. Usually, initial symptoms include a feeling of impending doom or fear, weakness, sweating, sneezing, shortness of breath, nasal pruritus, urticaria, and angioedema. These are followed rapidly by signs and symptoms in one or more target organs.

Cardiovascular signs and symptoms include hypotension, shock, and sometimes cardiac arrhythmias, which, if untreated, may precipitate circulatory collapse.

Respiratory signs and symptoms include nasal mucosal edema, profuse watery rhinorrhea, itching, nasal congestion, and sudden sneezing attacks. Edema of the upper respiratory tract (causing hoarseness, stridor, and dyspnea) is an early sign of acute respiratory failure.

GI and *genitourinary signs and symptoms* include severe stomach cramps, nausea, diarrhea, and urinary urgency and incontinence.

DIAGNOSTIC TESTS

Anaphylaxis can be diagnosed by the rapid onset of severe respiratory or cardiovascular reactions after exposure to a drug, vaccine, diagnostic agent, food, or food additive or after an insect sting. If these reactions occur without a known allergic stimulus, other possible causes of shock (acute heart attack, status asthmaticus, heart failure) must be ruled out.

TREATMENT

Anaphylaxis is always an emergency, requiring an *immediate* injection of epinephrine. In case of cardiac arrest,

the standard response requires cardiopulmonary resuscitation. Other therapy depends on the patient's response. Circulatory volume is maintained with volume expanders as needed. Blood pressure may be stabilized with I.V. vasopressors.

After the initial emergency, other medications, such as subcutaneous epinephrine, longer-acting epinephrine, and corticosteroids, are given for long-term management.

SPECIAL CONSIDERATIONS

● Airway patency must be maintained.

● The patient must be observed for signs of hypotension and shock.

 TEACHING TIP: Patient education can help to prevent anaphylaxis. Teach the patient to avoid exposure to known allergens and to wear a medical identification bracelet identifying allergies. (See *Teaching patients how to use an anaphylaxis kit,* page 15.)

Ankylosing spondylitis

This chronic, usually progressive inflammatory disease typically begins in the sacroiliac joints and gradually progresses to the lumbar, thoracic, and cervical regions of the spine. Bone and cartilage deterioration can lead to fibrous tissue formation and eventual fusion of the spine or peripheral joints.

CAUSES

Recent evidence strongly suggests a familial tendency in ankylosing spondylitis. The presence of histocompatibility antigen human leukocyte antigen (HLA/B27) and circulating immune complexes suggests immunologic activity.

SIGNS AND SYMPTOMS

The first symptom is intermittent lower-back pain that's usually most severe in the morning or after a period of inactivity. Other symptoms vary. (See *Identifying signs and symptoms of ankylosing spondylitis*.)

DIAGNOSTIC TESTS

Typical symptoms, family history, and blood tests showing HLA/B27 strongly suggest ankylosing spondylitis. Confirmation requires additional blood tests as well as X-rays.

TREATMENT

Because disease progression can't be stopped, treatment aims to delay further deformity through good posture, stretching and deep-breathing exercises and, in some patients, braces and lightweight supports. Anti-inflammatory analgesics help control pain and inflammation.

Severe hip involvement usually necessitates surgical hip replacement. Severe spinal involvement may require a spinal wedge osteotomy to separate and reposition the vertebrae. (This surgery is performed only on selected patients.)

SPECIAL CONSIDERATIONS

• Local heat application and massage may relieve pain.
• Mobility and degree of discomfort are assessed frequently.
• Take every measure to promote patient comfort; ankylosing spondylitis can be extremely painful and crippling. Keep in mind that limited range of motion makes simple tasks difficult.
• Comprehensive treatment should include counseling by a social worker, visiting nurse, and dietitian.
• The patient's height is measured every 3 to 4 months to detect any tendency toward kyphosis.

 TEACHING TIP: Teach the patient how to perform exercises that maintain strength and function. Stress the importance of maintaining good posture. To minimize deformities, instruct him to avoid physical activities that place undue stress on the back, such as lifting heavy objects. Instruct him to sleep in a prone position on a hard mattress and avoid using pillows under the neck or knees. Advise him to avoid prolonged walking, standing, sitting, or driving. Recommend that he seek vocational counseling if his job requires standing or prolonged sitting at a desk. Tell him to contact the local Arthritis Foundation chapter for a support group.

Identifying signs and symptoms of ankylosing spondylitis

Clinical features of ankylosing spondylitis may include:
• stiffness and limited motion of the lumbar spine
• pain and limited expansion of the chest (from involvement of the costovertebral joints)
• peripheral arthritis involving the shoulders, hips, and knees
• kyphosis (in advanced stages), caused by chronic stooping to relieve symptoms
• hip deformity and associated limited range of motion
• tenderness over the inflammation site
• mild fatigue, fever, anorexia, or weight loss
• aortic insufficiency and cardiomegaly
• upper lobe pulmonary fibrosis.
   These signs and symptoms progress unpredictably, and the disease may go into remission, exacerbation, or arrest at any stage.

Anorectal abscess and fistula

An anorectal abscess is a localized collection of pus caused by inflammation of the soft tissue near the rectum or anus. Such inflammation may produce an anal fistula — an abnormal opening in the anal skin — that may communicate with the rectum.

CAUSES

The inflammatory process that leads to abscess may begin with an abrasion or tear in the lining of the anal canal, rectum, or perianal skin, and subsequent infection by *Escherichia coli*, staphylococci, or streptococci. Such trauma may result from injections for treatment of internal hemorrhoids, enema-tip abrasions, puncture wounds from ingested eggshells or fish bones, or insertion of foreign objects.

As the abscess produces more pus, a fistula may form in the soft tissue beneath the muscle fibers of the sphincter, usually extending into the perianal skin. The internal (primary) opening of the abscess or fistula is usually near the anal glands and crypts; the external (secondary) opening is in the perianal skin.

SIGNS AND SYMPTOMS

Characteristics are throbbing pain and tenderness at the abscess site. A hard, painful lump develops on one side, preventing comfortable sitting.

DIAGNOSTIC TESTS

Anorectal abscess is detectable on physical examination. *Perianal abscess* is a red, tender, localized, oval swelling close to the anus. Sitting or coughing increases pain, and pus may drain from the abscess. *Ischiorectal abscess* involves the entire perianal region on the affected side of the anus. It's tender but may not produce drainage. *Submucous or high intermuscular abscess* may produce a dull, aching pain in the rectum, tenderness and, occasionally, induration. *Pelvirectal abscess* (rare) produces fever, malaise, and myalgia but no local anal or external rectal signs or pain.

If the abscess drains by forming a fistula, the pain usually subsides; major signs are pruritic drainage and subsequent perianal irritation. The external opening of a fistula generally appears as a pink or red, elevated, discharging sinus or ulcer on the skin near the anus. The patient may have chills, fever, nausea, vomiting, and malaise. Sigmoidoscopy, barium studies, and colonoscopy may be done to rule out other conditions.

TREATMENT

Anorectal abscesses require surgical incision under caudal anesthesia to promote drainage. Fistulas require a fistulotomy — removal of the fistula and associated granulation tissue — under caudal anesthesia. If the fistula tract is epithelialized, treatment requires fistulectomy — removal of the fistulous tract — followed by insertion of drains, which remain in place for 48 hours.

SPECIAL CONSIDERATIONS

After an incision is made to drain an anorectal abscess:
- The wound is examined frequently to assess proper healing.
- The patient may need a stool-softening laxative to avoid constipation, which might stress the incision.

 TEACHING TIP: Inform the patient that complete recovery takes time. Stress the importance of perianal cleanliness to help avoid another infection.

Anorectal stricture

In anorectal stricture (stenosis, contracture), anorectal lumen size decreases. Stenosis prevents dilation of the sphincter.

CAUSES

Anorectal stricture results from scarring after anorectal surgery or inflammation, inadequate postoperative care, or laxative abuse.

SIGNS AND SYMPTOMS

The patient with anorectal stricture strains excessively when defecating and is unable to completely evacuate his bowel. Other clinical effects include pain, bleeding, and pruritus ani.

DIAGNOSTIC TESTS

Visual inspection reveals narrowing of the anal canal. Digital examination reveals tenderness and tightness.

TREATMENT

Surgical removal of scar tissue is the most effective treatment. Digital or instrumental dilation may be beneficial but may cause additional tears and splits. If the cause of stricture is inflammation, the underlying inflammatory process must be corrected.

SPECIAL CONSIDERATIONS

● If surgery was performed under spinal anesthesia, the patient is kept flat for 6 to 8 hours after surgery.
● When the patient's condition is stable, his normal diet is resumed. Stool softeners, sitz baths, and analgesics are given as necessary.

Aplastic and hypoplastic anemias

In these blood disorders, the patient experiences pancytopenia — deficiencies in the levels of all blood cells — as well as impeded bone marrow development. Aplastic and hypoplastic anemias generally produce fatal bleeding or infection. Patients with severe blood cell deficiencies have a mortality of 80% to 90%.

CAUSES

Aplastic anemias usually result from neoplastic disease of the bone marrow or bone marrow destruction caused by exposure to drugs (antibiotics, anticonvulsants), toxic agents (such as benzene and chloramphenicol), or ionizing radiation. Anemias with no known cause may be congenital, as in anemia of Blackfan and Diamond and Fanconi's syndrome.

SIGNS AND SYMPTOMS

Clinical features vary with the severity of blood cell deficiencies, but they often develop gradually. Anemic symptoms include progressive weakness and fatigue, shortness of breath, headache, pallor and, ultimately, tachycardia and congestive heart failure. Also expect ecchymosis, petechiae, and hemorrhage, especially from the mucous membranes or into the retina or central nervous system.

Neutropenia may lead to infection (fever, oral and rectal ulcers, sore throat).

DIAGNOSTIC TESTS

Blood tests that measure the number and size of red blood cells (RBCs), the number of white blood cells, iron levels, clotting time, and other factors can confirm aplastic anemia. Bone marrow aspiration from several sites may provide additional data.

TREATMENT

Identifiable causes must be eliminated and vigorous supportive measures (transfusions of packed RBCs, platelets, or experimental human leukocyte antigen–matched leukocytes) are provided. Even after elimination of the cause, though, recovery can take months.

Bone marrow transplantation is the treatment of choice for anemia due to severe aplasia and for patients who need constant RBC transfusions. (See *Understanding bone marrow transplantation,* page 20.)

Patients with low leukocyte counts need special measures to prevent infection. Those with low hemoglobin counts may need respiratory support with oxygen in addition to blood transfusions.

Other treatments may include corticosteroids to stimulate erythroid production, marrow-stimulating agents, antilymphocyte globulin (experimental), immunosuppressive agents, and colony-stimulating factors to encourage growth of specific cellular components.

SPECIAL CONSIDERATIONS

● The patient is monitored for life-threatening hemorrhage, infection, adverse drug reactions, and blood transfusion reactions.
● Help prevent infection by washing your hands thoroughly before entering the patient's room.

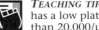 *TEACHING TIP:* If the patient has a low platelet count (less than 20,000/μl), teach him to avoid I.M. injections, use an electric razor and soft toothbrush, use a stool

Understanding bone marrow transplantation

In bone marrow transplantation, usually 500 to 700 ml of marrow are aspirated from the pelvic bones of a human leukocyte antigen–compatible donor (allogeneic) or of the recipient himself during periods of complete remission (autologous). The aspirated marrow is filtered and then infused into the recipient in an attempt to repopulate the patient's marrow with normal cells.

This procedure has brought about long-term, healthy survivals in about half the patients with severe aplastic anemia. It may also be effective in treating patients with acute leukemia, certain immunodeficiency diseases, and solid-tumor cancers.

Because bone marrow transplantation carries serious risks, it requires strict adherence to infection protection techniques and strict aseptic technique, and a primary caregiver to provide consistent care and continuous monitoring of patient status.

softener, and maintain a proper diet to prevent constipation. If he has a low hemoglobin count, recommend frequent rest periods to reduce fatigue. To decrease the risk of infection, advise him to consume a nutritious diet and practice meticulous mouth and perianal care. Also teach him to recognize signs of infection and to report them immediately.
• Support efforts to educate the public about the hazards of toxic agents. Urge people who work with radiation to wear protective clothing and a radiation-detecting badge and to observe plant safety precautions. Those who work with the solvent benzene should know that 10 parts/million is the highest safe environmental level.

Appendicitis

The most common disease requiring major surgery, appendicitis is an inflammation of the vermiform appendix. Since the advent of antibiotics, the incidence and death rate of appendicitis have declined. However, if untreated, this disease is invariably fatal.

CAUSES
Appendicitis probably results from an obstruction of the intestinal lumen caused by a fecal mass, stricture, barium ingestion, or viral infection. The obstruction triggers an inflammatory process that can lead to infection, thrombosis, necrosis, and perforation. If the appendix ruptures or perforates, the infected contents spill into the abdominal cavity, causing peritonitis — the most common and most perilous complication.

SIGNS AND SYMPTOMS
Typically, appendicitis begins with generalized or localized abdominal pain in the upper right part of the abdomen, followed by anorexia, nausea, and vomiting. Pain eventually localizes in the lower right part of the abdomen, with abdominal "board-like" rigidity, retractive respirations, increasing tenderness, increasingly severe abdominal spasms, and rebound tenderness.

Later signs and symptoms include constipation (although diarrhea is also possible), slight fever, and tachycardia. Sudden cessation of abdominal pain indicates a perforation or infarction of the appendix.

DIAGNOSTIC TESTS
Physical signs and symptoms, including tenderness and mild fever, and a moderately high white blood cell count generally support the diagnosis. Physical findings and blood test results rule out illnesses with similar symptoms.

TREATMENT

Appendectomy is the only effective treatment. Laparoscopic appendectomies, which decrease recovery time, are now being done. I.V. fluids are given to prevent dehydration.

If peritonitis develops, treatment may include GI intubation, parenteral replacement of fluids and electrolytes, and antibiotics.

SPECIAL CONSIDERATIONS

• Analgesics are given judiciously because they may mask symptoms.
• Placing the patient in Fowler's position may reduce pain.
• Continuing pain and fever may signal an abscess. If an abscess or peritonitis develops, incision and drainage may be necessary.
• Cathartics or enemas should never be used in a patient with appendicitis because they may rupture the appendix. Heat applied to the lower right abdomen may also cause rupture.

 PREVENTION: To help avert pulmonary complications, teach the patient to cough, breathe deeply, and turn frequently.

Arterial occlusive disease

In this disorder, obstruction or narrowing of the lumen of the aorta and its major branches causes an interruption of blood flow, usually to the legs and feet. Arterial occlusive disease may affect the carotid, vertebral, innominate, subclavian, mesenteric, or celiac arteries. (See *Possible sites of major artery occlusion,* page 22.)

CAUSES

Arterial occlusive disease is a frequent complication of atherosclerosis. Occlusion may result from emboli formation, thrombosis, or trauma.

SIGNS AND SYMPTOMS

Evidence of this disease varies with the occlusion site.
• *Carotid artery occlusion* typically causes neurologic dysfunction (such as transient ischemic attacks or transient blindness) and an auscultatory bruit over the affected vessel.
• *Vertebrobasilar and brachiocephalic artery occlusion* may lead to neurologic dysfunction; brachiocephalic occlusion may also cause right arm ischemia and a bruit over the right side of the neck.
• *Subclavian artery occlusion* may cause subclavian steal syndrome (backflow of blood from the brain into the subclavian artery distal to the occlusion), exercise-induced claudication and, possibly, gangrene.
• *Mesenteric artery occlusion* may cause bowel ischemia, sudden acute abdominal pain, nausea and vomiting, diarrhea, and shock.
• *Aortic bifurcation* may cause sensory and motor deficits and signs and symptoms of ischemia (sudden pain, and cold pale legs with decreased or absent peripheral pulses in both legs).
• *Iliac artery occlusion* may lead to intermittent claudication of the lower back, buttocks, and thighs.
• *Femoral and popliteal artery occlusion* may cause intermittent claudication of the calves on exertion, ischemia, foot pain, leg pallor and coolness, gangrene, and no palpable pulses in the ankles and feet.

DIAGNOSTIC TESTS

Diagnosis usually rests on history and physical findings. Supportive tests include arteriography and an ultrasound scan.

TREATMENT

Treatment depends on the cause, location, and size of the obstruction. For mild chronic disease, supportive measures include smoking cessation, hypertension control, and walking. For carotid artery occlusion, antiplatelet therapy may begin with dipyridamole and aspirin. For intermittent claudication of chronic occlusive disease, pentoxifylline may improve blood flow.

Acute arterial occlusive disease usually warrants surgery to restore circulation to the affected area. Possible procedures include embolectomy, thromboendarterectomy, patch graft-

Possible sites of major artery occlusion

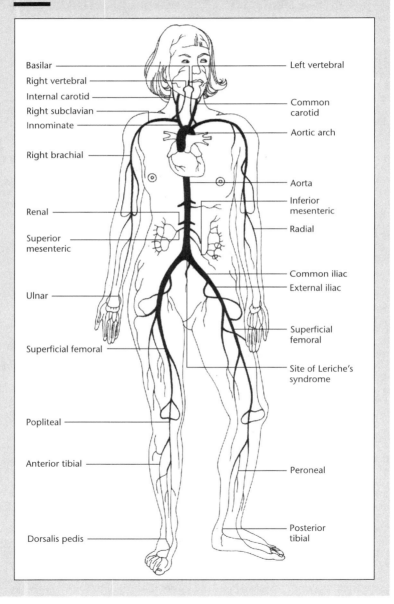

ing, and bypass graft, thrombolytic therapy, atherectomy, balloon or laser angioplasty, stent insertion, or a combination of these techniques.

Amputation is necessary if arterial reconstructive surgery fails or if gangrene, persistent infection, or intractable pain occurs.

SPECIAL CONSIDERATIONS
• The affected foot should be encased in soft cotton batting and repositioned frequently to prevent pressure on any one area. Avoid elevating or applying heat to the affected leg.
• A patient with carotid, innominate, vertebral, or subclavian artery occlusion should be monitored for signs of cerebrovascular accident, such as numbness in an arm or leg.
• In femoral and popliteal artery occlusion, the patient should be assisted to walk as soon as possible and should be discouraged from prolonged sitting.

 TEACHING TIP: Patient-teaching topics include proper foot care, the importance of smoking cessation, compliance with the prescribed regimen, and avoiding tight clothing. Instruct the patient to watch for and report signs and symptoms of recurrence (pain, pallor, numbness, paralysis, absence of pulse).

Asbestosis

Asbestosis is a chronic lung disease that leads to diffuse interstitial fibrosis. It can take as long as 15 to 20 years to develop after regular exposure to asbestos has ended. The disease aggravates the risk of lung cancer in cigarette smokers.

CAUSES
Asbestosis results from inhaling asbestos fibers. Sources include the mining and milling of asbestos, the construction industry (where asbestos is used in a prefabricated form), and the fireproofing and textile industries. Asbestos is also used to produce paints, plastics, and brake and clutch linings.

Asbestos-related diseases develop in families of asbestos workers as a result of exposure to fibrous dust shaken off workers' clothing at home. In the general public, such diseases result from exposure to fibrous dust or waste piles from nearby asbestos plants.

SIGNS AND SYMPTOMS
The first symptom is usually dyspnea on exertion, typically after 10 years' exposure to asbestos. As fibrosis extends, dyspnea on exertion increases until, eventually, dyspnea occurs even at rest. Advanced disease also causes a dry cough (which may be productive in smokers), chest pain, recurrent respiratory infections, and tachypnea.

Cardiovascular complications include pulmonary hypertension, right ventricular hypertrophy, and cor pulmonale. Finger clubbing commonly occurs.

DIAGNOSTIC TESTS
A physical examination reveals dry crackles at the lung bases. Arterial blood gas studies reveal decreases in the partial pressure of arterial oxygen (PaO_2) and carbon dioxide. Chest X-rays and pulmonary function studies aid diagnosis.

TREATMENT
Respiratory symptoms may be relieved by chest physiotherapy, aerosol therapy, inhaled mucolytics, and increased fluid intake. Respiratory infections call for prompt antibiotic administration.

Hypoxia requires oxygen administration by cannula or mask or by mechanical ventilation if PaO_2 can't be maintained above 40 mm Hg.

SPECIAL CONSIDERATIONS
 PREVENTION: To help the patient avoid infections, teach him to stay away from crowds and persons with infections

PATHOPHYSIOLOGY
Types of aspergillosis

The four major types of aspergillosis include:
- aspergilloma, which produces a fungus ball in the lungs
- allergic aspergillosis, a hypersensitive asthmatic reaction to *Aspergillus* antigens
- aspergillosis endophthalmitis, an infection of the eye that can lead to blindness
- disseminated aspergillosis, a rapidly fatal infection that causes septicemia, thrombosis, and infarction of virtually any organ.

and to receive influenza and pneumococcal vaccines. To improve his ventilatory efficiency, encourage physical reconditioning, energy conservation in daily activities, and relaxation techniques.

Aspergillosis

This opportunistic infection is caused by fungi of the genus *Aspergillus,* usually *A. fumigatus, A. flavus,* or *A. niger.* It occurs in several forms. (See *Types of aspergillosis.*) The prognosis varies with each form.

Aspergillosis may cause an infection of the ear, cornea, and prosthetic heart valves; pneumonia; sinusitis; and brain abscesses.

CAUSES

Aspergillus is found worldwide, often in fermenting compost piles and damp hay. It's transmitted by inhaling fungal spores or, in aspergillosis endophthalmitis, by the invasion of spores through a wound or other tissue injury.

Aspergillus causes clinical infection only in persons who become especially vulnerable to it. Such vulnerability can result from excessive or prolonged use of antibiotics or immunosuppressive agents; from radiation; from such conditions as AIDS, Hodgkin's disease, leukemia, alcoholism, sarcoidosis, bronchitis, or bronchiectasis; from organ transplantation; and, in aspergilloma, from tuberculosis or another cavitary lung disease.

SIGNS AND SYMPTOMS

- *Aspergilloma* typically either causes no symptoms or mimics tuberculosis, leading to a productive cough and purulent or blood-tinged sputum, dyspnea, empyema, and lung abscesses.
- *Allergic aspergillosis* causes wheezing, dyspnea, cough with some sputum production, pleural pain, and fever.
- *Aspergillosis endophthalmitis* usually appears 2 to 3 weeks after an eye injury or surgery, causing clouded vision, eye pain, and reddened conjunctivae.
- *Disseminated aspergillosis* causes thrombosis, infarctions, and signs and symptoms of septicemia (chills, fever, hypotension, delirium), with azotemia, hematuria, urinary tract obstruction, headaches, seizures, bone pain and tenderness, and soft-tissue swelling.

DIAGNOSTIC TESTS

A chest X-ray may help detect aspergilloma. In aspergillosis endophthalmitis, a history of eye injury or surgery and laboratory tests showing *Aspergillus* confirm the diagnosis. In allergic aspergillosis, sputum analysis shows eosinophils.

TREATMENT

Treatment of aspergilloma calls for local excision of the lesion. Allergic aspergillosis requires desensitization and, possibly, steroids.

Disseminated aspergillosis and aspergillosis endophthalmitis require a 2- to 3-week course of I.V. amphotericin B. However, disseminated aspergillosis often resists amphotericin B therapy.

SPECIAL CONSIDERATIONS

● Supportive therapy, such as chest physiotherapy and coughing, can improve pulmonary function.

Asthma

A reversible lung disease, asthma is characterized by obstruction or narrowing of the airways, which are typically inflamed and overrespond to various stimuli. Asthma may resolve spontaneously or require treatment.

CAUSES

Causes of asthma vary with the form of the disease. *Extrinsic (atopic) asthma* results from sensitivity to specific external allergens, such as pollen, animal dander, house dust or mold, feather pillows, or food additives containing sulfites.

In *intrinsic asthma,* no extrinsic allergen can be identified. Most cases follow a severe respiratory infection. Irritants, emotional stress, fatigue, exposure to noxious fumes, and endocrine, temperature, and humidity changes may aggravate intrinsic asthma attacks. In many asthmatics, intrinsic and extrinsic asthma coexist.

SIGNS AND SYMPTOMS

An asthma attack may begin dramatically, with simultaneous onset of many severe symptoms. Or it may start gradually, with slowly increasing respiratory distress. Symptoms typically include progressively worsening shortness of breath, cough, wheezing, and chest tightness, or a combination of these.

During an acute attack, the cough sounds tight and dry. As the attack subsides, tenacious mucoid sputum is produced (except in young children, who don't expectorate). Characteristic wheezing may be accompanied by coarse rhonchi. Accessory muscle use is particularly common in children. Acute attacks may be accompanied by tachycardia, tachypnea, and diaphoresis. In severe attacks, the patient may be unable to speak more than a few words without pausing for breath. Cyanosis, confusion, and lethargy indicate onset of life-threatening status asthmaticus and respiratory failure.

DIAGNOSTIC TESTS

Pulmonary function studies reveal signs of airway obstruction during an attack. Pulse oximetry may show decreased arterial oxygen saturation (SaO_2). Arterial blood gas (ABG) analysis best indicates attack severity. In acutely severe asthma, partial pressure of arterial oxygen measures less than 60 mm Hg, partial pressure of arterial carbon dioxide is 40 mm Hg or more, and pH usually decreases. Complete blood count with white blood cell differential reveals an increased eosinophil count. Chest X-rays may show overinflated lungs with areas of collapsed air sacs.

TREATMENT

Acute asthma requires measures that decrease bronchoconstriction, reduce bronchial airway edema, and improve pulmonary ventilation. If asthma results from an infection, antibiotics are prescribed. Drug therapy usually includes:

● bronchodilators to decrease bronchoconstriction, for example, methylxanthines and $beta_2$-adrenergic agonists

● corticosteroids for their anti-inflammatory and immunosuppressive effects

● cromolyn and nedocromil to help avert release of chemical mediators that cause bronchoconstriction

● anticholinergic bronchodilators. Medical treatment of asthma attacks is tailored to each patient. For information on general therapy, see *Asthma treatments,* page 26.)

SPECIAL CONSIDERATIONS

● ABG levels, pulmonary function test results, and SaO_2 values are important indicators of patient status.
● High Fowler's position helps ease severity of the attack.
● Postural drainage and chest percussion can help clear secretions.

Asthma treatments

Treatment depends on the pattern and severity of the patient's asthma. General treatments are described below.

Chronic moderate asthma

Initial treatment may include an inhaled beta-adrenergic bronchodilator, an inhaled corticosteroid, and cromolyn.

Chronic severe asthma

Initially, around-the-clock oral bronchodilator therapy with a long-acting theophylline or a $beta_2$-adrenergic agonist may be required, supplemented with an inhaled $beta_2$-adrenergic agonist and an inhaled corticosteroid with or without cromolyn.

Acute asthma attack

Acute attacks that don't respond to self-treatment may require hospital care, $beta_2$-adrenergic agonists and, possibly, oxygen. I.V. aminophylline may be added and I.V. fluid therapy is started. Patients who don't respond to this treatment, whose airways remain obstructed, and who have increasing respiratory difficulty are at risk for status asthmaticus and may require mechanical ventilation.

Status asthmaticus

Treatment consists of aggressive drug therapy: a $beta_2$-adrenergic agonist by nebulizer every 30 to 60 minutes, possibly supplemented with subcutaneous epinephrine, I.V. corticosteroids, I.V. aminophylline, oxygen administration, I.V. fluid therapy, and intubation and mechanical ventilation.

 TEACHING TIP: Instruct the patient to avoid known allergens and irritants. Supply information about names, dosages, actions, and adverse effects of all drugs and special instructions for their use; special breathing techniques; and effective coughing. Teach the patient how to use a metered-dose inhaler. Emphasize the importance of immediately reporting a fever higher than 100° F (37.8° C), chest pain, shortness of breath without coughing or exercising, or uncontrollable coughing.

Atelectasis

In this condition, clusters of alveoli or lung segments fail to expand completely, possibly leading to partial or complete lung collapse. The collapsed areas are unavailable for gas exchange; unoxygenated blood passes through these areas unchanged, causing hypoxia.

Atelectasis may be chronic or acute and occurs to some degree in many patients undergoing upper abdominal or thoracic surgery. The prognosis depends on prompt removal of any airway obstruction, relief of hypoxia, and lung reexpansion.

CAUSES

Atelectasis is frequently a problem in patients with chronic obstructive pulmonary disease, bronchiectasis, or cystic fibrosis and in those who smoke heavily. Atelectasis may also result from occlusion by foreign bodies, bronchogenic carcinoma, and inflammatory lung disease.

Other causes include respiratory distress syndrome of the newborn, oxygen toxicity, pulmonary edema, conditions that cause external compression or that make deep breathing painful (such as upper abdominal surgical incisions, rib fractures, or obesity), prolonged immobility, and mechanical ventilation using constant small tidal volumes without intermittent deep breaths.

SIGNS AND SYMPTOMS
Clinical effects vary, but generally include dyspnea. Atelectasis of a small lung area may cause only mild symptoms that subside without specific treatment. Massive collapse can produce severe dyspnea, anxiety, cyanosis, diaphoresis, peripheral circulatory collapse, tachycardia, and substernal or intercostal retraction. Also, atelectasis may result in compensatory hyperinflation of unaffected lung areas, mediastinal shift to the affected side, and elevation of the ipsilateral hemidiaphragm.

DIAGNOSTIC TESTS
Auscultation reveals diminished or bronchial breath sounds; percussion reveals lung collapse. In widespread atelectasis, chest X-rays show characteristic lung changes. If the cause is unknown, bronchoscopy may be done to rule out an obstruction.

TREATMENT
Appropriate treatment includes incentive spirometry, mucolytics, chest percussion, postural drainage, analgesics, adequate fluid intake, humidified air, and frequent coughing and deep-breathing exercises. If these measures fail, bronchoscopy may help remove secretions. Humidity and bronchodilators can improve mucociliary clearance and dilate airways.

SPECIAL CONSIDERATIONS
• To prevent atelectasis, encourage postoperative and other high-risk patients to cough and deep-breathe every 1 to 2 hours.
• A pillow held tightly over the incision can reduce pain during coughing in postoperative patients. These patients should be gently repositioned often and helped to walk as soon as possible.
• Provide reassurance and emotional support because the patient may be frightened by his limited breathing capacity.

 TEACHING TIP: To encourage deep breathing, teach the patient to use an incentive spirometer every 1 to 2 hours. Also urge him to stop smoking, to lose weight, or both, as needed.

Atopic dermatitis
This chronic skin disorder is characterized by superficial skin inflammation and intense itching. Although atopic dermatitis may appear at any age, it typically begins during infancy or early childhood. It may then subside spontaneously, followed by exacerbations in late childhood, adolescence, or early adulthood. Atopic dermatitis affects less than 1% of the population.

CAUSES
Several theories attempt to explain the pathogenesis of this disorder, which has an unknown cause. One theory suggests an underlying metabolically or biochemically induced skin disorder that's genetically linked to elevated serum immunoglobulin E (IgE) levels. Another theory suggests defective T-cell function.

Factors that may exacerbate atopic dermatitis include irritants, infections (commonly caused by *Staphylococcus aureus),* and some allergens. Although no reliable link exists between atopic dermatitis and exposure to inhaled allergens (such as house dust and animal dander), exposure to food allergens (such as soybeans, fish, or nuts) may coincide with flare-ups of atopic dermatitis.

SIGNS AND SYMPTOMS
Scratching the skin causes vasoconstriction and intensifies pruritus, resulting in erythematous, weeping lesions. Eventually, the lesions become scaly and lichenified. Usually, they're located in areas of flexion and extension, such as the neck, antecubital fossa, popliteal folds, and behind the ears.

DIAGNOSTIC TESTS
Typically, the patient has a history of atopy, such as asthma, hay fever, or urticaria; family members may have a similar history. Laboratory tests re-

veal eosinophilia and elevated serum
IgE levels.

TREATMENT

Measures to ease this chronic disorder include meticulous skin care, environmental control of offending allergens, and drug therapy. Because
dry skin aggravates itching, frequent
application of nonirritating topical
lubricants is important, especially after bathing or showering. Minimizing
exposure to allergens and irritants
also helps control symptoms.

Drug therapy involves corticosteroids and antipruritics. Active dermatitis responds well to topical corticosteroids such as fluocinolone ace-
tonide; these drugs should be applied
immediately after bathing for optimal penetration. Oral antihistamines
help control itching. A bedtime dose
of antihistamines may reduce involuntary scratching during sleep. If a
secondary infection develops, antibiotics are necessary.

Because this disorder may frustrate
the patient and strain family ties,
counseling may play a role in treatment.

SPECIAL CONSIDERATIONS

• The patient should avoid using
laundry additives.

 TEACHING TIP: Emphasize
the importance of good personal hygiene. Also, teach
the patient how to recognize signs
and symptoms of secondary infection.

Basal cell epithelioma

A slow-growing, destructive skin tumor, basal cell epithelioma, or carcinoma, usually occurs in persons over age 40. More prevalent in blond, fair-skinned males, it's the most common malignant tumor affecting whites.

CAUSES

Prolonged sun exposure is the most common cause of basal cell epithelioma. Other causes are arsenic ingestion, radiation exposure, burns, immunosuppression and, rarely, vaccinations.

SIGNS AND SYMPTOMS

Three types of basal cell epithelioma occur:
• *Noduloulcerative lesions* occur most often on the face. In early stages, these lesions are small, smooth, pinkish, translucent papules. As they enlarge, their centers become depressed and their borders become firm and elevated. Ulceration and local invasion eventually occur. These tumors rarely metastasize. However, if untreated, they can spread to vital areas and become infected.
• *Superficial basal cell epitheliomas* are often numerous and commonly occur on the chest and back. These oval or irregularly shaped, lightly pigmented plaques have sharply defined and slightly elevated threadlike borders. The lesions appear scaly; small, atrophic areas in the center resemble psoriasis or eczema. Usually chronic, they rarely invade other areas.
• *Sclerosing basal cell epitheliomas* are waxy, sclerotic, yellow to white plaques without distinct borders. Occurring on the head and neck, these lesions often look like small patches of scleroderma. They seldom invade other areas.

DIAGNOSTIC TESTS

Basal cell cancer is diagnosed by clinical appearance, biopsy, and cell microstructure studies.

TREATMENT

Treatment depends on lesion size, location, and depth. Curettage and electrodesiccation offer good cosmetic results for small lesions. Topical fluorouracil is often used for superficial lesions to produce marked local irritation or inflammation in the involved tissue.

Microscopically controlled surgical excision carefully removes recurrent lesions until a tumor-free plane is achieved. Irradiation is used if the tumor location requires it, and for elderly or debilitated patients who might not withstand surgery.

Cryotherapy with liquid nitrogen freezes and kills the cells. Chemosurgery (often necessary for persistent or recurrent lesions) consists of periodic applications of a fixative paste and subsequent removal of fixed pathologic tissue.

SPECIAL CONSIDERATIONS

• Local inflammation from topical fluorouracil can be relieved with cool compresses or corticosteroid ointment.
• The patient should eat frequent, small, high-protein meals. Eggnog, pureed foods, and liquid protein supplements are good choices if the lesion has invaded the oral cavity and is causing eating problems.
• A patient with noduloulcerative basal cell epithelioma should wash gently when ulcerations and crusting occur. Scrubbing too vigorously may cause bleeding.

 PREVENTION: To help prevent disease recurrence, teach the patient to avoid excessive sun exposure and to use a strong sunscreen or sunshade to guard against skin damage from ultraviolet rays.

Bell's palsy

This neurologic disorder affects the seventh cranial (facial) nerve, producing unilateral facial weakness or paralysis. Onset is rapid.

Bell's palsy occurs in all age-groups but is most common in persons under age 60. In 80% to 90% of patients, it subsides spontaneously, with complete recovery in 1 to 8 weeks; however, recovery may be delayed in older adults. If recovery is partial, contractures may develop on the paralyzed side of the face. Bell's palsy may recur on the same or opposite side of the face.

CAUSES

The seventh cranial nerve is responsible for motor innervation of the facial muscles. In Bell's palsy, the nerve is blocked by an inflammatory reaction around the nerve. This is commonly associated with infections and can result from hemorrhage, tumor, meningitis, or local trauma.

SIGNS AND SYMPTOMS

Bell's palsy usually produces unilateral facial weakness, occasionally with aching pain around the angle of the jaw or behind the ear. On the weak side, the mouth droops, causing the patient to drool saliva from the corner of his mouth. Taste perception is distorted over the affected anterior portion of the tongue.

The forehead appears smooth, and the patient's ability to close his eye on the weak side is markedly impaired. When he tries to close this eye, it rolls upward (Bell's phenomenon) and shows excessive tearing.

DIAGNOSTIC TESTS

Diagnosis depends on clinical presentation: distorted facial appearance and inability to raise the eyebrow, close the eyelid, smile, show the teeth, or puff out the cheek. After 10 days, electromyography helps predict the level of expected recovery by distinguishing a temporary conduction defect from pathologic inflammation of nerve fibers.

TREATMENT

Typically, patients receive prednisone, an oral corticosteroid that reduces facial nerve edema and improves nerve conduction and blood flow. After the 14th day of prednisone therapy, electrotherapy may help prevent atrophy of facial muscles.

SPECIAL CONSIDERATIONS

• If the patient experiences GI distress during prednisone treatment, a concomitant antacid usually provides relief. With a diabetic patient, prednisone must be used with caution.
• To reduce pain, moist heat is applied to the affected side of the face.
• To help maintain muscle tone, the patient's face is massaged with a gentle upward motion two to three times daily for 5 to 10 minutes.
• A facial sling may be applied to improve lip alignment.
• To prevent excessive weight loss, the patient is instructed to chew on the unaffected side of his mouth.

 TEACHING TIP: Advise the patient to protect his eye by covering it with an eyepatch, especially when outdoors. Tell him to keep warm and avoid exposure to dust and wind. When exposure is unavoidable, instruct him to cover his face.

Benign prostatic hyperplasia

In benign prostatic hyperplasia or hypertrophy (BPH), the prostate gland enlarges sufficiently to compress the urethra, causing overt urinary obstruction. (See *How an enlarged prostate blocks urine flow.*)

BPH may also cause formation of a pouch in the bladder, which retains urine when the rest of the bladder empties. The retained urine may lead to calculus formation or cystitis.

PATHOPHYSIOLOGY

How an enlarged prostate blocks urine flow

These illustrations contrast a normal prostate gland with an enlarged one. Enlargement narrows the urethra, interfering with urine flow. This may lead to urine retention and eventually may damage the kidneys.

Normal prostate gland

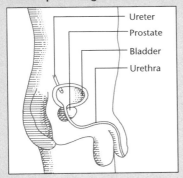

- Ureter
- Prostate
- Bladder
- Urethra

Enlarged prostate gland

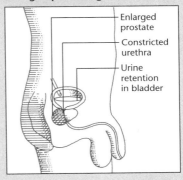

- Enlarged prostate
- Constricted urethra
- Urine retention in bladder

CAUSES

Recent evidence suggests a link between BPH and hormonal activity. As men age, production of androgenic hormones decreases, causing an imbalance in androgen and estrogen levels, along with high levels of dihydrotestosterone, the main prostatic intracellular androgen.

SIGNS AND SYMPTOMS

Typically, BPH starts with a group of symptoms known as *prostatism:* reduced urinary stream caliber and force, difficulty starting the urine flow, a feeling of incomplete voiding and, occasionally, urine retention. As obstruction increases, urination becomes more frequent, with nocturia, incontinence and, possibly, hematuria.

As BPH worsens, complete urinary obstruction may follow infection or use of decongestants, tranquilizers, alcohol, antidepressants, or anticholinergics. Possible complications

include infection, renal insufficiency, hemorrhage, and shock.

DIAGNOSTIC TESTS

Physical examination reveals symptoms of an enlarged prostate. Laboratory tests to confirm the condition include:
- fluoroscopy with dye to locate urinary tract blockage and bladder pouches
- blood test results that suggest poor kidney function
- urinalysis and urine culture to identify bacteria causing a urinary tract infection.

TREATMENT

Depending on the size of the enlarged prostate, the patient's age and health, and the extent of obstruction, BPH is treated symptomatically or surgically. Conservative therapy includes prostate massages, sitz baths, fluid restriction for bladder distention, and antimicrobials for infection. Regular ejaculation may help relieve prostatic congestion.

Urine flow rates can be improved with alpha₁-adrenergic blockers, such as terazosin and prazosin. Finasteride, which may reduce the size of the prostate in some patients, is under investigation.

Surgery is the only effective therapy to relieve acute urine retention, hydronephrosis, and other intolerable symptoms. A transurethral resection may be performed if the prostate weighs less than 2 oz (56.7 g). Some patients undergo open surgical removal through such procedures as suprapubic or retropubic resection. Balloon dilatation of the prostate is being investigated.

SPECIAL CONSIDERATIONS

• After prostate surgery, take measures to maintain patient comfort and prevent postoperative complications.

 ACTION STAT: If the patient develops sudden fever, severe chills, tachycardia, or hypotension, get assistance immediately. These signs and symptoms suggest septic shock — the most serious complication of prostate surgery.

• Shock and hemorrhage are signs of prostatic bleeding. Frequent checks of the catheter for patency and urine color and of dressings for bleeding can avert serious complications.

• After a urinary catheter is removed, the patient may experience frequency, dribbling, and occasional hematuria. Explain to the patient and family that urinary control will return.

 TEACHING TIP: Reinforce prescribed limits on activities. Advise the patient to restrict sexual activity for at least several weeks after discharge. Instruct him to follow the prescribed oral antibiotic drug regimen. Tell him to report inability to void, passage of bloody urine, or fever.

Berylliosis

A form of pneumoconiosis, berylliosis (beryllium poisoning) is a systemic

granulomatous disorder marked mainly by pulmonary manifestations. Most patients with chronic berylliosis become only slightly to moderately disabled by impaired lung function and other symptoms. However, with each acute exacerbation, the prognosis worsens.

CAUSES

Berylliosis results from beryllium inhalation or absorption through the skin. Severity varies with the amount inhaled. The disease occurs among beryllium alloy workers, cathode ray tube makers, gas mantle makers, fluorescent light workers, missile technicians, and nuclear reactor workers. Families of beryllium workers and people who live near plants where beryllium alloy is used are also at risk.

SIGNS AND SYMPTOMS

Absorption of beryllium through broken skin causes an itchy rash that usually subsides within 2 weeks after exposure. A "beryllium ulcer" results from accidental implantation of beryllium metal in the skin.

Respiratory features

Acute berylliosis may cause swelling and ulceration of nasal mucosa, which may progress to septal perforation, tracheitis, and bronchitis. Acute pulmonary disease may develop within a few days or weeks later, producing a progressive dry cough, chest tightness, substernal pain, tachycardia, and signs and symptoms of bronchitis.

About 10% of patients with acute berylliosis develop chronic disease 10 to 15 years after exposure. The chronic form causes increasing dyspnea that becomes progressively worse, along with mild chest pain, dry unproductive cough, and tachypnea.

Other clinical features

Some patients experience pulmonary hypertension, right ventricular hypertrophy, cor pulmonale, hepatosplenomegaly, renal calculi, lymphadenopathy, anorexia, and fatigue.

DIAGNOSTIC TESTS

The patient history reveals occupational, family, or neighborhood exposure to beryllium dust, fumes, or mist. Chest X-rays show characteristic findings in both acute and chronic berylliosis.

Pulmonary function studies show decreases in vital capacity, forced vital capacity, and compliance, among other findings. Arterial blood gas analysis reveals decreases in the partial pressures of arterial oxygen (PaO_2) and carbon dioxide.

TREATMENT

Beryllium ulcer requires excision or curettage. Acute berylliosis calls for prompt corticosteroid therapy. Hypoxia may require oxygen administration by nasal cannula or mask. Severe respiratory failure warrants mechanical ventilation if PaO_2 can't be maintained above 40 mm Hg.

Chronic berylliosis is usually treated with corticosteroids; lifelong maintenance therapy may be necessary. Respiratory signs and symptoms may be treated with bronchodilators, increased fluid intake, and chest physiotherapy.

SPECIAL CONSIDERATIONS

 TEACHING TIP: Encourage the patient to practice physical reconditioning, energy conservation in daily activities, and relaxation techniques. To help prevent infection, instruct him to avoid crowds and persons with infection and to receive influenza and pneumococcal vaccines.

Bladder cancer

Bladder tumors can develop on the surface of the bladder wall or grow within the bladder wall and quickly invade underlying muscles. Most bladder tumors (90%) are transitional cell carcinomas.

CAUSES

Certain environmental carcinogens, such as 2-naphthylamine, benzidine, tobacco, and nitrates, predispose people to transitional cell tumors. Thus, rubber workers, weavers, leather finishers, aniline dye workers, hairdressers, petroleum workers, and spray painters are at high risk. The period between exposure to the carcinogen and development of signs and symptoms is about 18 years.

SIGNS AND SYMPTOMS

In early stages, approximately 25% of patients have no signs or symptoms. Commonly, the first sign is gross, painless, intermittent hematuria. An invasive lesion may cause suprapubic pain after voiding. Other signs and symptoms include bladder irritability, urinary frequency, nocturia, and dribbling.

DIAGNOSTIC TESTS

Bladder cancer is confirmed with biopsy and cystoscopy. Additional tests may be needed to determine if the tumor has invaded the prostate gland or nearby lymph nodes. These tests may include urinalysis, urinary tract X-rays, computed tomography scan, and ultrasonography.

TREATMENT

Appropriate treatment for bladder cancer varies.

Superficial tumors that haven't invaded the muscle are removed by transurethral resection and fulguration (electrical destruction). Intravesicular chemotherapy (washing the bladder directly with antineoplastic drugs) is also used. Superficial tumors too large to be treated through a cystoscope require segmental bladder resection. This procedure is feasible only if the tumor isn't near the bladder neck or ureteral orifices.

Radical cystectomy is the treatment of choice for *infiltrating tumors.* The surgeon forms a urinary diversion, usually an ileal conduit. The patient must then wear an external pouch continuously. Other types of urinary diversion include ureterostomy, nephrostomy, vesicostomy, ileal bladder, ileal loop, and sigmoid conduit.

For *advanced bladder cancer,* treatment includes cystectomy to remove

Caring for a urinary stoma

If your responsibilities include patient teaching, provide these instructions to a patient with a urinary stoma.

Preparing and applying the pouch

• Show the patient how to prepare and apply the pouch, which may be reusable or disposable. If he chooses the reusable type, he'll need at least two.

• To select the right pouch size, tell the patient to measure the stoma and order a pouch with an opening that clears the stoma with a ⅛" margin. Instruct him to remeasure the stoma after he goes home, in case the size changes. The pouch should have a drainage valve at the bottom. Tell him to empty the pouch when it's one-third full or every 2 to 3 hours.

• To ensure a good skin seal, advise the patient to select a skin barrier that contains synthetics and little or no karaya. He should check the pouch frequently to make sure that the skin seal remains intact. A good skin seal with a skin barrier may last for 3 to 6 days, so the pouch should be changed only that often. Tell the patient he can wear a loose-fitting elastic belt to help secure the pouch.

• The ileal conduit stoma reaches its permanent size 2 to 4 months after surgery. Because the intestine normally produces mucus, tell the patient not to be alarmed by mucus that appears in the draining urine.

Cleaning the skin near the stoma

Instruct the patient to keep the skin around the stoma clean and free from irritation, as follows:

• After removing the pouch, wash the skin with water and mild soap. Rinse well with clear water to remove soap residue, and then gently pat the skin dry; don't rub.

• Place a gauze sponge soaked with vinegar-water (1 part: 3 parts) over the stoma for a few minutes to prevent uric acid crystal buildup. While preparing the skin, place a rolled-up dry sponge over the stoma to collect draining urine.

• Coat the skin with a silicone skin protector, and cover with the collection pouch. If skin irritation or breakdown occurs, apply a layer of antacid precipitate to the clean, dry skin before coating with the skin protector.

Other instructions

Advise the patient that he can level uneven surfaces on his abdomen with a variety of specially prepared products or skin barriers.

---

the tumor, radiation therapy, and systemic chemotherapy.

Investigational treatments for bladder cancer include photodynamic therapy and intravesicular administration of interferon alfa and tumor necrosis factor.

SPECIAL CONSIDERATIONS

• After surgery, the patient with a urinary stoma should be encouraged to look at it.

• Males are impotent after radical cystectomy and urethrectomy. Later, the patient may desire a penile implant to make sexual intercourse (without ejaculation) possible.

• When a patient with a urinary diversion is discharged, follow-up home health care providers or enterostomal therapists help coordinate his care.

• Encourage the patient's spouse, friend, or relative to attend teaching

sessions regarding the urinary stoma. (See *Caring for a urinary stoma.*) However, warn this person beforehand that a negative reaction to the stoma can impede the patient's adjustment.
• Chemical workers and people with a history of benign bladder tumors or persistent cystitis should have periodic cytologic examinations and learn about the dangers of disease-causing agents.
• The American Cancer Society and the United Ostomy Association are valuable resources for people with urinary stomas.

Blastomycosis

Also called Gilchrist's disease, blastomycosis is caused by the yeastlike fungus *Blastomyces dermatitidis,* which usually infects the lungs and causes bronchopneumonia. Less frequently, this fungus may spread through the bloodstream and cause osteomyelitis and central nervous system (CNS), skin, and genital disorders. Untreated blastomycosis is slowly progressive and usually fatal. However, spontaneous remissions occasionally occur.

CAUSES
Blastomycosis is generally found in North America (where *B. dermatitidis* normally inhabits the soil) and is endemic to the southeastern United States. *B. dermatitidis* is probably inhaled by people in close contact with the soil. The incubation period may range from weeks to months.

SIGNS AND SYMPTOMS
Initial signs and symptoms of *pulmonary blastomycosis* mimic those of a viral upper respiratory infection — a dry, hacking, or productive cough; pleuritic chest pain; fever; shaking chills; night sweats; malaise; anorexia; and weight loss.
Cutaneous blastomycosis causes small, painless, nonpruritic macules or papules on exposed body parts. These lesions become raised and reddened, and occasionally progress to draining skin abscesses or fistulas.

Skeletal involvement causes soft-tissue swelling, tenderness, and warmth over bony lesions, which generally occur in the thoracic, lumbar, and sacral regions; in the long bones of the legs; and, in children, in the skull.
CNS involvement may lead to meningitis or cerebral abscesses, resulting in a decreased level of consciousness (LOC), lethargy, and change in mood or affect.

DIAGNOSTIC TESTS
Diagnosis of blastomycosis requires:
• culture of *B. dermatitidis* from skin lesions, pus, sputum, or lung secretions
• microscopic examination and analysis of tissue removed from the skin or the lungs, or of bronchial washings, sputum, or pus
• immunologic tests to detect antibodies to the fungus.
  A chest X-ray is usually ordered if lung infection is suspected.

TREATMENT
All forms of blastomycosis respond to amphotericin B. Ketoconazole or fluconazole may be used as an alternative. Patient care is mainly supportive.

SPECIAL CONSIDERATIONS

ACTION STAT: Report any hearing loss, tinnitus, or dizziness immediately. These symptoms are adverse effects of amphotericin B.
• In severe pulmonary blastomycosis, hemoptysis is a risk. If the patient has a fever, a cool room and tepid sponge baths can provide relief.
• If blastomycosis causes joint pain or swelling, the joint should be elevated and heat applied.
• In CNS infection, the patient should be monitored carefully for decreasing LOC.

Blepharitis

A common inflammation, blepharitis produces a red-rimmed appearance of the margins of the eyelids. Commonly chronic and bilateral, it can affect both the upper and lower lids. Seborrheic blepharitis, characterized by waxy scales, is common in older adults and in persons with red hair. Staphylococcal (ulcerative) blepharitis is characterized by dry scales, with tiny ulcerated areas along the lid margins. Both types may coexist.

Blepharitis tends to recur and become chronic. It can be controlled if treatment begins before the onset of ocular involvement.

CAUSES

Seborrheic blepharitis generally results from seborrhea of the scalp, eyebrows, and ears. Ulcerative blepharitis is caused by *Staphylococcus aureus* infection. (People with this infection may also tend to develop chalazions and styes.)

SIGNS AND SYMPTOMS

Clinical features of blepharitis include itching, burning, a foreign-body sensation, and sticky, crusted eyelids on waking. This constant irritation results in unconscious rubbing of the eyes (causing reddened rims) or continual blinking. Other signs include waxy scales in seborrheic blepharitis, flaky scales on lashes, loss of lashes, and ulcerated areas on lid margins in ulcerative blepharitis.

DIAGNOSTIC TESTS

Diagnosis depends on the patient history and characteristic signs and symptoms. In ulcerative blepharitis, a culture of the ulcerated lid margin shows *S. aureus.*

TREATMENT

Early treatment is essential to prevent recurrence or complications. Treatment depends on the type of blepharitis:

• *seborrheic blepharitis:* daily shampooing of eyelashes (using a mild shampoo on a damp applicator stick or a washcloth) to remove scales from the lid margins; also, frequent shampooing of the scalp and eyebrows

• *ulcerative blepharitis:* warm com-

presses applied to the eye and a sulfonamide eye ointment or an appropriate antibiotic

• *blepharitis resulting from pediculosis:* removal of nits (with forceps) or application of ophthalmic physostigmine or other ointment as an insecticide.

SPECIAL CONSIDERATIONS

• The patient should gently remove scales from the lid margins daily with an applicator stick or a clean washcloth.

 TEACHING TIP: Teach the patient to use the following method to apply warm compresses: First, run warm water into a clean bowl. Then immerse a clean cloth in the water and wring it out. Place the warm cloth against the closed eyelid. (Be careful not to burn the skin.) Hold the compress in place until it cools. Continue this procedure for 15 minutes.

• Antibiotic ophthalmic ointment should be applied after a 15-minute application of warm compresses.

Bone tumors, primary malignant

A rare type of bone cancer, primary malignant bone tumors (sarcomas of the bone) constitute less than 1% of all malignant tumors. They may originate in osseous or nonosseous tissue. Osseous tumors arise from the bony structure itself and include osteogenic sarcoma (the most common), parosteal osteogenic sarcoma, chondrosarcoma, and malignant giant cell tumor. Nonosseous tumors arise from hematopoietic, vascular, and neural tissues and include Ewing's sarcoma, fibrosarcoma, and chordoma.

CAUSES

Primary malignant bone tumors have no known cause. Some researchers suggest that they arise in areas of rapid growth because children and young adults with such tumors seem to be much taller than average. Other theories point to heredity, trauma, and excessive radiation therapy.

SIGNS AND SYMPTOMS

Bone pain is the most common feature of primary malignant bone tumors. Often more intense at night, it usually isn't associated with mobility. The pain is dull and typically localized. Presence of a mass or tumor is also common.

The tumor site may be tender and swollen; the tumor itself is often palpable. Pathologic fractures are common.

DIAGNOSTIC TESTS

A biopsy is essential to confirm a primary malignant bone tumor. Bone X-rays, radioisotope bone scans, and computed tomography scans show tumor size.

TREATMENT

Excision of the tumor along with a 3" (7.6 cm) margin is the treatment of choice. This procedure may be combined with preoperative chemotherapy.

In some patients, radical surgery (such as hemipelvectomy or interscapulothoracic amputation) is necessary. However, surgical tumor resection has saved limbs from amputation.

Intensive chemotherapy includes administration of doxorubicin, vincristine, cyclophosphamide, cisplatin, and dacarbazine. Chemotherapy may be infused intra-arterially into the long bones of the legs.

SPECIAL CONSIDERATIONS

• The foot of the patient's bed should be elevated or the stump placed on a pillow for the first 24 hours after surgery. The stump shouldn't be elevated for more than 48 hours because this may lead to contractures.
• If necessary, pillows can be used as braces, allowing the affected part to remain at rest.
• If surgery will affect the patient's lower extremities, a physical therapist can provide instruction in the use of assistive devices preoperatively.
• Early rehabilitation for amputees usually calls for the start of physical therapy 24 hours postoperatively.

• To avoid contractures and promote wound healing, the patient should avoid dangling the stump over the edge of the bed; sitting in a wheelchair with the stump flexed; placing a pillow under his hip, knee, or back or between his thighs; lying with knees flexed; resting an above-the-knee stump on the crutch handle; or abducting an above-the-knee stump.
• In selecting a prosthesis, the patient's needs, financial resources, age, and possible vision problems and the types of prostheses available are considered. The rehabilitation staff helps him make the final decision.

 TEACHING TIP: Provide instructions and demonstrations in readjusting body weight to make it easier for the patient to get in and out of the bed and the wheelchair.

Botulism

A life-threatening paralytic illness, botulism results from an exotoxin produced by the gram-positive, anaerobic bacillus *Clostridium botulinum.* It occurs as botulism food poisoning, wound botulism, and infant botulism. (See *Botulism in infants,* page 38.) Mortality rate is about 25%, with death most often caused by respiratory failure during the first week of illness.

CAUSES

Botulism usually results from ingestion of inadequately cooked contaminated foods — especially those with low acid content, such as home-canned fruits and vegetables, sausages, and smoked or preserved fish or meat. Rarely, it results from wound infection with *C. botulinum.*

SIGNS AND SYMPTOMS

The disease usually presents within 12 to 36 hours after ingestion of contaminated food. Severity varies with the amount of toxin ingested and the patient's immunologic status. Generally, early onset (within 24 hours) signals critical and potentially fatal illness. Initial signs and symptoms in-

Botulism in infants

Recent findings show that an infant's GI tract can become colonized with *Clostridium botulinum* from some unknown source. Infant botulism usually afflicts infants ages 3 to 20 weeks.

Clinical features

Infant botulism can cause hypotonic (floppy) infant syndrome, which may lead to constipation, feeble cry, depressed gag reflex, and inability to suck. Cranial nerve deficits may occur, causing a flaccid facial expression, ptosis, ophthalmoplegia, generalized muscle weakness, hypotonia, and areflexia. Loss of head control may be striking. Respiratory arrest is likely.

• Before giving botulinum antitoxin, an accurate patient history of allergies, especially to horses, must be taken and a skin test performed. Because anaphylaxis or other hypersensitivity and serum sickness are risks, epinephrine and emergency airway equipment should be available.

 TEACHING TIP: If the patient returns home, tell the family to watch for weakness, blurred vision, and slurred speech, and to return the patient to the hospital immediately if such signs or symptoms appear.

• Botulism prevention calls for proper techniques during food processing and preserving. People must avoid even *tasting* food from a bulging can or one with a peculiar odor, and should sterilize by boiling any utensil that comes in contact with suspected food. Ingestion of even a small amount of food contaminated with botulism toxin can prove fatal.

clude dry mouth, sore throat, weakness, vomiting, and diarrhea.

The cardinal sign of botulism, though, is acute symmetrical cranial nerve impairment (ptosis, diplopia, dysarthria), followed by descending weakness or paralysis of muscles in the extremities or trunk and dyspnea from respiratory muscle paralysis.

DIAGNOSTIC TESTS

Identification of the offending poison in the patient's blood, stools, stomach contents, or the suspected food confirms the diagnosis. Diagnosis must rule out other diseases often confused with botulism.

TREATMENT

Botulinum antitoxin (available through the Centers for Disease Control and Prevention) is the treatment of choice.

SPECIAL CONSIDERATIONS

• Induced vomiting, gastric lavage, and a high enema can purge any unabsorbed toxin from the bowel if ingestion has occurred within several hours.

Brain abscess

This intracranial abscess is a free or encapsulated collection of pus that usually occurs in the temporal lobe, cerebellum, or frontal lobes. It can vary in size and may occur singly or multilocularly. About 30% of patients develop focal seizures.

An untreated brain abscess is usually fatal; with treatment, the prognosis is only fair.

CAUSES

A brain abscess usually occurs secondary to some other infection, especially otitis media, sinusitis, dental abscess, and mastoiditis. Other causes include subdural empyema; bacterial endocarditis; human immunodeficiency virus infection; bacteremia; pulmonary or pleural infection; pelvic, abdominal, and skin infections; and cranial trauma, such as a penetrating head wound or compound skull fracture.

SIGNS AND SYMPTOMS

Generally, brain abscess produces clinical effects similar to those of a brain tumor. Early symptoms result from increased intracranial pressure (ICP) and include constant intractable headache, worsened by straining; nausea; vomiting; and focal or generalized seizures. Typical later symptoms include ocular disturbances, such as nystagmus and decreased vision.

Other features differ with the abscess site. Depending on abscess size and location, level of consciousness varies from drowsiness to deep stupor.

DIAGNOSTIC TESTS

A history of infection — especially of the middle ear, mastoid, nasal sinuses, heart, or lungs — or a history of congenital heart disease, along with such clinical features as increased ICP, point to a brain abscess. A computed tomography (CT) scan and, occasionally, arteriography help locate the site.

A CT-guided stereotactic biopsy may be done to drain and culture the abscess. Other tests include culture and sensitivity of drainage to identify the causative organism, skull X-rays, and a radioisotope scan.

TREATMENT

Therapy consists of antibiotics to combat the underlying infection and surgical aspiration or drainage of the abscess. However, surgery is delayed until the abscess becomes encapsulated and is contraindicated in patients with debilitating cardiac conditions. A penicillinase-resistant antibiotic given for at least 2 weeks before surgery can reduce the risk of spreading infection. Other treatments during the acute phase may include mechanical ventilation, I.V. fluids, diuretics, glucocorticoids, and anticonvulsants.

SPECIAL CONSIDERATIONS

 ACTION STAT: Report signs and symptoms of meningitis (nuchal rigidity, headaches, chills, sweats) — an ever-present threat.

• The patient with an acute brain ab-scess requires intensive care monitoring, with frequent assessment of neurologic status.

• To promote drainage and prevent reaccumulation of the abscess, the patient is positioned on the operative side.

 PREVENTION: To help prevent brain abscess, stress the need for prompt treatment of otitis media, mastoiditis, dental abscess, and other infections.

Brain tumors, malignant

Malignant brain tumors (gliomas, meningiomas, and schwannomas) are common, with an incidence of 4.5 per 100,000. In adults, the most common tumor types are gliomas and meningiomas; these tumors are usually supratentorial (above the covering of the cerebellum). In children, the most common tumors are astrocytomas, medulloblastomas, ependymomas, and brain stem gliomas.

CAUSES

The cause of brain tumors is unknown.

SIGNS AND SYMPTOMS

Brain tumors cause central nervous system changes by invading and destroying tissues and by secondary effect — mainly compression of the brain, cranial nerves, and cerebral vessels; cerebral edema; and increased intracranial pressure (ICP). Generally, clinical features result from increased ICP and vary with the type of tumor, its location, and the degree of invasion.

Glioblastoma multiforme

Glioblastoma multiforme causes increased ICP with resulting nausea, vomiting, headache, and papilledema. The patient may also show mental and behavioral changes, altered vital signs, and speech and sensory disturbances. Other signs and symptoms depend on the tumor's location. For instance, a tumor in the temporal lobe may cause psychomotor seizures, whereas one in the frontal lobe may produce abnormal reflexes and motor responses.

Astrocytoma
The patient with an astrocytoma typically experiences headache, changes in mental activity, decreased motor strength and coordination, seizures, and altered vital signs. Other clinical features vary with tumor location. An astrocytoma in the thalamus or hypothalamus, for instance, causes various endocrine, metabolic, autonomic, and behavioral changes. An astrocytoma affecting the third ventricle produces changes in mental activity and level of consciousness, nausea, pupillary dilation, and a sluggish light reflex.

Oligodendroglioma
An oligodendroglioma results in increased ICP along with visual disturbances and mental and behavior changes. Depending on the tumor's location, the patient may also have hallucinations, seizures, ataxia, dizziness, poor balance, and cranial nerve palsies.

Ependymoma
Signs and symptoms of an ependymoma resemble those of an oligodendroglioma. Depending on the tumor's size, the patient may also have obstructive hydrocephalus and increased ICP.

Medulloblastoma
A medulloblastoma causes signs and symptoms of increased ICP. If the tumor is in the brain stem or cerebrum, the patient may also experience nystagmus, hearing loss, visual disturbances, dizziness, ataxia, facial paresthesia, and cranial nerve palsies.

Meningioma
Two-thirds of patients with meningiomas experience seizures. Other signs and symptoms include headache, vomiting, changes in mental activity and, possibly, skull changes such as a bony bulge over the tumor. Other clinical features vary with the tumor's location. For instance, if both optic nerves and frontal lobes are compressed, headaches and bilateral vision loss may occur.

Schwannoma
A schwannoma may cause unilateral hearing loss, stiff neck, hydrocephalus, ataxia, and uncoordinated arm movements. Because this tumor affects the cranial nerve sheath, it may disturb functions controlled by cranial nerves. For instance, a schwannoma affecting cranial nerve VI may cause double vision; a schwannoma affecting cranial nerve X may cause weakness of the palate, tongue, and nerve muscles on the same side as the tumor.

DIAGNOSTIC TESTS
In many cases, a brain tumor is diagnosed by performing a tissue biopsy during stereotactic surgery. Additional studies include neurologic assessment, skull X-rays, a brain scan, computed tomography scans, magnetic resonance imaging, and cerebral angiography. Lumbar puncture shows increased pressure and protein levels in the cerebrospinal fluid (CSF).

TREATMENT
Remedial approaches include removing a resectable tumor; reducing a nonresectable tumor; relieving cerebral edema, increased ICP, and other symptoms; and preventing further neurologic damage.

Treatments may include surgery, radiation, chemotherapy, or reduction of increased ICP with diuretics, corticosteroids, or possibly CSF shunting. Chemotherapy for malignant brain tumors includes nitrosoureas; intrathecal and intra-arterial administration maximize drug actions.

SPECIAL CONSIDERATIONS
• After infratentorial craniotomy, the patient is kept flat for 48 hours, but logrolled every 2 hours to minimize complications of immobilization.

PREVENTION: Warn the patient to avoid Valsalva's maneuver or isometric muscle contractions when moving or sitting up in bed; these motions can increase ICP.

• Because brain tumors may cause residual neurologic deficits that cause physical or mental handicaps, rehabilitation should begin early. Occupational and physical therapists can provide instructions and exercises to help the patient retain independence in daily activities and provide aids for self-care and mobilization.

• If the patient is aphasic, consultation with a speech pathologist should be scheduled.

Breast cancer

The most common cancer affecting women, breast cancer is the number two killer (after lung cancer) of women ages 35 to 54. It occurs in men, but rarely. The 5-year survival rate has improved because of earlier diagnosis and the variety of treatments now available.

CAUSES
The cause of breast cancer isn't known, but its high incidence in women implicates estrogen. Certain predisposing factors are clear. (See *Risk factors for breast cancer*.)

SIGNS AND SYMPTOMS
Warning signs of possible breast cancer include a lump or mass in the breast, a change in breast symmetry or size, a change in breast skin or skin temperature, unusual nipple drainage or discharge or a change in the nipple, and edema of the arm.

DIAGNOSTIC TESTS
The most reliable way to detect breast cancer is by monthly self-examination, with immediate evaluation of any abnormality. Other tests include mammography and biopsy. Because mammography can produce a false-negative result, most doctors do a fine-needle aspiration or surgical biopsy if the woman has a suspicious

---

Risk factors for breast cancer

The following factors seem to increase a woman's risk of breast cancer:
• family history of breast cancer
• long menstrual cycle (began menses early or menopause late)
• no pregnancies
• first pregnancy after age 31
• history of unilateral breast cancer
• history of endometrial or ovarian cancer
• exposure to low-level ionizing radiation.

Many other possible predisposing factors have been investigated, including estrogen therapy, antihypertensives, high-fat diet, obesity, and fibrocystic tissue of the breasts.

---

mass. Ultrasound, which can distinguish a fluid-filled cyst from a tumor, can be used instead of a surgical biopsy.

Bone scans, computed tomography scans, alkaline phosphatase levels, liver function studies, and a liver biopsy can detect the spread of cancer to distant sites. A hormonal receptor assay is done to determine if the tumor is estrogen- or progesterone-dependent; this test guides decisions to use therapy that blocks the action of estrogen.

TREATMENT
In choosing therapy, the patient and doctor consider the disease stage, the woman's age and menopausal status, and the disfiguring effects of surgery. Treatment for breast cancer may include one or any combination of the following.

Surgery
Surgery involves either mastectomy or lumpectomy. A *lumpectomy* may be the only surgery needed, especially if

the tumor is small and there's no evidence of axillary node involvement. Radiation therapy is often combined with this surgery.

In *lumpectomy and dissection of the axillary lymph nodes,* the tumor and axillary lymph nodes are removed, leaving the breast intact.

A *simple mastectomy* removes the breast but not the lymph nodes or pectoral muscles. A *modified radical mastectomy* removes the breast and axillary nodes. A *radical mastectomy* removes the breast, pectoralis major and minor, and axillary lymph nodes.

Chemotherapy, tamoxifen, and peripheral stem cell therapy

Various cytotoxic drug combinations may be used as adjuvant or primary therapy. Tamoxifen, an estrogen antagonist, is the adjuvant treatment of choice for postmenopausal patients with positive estrogen receptor status. Peripheral stem cell therapy may be used for advanced breast cancer.

Primary radiation therapy

Used before or after tumor removal, primary radiation is effective for small tumors in early stages with no evidence of distant metastasis.

SPECIAL CONSIDERATIONS

• Showing the patient where the incision will be can help to alleviate anxiety and reduce her fears about postoperative appearance. After surgery, the patient and her partner should be encouraged to look at the incision as soon as feasible.
• The patient is encouraged to get out of bed as soon as possible (even as soon as the anesthesia wears off or the first evening after surgery).

 PREVENTION: To help prevent lymphedema of the arm, instruct the patient to exercise her hand and arm regularly and to avoid activities that might cause infection in this hand or arm.
• Depression after mastectomy is a risk. Refer the patient to an appropri-

ate organization, such as the American Cancer Society's Reach to Recovery.

Bronchiectasis

A condition marked by chronic abnormal dilation of bronchi and destruction of bronchial walls, bronchiectasis is usually bilateral and involves the basilar segments of the lower lung lobes. This disease has three forms: cylindrical (fusiform), varicose, and saccular (cystic).

The availability of antibiotics to treat acute respiratory tract infections has dramatically decreased the incidence of bronchiectasis in the past 20 years. However, once established, the disease is irreversible.

CAUSES

This disease results from conditions associated with repeated damage to bronchial walls and abnormal mucociliary clearance, which cause breakdown of supporting tissue adjacent to airways. (See *Understanding the causes of bronchiectasis.*)

SIGNS AND SYMPTOMS

Initially, bronchiectasis may be asymptomatic. When symptoms arise, they're often attributed to other illnesses.

The classic sign is a chronic cough that produces copious, foul-smelling, mucopurulent secretions. Other typical findings include coarse crackles during inspiration over involved lobes or segments, occasional wheezes, dyspnea, sinusitis, weight loss, anemia, malaise, clubbing, recurrent fever, chills, and other signs and symptoms of infection.

DIAGNOSTIC TESTS

A history of recurrent bronchial infections, pneumonia, and a bloody cough in a patient whose chest X-rays show peribronchial thickening, collapsed lung areas, and scattered cystic changes suggest bronchiectasis. A computed tomography scan and bronchoscopy can help to pinpoint a bleeding site.

PATHOPHYSIOLOGY

Understanding the causes of bronchiectasis

The following conditions can lead to bronchiectasis:
- cystic fibrosis
- immunologic disorders such as agammaglobulinemia
- recurrent, inadequately treated bacterial respiratory tract infections, such as tuberculosis and complications of measles, pneumonia, pertussis, or influenza
- obstruction related to recurrent infection
- inhalation of corrosive gas or repeated aspiration of gastric juices into the lungs
- congenital anomalies (rare).

TREATMENT

Typically, antibiotics are given orally or I.V. for 7 to 10 days or until sputum production decreases. Bronchodilators, combined with postural drainage and chest percussion, help remove secretions if the patient has bronchospasm and thick, tenacious sputum. Bronchoscopy may be used to help mobilize secretions. Hypoxia calls for oxygen therapy.

SPECIAL CONSIDERATIONS

- Supportive care helps the patient adjust to the permanent lifestyle changes that irreversible lung damage necessitates. Thorough teaching is vital, including an explanation of scheduled diagnostic tests, effective coughing and deep-breathing techniques, and the importance of smoking cessation.
- Chest physiotherapy is performed several times a day. The patient must maintain each position for 10 minutes; then percussion is performed and the patient instructed to cough.
- Balanced, high-protein meals promote good health and tissue healing; high fluid intake aids expectoration. Frequent mouth care helps to remove foul-smelling sputum.
- To reduce the risk of infection, the patient should dispose of all secretions properly.

TEACHING TIP: Instruct the patient to take medications exactly as prescribed and to avoid air pollutants and people with upper respiratory tract infections.
- Prevention efforts include treating bacterial pneumonia vigorously and stressing the need for immunization to prevent childhood diseases.

Buerger's disease

Also called *thromboangiitis obliterans,* this inflammatory, nonatheromatous occlusive condition causes segmental lesions and subsequent thrombus formation in the small and medium arteries (and sometimes the veins). The result is decreased blood flow to the feet and legs. Buerger's disease may cause ulceration and, eventually, gangrene.

CAUSES

Although the cause of Buerger's disease is unknown, a definite link exists to smoking, suggesting a hypersensitivity reaction to nicotine. Incidence is highest among men of Jewish ancestry, ages 20 to 40, who smoke heavily. Precipitating factors include emotional stress, exposure to extreme temperatures, and trauma.

SIGNS AND SYMPTOMS

Buerger's disease typically causes intermittent claudication of the instep, which is aggravated by exercise and relieved by rest. During exposure to low temperatures, the feet become cold, cyanotic, and numb; later, they redden, become hot, and tingle. Occasionally, Buerger's disease also affects the hands, possibly resulting in painful fingertip ulcerations.

Associated features may include impaired peripheral pulses, migratory superficial thrombophlebitis and, in later stages, ulceration, muscle atrophy, and gangrene.

DIAGNOSTIC TESTS

History and physical findings may strongly suggest Buerger's disease. Supportive diagnostic tests include arteriography and ultrasonography.

TREATMENT

Therapy may include an exercise program that uses gravity to fill and drain blood vessels. A patient with severe disease may undergo a lumbar sympathectomy to increase blood supply to the skin. Amputation may be necessary for nonhealing ulcers, intractable pain, or gangrene.

SPECIAL CONSIDERATIONS

• Comfort measures for a patient who has ulcers and gangrene include bed rest, use of a padded footboard or bed cradle to prevent pressure from bed linens, and protection of the feet with soft padding. The feet should be washed gently with a mild soap and tepid water, rinsed thoroughly, and patted dry.
• If the patient has undergone amputation, rehabilitative needs should be assessed. Physical therapists, occupational therapists, and social service agencies should provide instruction and guidance as needed.

 TEACHING TIP: To make treatment more effective, urge the patient to stop smoking permanently. Instruct him to wear well-fitting shoes and cotton or wool socks and to inspect his feet daily for cuts, abrasions, and signs of skin

breakdown. Urge him to seek medical attention immediately after any trauma.

Candidiasis

Candidiasis is usually a mild, superficial fungal infection. Most often, it infects the nails (onychomycosis), skin (diaper rash), or mucous membranes, especially the oropharynx (thrush), vagina (moniliasis), esophagus, and GI tract.

Rarely, these fungi enter the bloodstream and invade organs, causing serious infections. The prognosis varies with the patient's resistance.

CAUSES
Candidiasis is caused by the *Candida* genus. Most cases result from *C. albicans*. Other infective strains include *C. parapsilosis, C. tropicalis,* and *C. guilliermondii*.

Part of the normal flora of the GI tract, mouth, vagina, and skin, these fungi cause infection when some change in the body permits their sudden proliferation — rising glucose levels from diabetes mellitus, lowered resistance, or systemic introduction (for instance, during surgery). However, the most common predisposing factor is the use of broad-spectrum antibiotics, which decrease the number of normal flora and permit candidal organisms to proliferate.

SIGNS AND SYMPTOMS
Superficial candidiasis produces symptoms that correspond to the infection site:
• *skin:* scaly, erythematous, papular rash appearing below the breast, between the fingers, and at the axillae, groin, and umbilicus.
• *nails:* red, swollen, darkened nail bed
• *oropharyngeal mucosa (thrush):* cream-colored or bluish white patches of exudate on the tongue, mouth, or pharynx (see *Identifying thrush,* page 46).

• *esophageal mucosa:* dysphagia, retrosternal pain, regurgitation and, occasionally, scales in the mouth and throat
• *vaginal mucosa:* white or yellow discharge with pruritus and local excoriation, white or gray raised patches on vaginal walls with local inflammation, dyspareunia.

Systemic (generalized) infection causes chills; high, spiking fever; hypotension; prostration; occasional rash; and other symptoms that vary with the affected organs.

DIAGNOSTIC TESTS
Diagnosis of superficial candidiasis depends on evidence of *Candida* on a Gram stain of skin, vaginal scrapings, pus, or sputum. Systemic infections require specimen collection for a blood or tissue culture.

TREATMENT
Therapy aims to improve the underlying condition that predisposes the patient to candidiasis, such as controlling diabetes or discontinuing antibiotic therapy, if possible. Antifungal drugs are used; selection depends on the site and type of infection.

SPECIAL CONSIDERATIONS
• Mouth discomfort can be relieved by applying a topical anesthetic, such as lidocaine, at least 1 hour before meals. (However, this may suppress the gag reflex and cause aspiration.)
• A nonirritating mouthwash loosens tenacious secretions and a soft toothbrush avoids irritation.

 TEACHING TIP: Instruct a patient who's using nystatin solution to swish it around in the mouth for several minutes before swallowing.
• Cornstarch or dry padding in intertriginous areas of obese patients prevents irritation.

Identifying thrush

Candidiasis of the oropharyngeal mucosa (thrush) causes cream-colored or bluish white pseudomembranous patches on the tongue, mouth, or pharynx. Fungal invasion may extend to circumoral tissues.

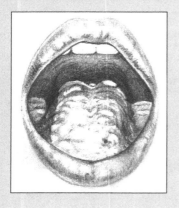

Cardiac arrhythmias

Cardiac arrhythmias are deviations in the heart's rhythm. They may involve a change in the rate or regularity of the heartbeat, the site of impulse origin, or the sequence of activation.

Arrhythmias are generally classified according to origin (ventricular or supraventricular). Their effect on cardiac output and blood pressure, partially influenced by the origin site, determines their clinical significance.

CAUSES

Arrhythmias may be congenital or may result from such factors as myocardial ischemia, myocardial infarction, or organic heart disease. Drug toxicity or degeneration of cardiac conductive tissue (sick sinus syndrome) can also trigger arrhythmias.

SIGNS AND SYMPTOMS

Arrhythmias vary in severity from mild, asymptomatic conditions that require no treatment (such as sinus arrhythmia) to catastrophic ventricular fibrillation, which necessitates immediate resuscitation.

DIAGNOSTIC TESTS

Cardiac arrhythmias are diagnosed from characteristic features on the electrocardiogram.

TREATMENT

Treatment varies with the type of arrhythmia. Many patients receive antiarrhythmic medications or other drugs that affect the heart. Patients with such arrhythmias as sinus bradycardia, sinus arrest, premature junctional rhythm, and heart block may receive a temporary or permanent artificial pacemaker. Also, any underlying condition is treated as appropriate.

Patients with immediately life-threatening arrhythmias, such as ventricular fibrillation or asystole, may need cardiopulmonary resuscitation (CPR), defibrillation, endotracheal intubation, and emergency medications.

SPECIAL CONSIDERATIONS

 ACTION STAT: A patient who develops a life-threatening arrhythmia must be rapidly assessed for level of consciousness, respirations, and pulse. Begin CPR, if indicated, and be prepared for resuscitative procedures, such as cardioversion, if indicated.

● To avert pacemaker malfunction, the patient's activity is restricted, the pulse is monitored regularly, and the patient is checked for signs of decreased cardiac output. He is warned about environmental hazards, as indicated by the manufacturer.

 TEACHING TIP: Advise the patient to report fainting spells and light-headedness, and stress the importance of regular checkups.

Cardiac tamponade

In this disorder, a rapid, unchecked rise in intrapericardial pressure impairs diastolic filling of the heart. The rise in pressure usually results from blood or fluid accumulation in the pericardial sac.

If fluid accumulates rapidly, cardiac tamponade is commonly fatal and necessitates emergency lifesaving measures. A slow accumulation and rise in pressure, as in pericardial effusion associated with cancer, may not cause immediate symptoms.

CAUSES

Increased intrapericardial pressure and cardiac tamponade may be idiopathic (Dressler's syndrome) or may result from such conditions as effusion, hemorrhage caused by heart trauma or rupture, acute myocardial infarction, or uremia.

SIGNS AND SYMPTOMS

Cardiac tamponade classically causes neck vein distention, reduced arterial blood pressure, muffled heart sounds, and pulsus paradoxus (an abnormal inspiratory drop in systemic blood pressure greater than 15 mm Hg). Ventricular end-systolic volume may fall and intracardiac pressures may rise.

Other signs and symptoms may include dyspnea, diaphoresis, pallor or cyanosis, anxiety, tachycardia, narrow pulse pressure, restlessness, and hepatomegaly. However, the lung fields remain clear.

DIAGNOSTIC TESTS

Chest X-ray, electrocardiography (ECG), pulmonary artery catheterization, and ultrasonography of the heart identify the effects of cardiac tamponade.

TREATMENT

Treatment aims to relieve intrapericardial pressure and cardiac compression by removing accumulated blood or fluid. Pericardiocentesis (needle aspiration of the pericardial cavity) or surgical creation of an opening dramatically improves systemic arterial pressure and cardiac output. Such treatment necessitates continuous hemodynamic and ECG monitoring in the intensive care unit.

Depending on the cause of tamponade, additional treatment may include blood transfusion, thoracotomy, or administration of protamine sulfate (a heparin antagonist) or vitamin K.

SPECIAL CONSIDERATIONS

• If the patient needs pericardiocentesis, a pericardial aspiration needle attached to a 50-ml syringe by a three-way stopcock, an ECG machine, and an emergency cart with a defibrillator (kept turned on) should be ready for immediate bedside use.

Cardiomyopathy

Cardiomyopathy is the general term applied to diseases of the heart's muscle fibers. It occurs in three main forms: dilated, hypertrophic, and restrictive. (See *Three types of cardiomyopathy,* page 48.)

CAUSES

The origin of most cardiomyopathies is unknown. However, hypertrophic cardiomyopathy is almost always inherited as a non-sex-linked autosomal dominant trait.

SIGNS AND SYMPTOMS

Dilated cardiomyopathy causes signs and symptoms of both left-sided and right-sided congestive heart failure (CHF) — shortness of breath, orthopnea, dyspnea on exertion, paroxysmal nocturnal dyspnea, fatigue, irritating dry cough at night, edema, and jugular vein distention.

Hypertrophic cardiomyopathy may cause angina pectoris, arrhythmias, dyspnea, orthopnea, syncope, CHF, and death.

Restrictive cardiomyopathy leads to fatigue, dyspnea, orthopnea, chest pain, generalized edema, liver engorgement, peripheral cyanosis, and pallor.

PATHOPHYSIOLOGY

Three types of cardiomyopathy

Dilated cardiomyopathy interferes with myocardial metabolism and grossly dilates all four heart chambers. It leads to intractable congestive heart failure (CHF), arrhythmias, and emboli. Commonly, it's not diagnosed until the advanced stages, making prognosis poor.

Hypertrophic cardiomyopathy is characterized by disproportionate, asymmetric thickening of the interventricular septum. Cardiac output may be low, normal, or high, depending on whether stenosis is obstructive or nonobstructive. Low cardiac output may lead to potentially fatal CHF. Some patients progressively deteriorate; others remain stable for years.

Restrictive cardiomyopathy is marked by restricted ventricular filling and endocardial fibrosis and thickening. If severe, it's irreversible.

DIAGNOSTIC TESTS

No single test confirms *dilated cardiomyopathy*. Diagnosis requires elimination of other possible causes of CHF and irregular heart rhythms. Thus, the patient may undergo electrocardiography (ECG), echocardiography, and a chest X-ray. To diagnose *hypertrophic cardiomyopathy*, the patient may undergo echocardiography, ECG, cardiac catheterization, and phonocardiography. Tests done to diagnose *restrictive cardiomyopathy* may include chest X-ray, echocardiography, ECG, arterial pulsation, and cardiac catheterization.

TREATMENT

Treatment varies with the type of cardiomyopathy.

Dilated cardiomyopathy

The underlying cause is corrected. To improve the heart's pumping ability, the patient typically receives digoxin, diuretics, oxygen, and a sodium-restricted diet. Other treatments include bed rest and steroids.

If these measures fail, heart transplantation may be recommended for carefully selected patients. For some patients, cardiomyoplasty is done to help the ventricle to pump blood effectively, or a cardiomyostimulator is used to deliver bursts of electrical impulses during systole to contract the muscle.

Hypertrophic cardiomyopathy

Propranolol may be given to ease angina, syncope, dyspnea, and arrhythmias. Atrial fibrillation necessitates cardioversion. If drug therapy fails, surgery (ventricular myotomy alone or combined with mitral valve replacement) is indicated.

Restrictive cardiomyopathy

Although no therapy currently exists for this form of the disease, digitalis glycosides, diuretics, and a restricted sodium diet ease CHF symptoms. Oral vasodilators may control intractable CHF. Anticoagulant therapy may be necessary to prevent thrombophlebitis in the patient on prolonged bed rest.

SPECIAL CONSIDERATIONS

For patients with dilated cardiomyopathy:
● If the patient is receiving vasodilators, blood pressure and heart rate are checked frequently. If he becomes hypotensive, the infusion is stopped and he's placed supine with legs elevated.

For patients with hypertrophic cardiomyopathy:
● Warn the patient to avoid strenuous physical activity, such as running.

Syncope or sudden death may follow even well-tolerated exercise. Instruct him to receive prophylaxis for subacute bacterial endocarditis before dental work or surgery.

For patients with restrictive cardiomyopathy:
• Advise the patient to watch for and report signs and symptoms of digoxin toxicity (anorexia, nausea, vomiting, yellow vision) and to record and report weight gain. If sodium restriction is ordered, teach him to avoid canned foods, pickles, smoked meats, and table salt.

For all patients:
• Psychosocial counseling can assist the patient and family in coping with a restricted lifestyle.
• Encourage family members to learn cardiopulmonary resuscitation.

Carpal tunnel syndrome

Carpal tunnel syndrome — sensory and motor changes in the median distribution of the hand — results from compression of the median nerve at the wrist, within the carpal tunnel. This nerve passes through (along with blood vessels and flexor tendons) to the fingers and thumb.

The syndrome poses a serious occupational health problem. Assembly-line workers and packers and persons who repeatedly use poorly designed tools are at the highest risk. Any strenuous use of the hands — sustained grasping, twisting, or flexing — aggravates the condition.

CAUSES
The carpal tunnel is formed by the carpal bones and the transverse carpal ligament. (See *Anatomy of the carpal tunnel.*) Inflammation or fibrosis of the tendon sheaths that pass through the tunnel can cause edema and compression of the median nerve.

Various conditions can make the carpal tunnel swell, pressing the median nerve against the transverse carpal ligament. Such conditions include rheumatoid arthritis, nerve

Anatomy of the carpal tunnel

This illustration shows the carpal tunnel. Note the median nerve, flexor tendons of fingers, and blood vessels passing through the tunnel on their way from the forearm to the hand.

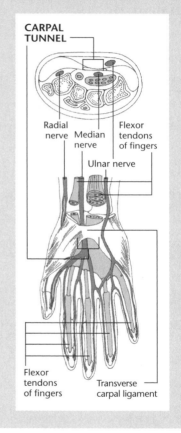

compression, pregnancy, renal failure, menopause, diabetes mellitus, hypothyroidism, myxedema, benign tumors, and tuberculosis. Another cause of carpal tunnel syndrome is dislocation or acute sprain of the wrist.

SIGNS AND SYMPTOMS

The patient typically complains of weakness, pain, burning, numbness, or tingling in one or both hands. Typically, these symptoms affect the thumb, forefinger, middle finger, and half of the fourth finger. The patient can't clench his hand into a fist. The pain may spread to the forearm and even as far as the shoulder.

DIAGNOSTIC TESTS

After losing feeling in affected fingers (diminished reaction to a light touch or pinprick), the patient may lose muscle strength as well. Other diagnostic indicators include:
• a tingling sensation in the hand when the wrist is tapped
• reproduction of symptoms when the patient holds the forearms vertically and allows both hands to drop down at the wrists for 1 minute
• pain and tingling in the wrist when a blood pressure cuff is inflated on the forearm for 1 to 2 minutes.

TREATMENT

The patient's wrist may be splinted in neutral extension for 1 to 2 weeks. Effective treatment may also require correction of an underlying disorder. If carpal tunnel syndrome is clearly linked with the patient's occupation, he may have to seek other work.

When conservative treatment fails, the only alternative is surgical nerve decompression by resecting the entire transverse carpal tunnel ligament or by using endoscopic surgical techniques. Neurolysis (freeing of nerve fibers) may also be necessary.

SPECIAL CONSIDERATIONS

• The patient should try to use his hands as much as possible. If his dominant hand is affected, he may need assistance with eating and bathing.
• After surgery, exercising the hands in warm water and removing the sling (if present) to perform exercises for the elbow and shoulder may be helpful.

 TEACHING TIP: Show the patient how to apply a splint, if recommended. Emphasize that the splint shouldn't be too tight.
• Occupational counseling may be useful if the patient has to change jobs because of carpal tunnel syndrome.

Cataract

A common cause of vision loss, a cataract is a gradually developing opacity of the lens or lens capsule of the eye. Cataracts commonly occur in both eyes, each one progressing independently. Cataracts are most prevalent in people over age 70. The prognosis is generally good; surgery improves vision in 95% of affected people.

CAUSES

Senile cataracts develop in elderly patients, probably from degenerative changes in lens proteins. *Congenital cataracts* occur in neonates as genetic defects or as a result of maternal rubella. *Traumatic cataracts* develop after a foreign body injures the lens with such force that aqueous or vitreous humor enters the lens capsule.

Complicated cataracts arise as secondary effects in patients with uveitis, glaucoma, retinitis pigmentosa, or a detached retina or during the course of a systemic disease such as diabetes. They can also result from exposure to ionizing radiation or infrared rays.

Toxic cataracts result from toxicity with prednisone, ergot alkaloids, dinitrophenol, naphthalene, or phenothiazines.

SIGNS AND SYMPTOMS

Typically, the patient experiences painless, gradual blurring and vision loss. As the cataract progresses, the pupil turns milky white. Some patients complain of blinding glare from headlights when they drive at night. Others report poor reading vision and an unpleasant glare and poor vision in bright sunlight.

DIAGNOSTIC TESTS
Shining a penlight into the eye reveals the white area of an advanced cataract behind the pupil. Confirming the diagnosis requires ophthalmoscopic and slit-lamp examinations.

TREATMENT
Cataracts require surgical extraction of the opaque lens and postoperative correction of visual deficits.

Surgical procedures
• *Extracapsular cataract extraction* removes the anterior lens capsule and cortex, leaving the posterior capsule intact. A posterior chamber intraocular lens is implanted.
• *Phacoemulsification* fragments the lens with ultrasonic vibrations and aspirates the pieces.
• *Intracapsular cataract extraction* (rarely performed today) removes the entire lens within the intact capsule by cryoextraction (the moist lens sticks to a cold metal probe for removal with gentle traction).

Correction of visual deficits
A patient with an intraocular lens implant may have improved vision once the eye patch is removed; however, the intraocular lens corrects distance vision only. The patient will also need corrective reading glasses or a corrective contact lens.

Where no intraocular lens has been implanted, the patient may be given temporary aphakic cataract glasses; in about 4 to 8 weeks, he'll be refracted for his own glasses.

SPECIAL CONSIDERATIONS
• To help prevent accidental eye injury, advise the patient to wear an eye shield or glasses during the day and an eye shield at night.

 TEACHING TIP: Provide instructions on correct eyedrop instillation and activity restrictions. Advise the patient to immediately report any sharp eye pain. If he has had surgery, warn him to avoid activities that increase intraocular pressure such as straining.

Cerebral aneurysm

In this type of aneurysm, a weakness in the wall of a cerebral artery leads to localized dilation of the artery. The most common form is the *berry aneurysm,* a saclike outpouching in a cerebral artery.

Cerebral aneurysms usually arise at an arterial junction in the circle of Willis located at the base of the brain. They often rupture and cause subarachnoid hemorrhage.

Generally, a cerebral aneurysm poses three major threats: death from increased intracranial pressure (ICP), bleeding episodes, and vasospasm. Other complications include acute hydrocephalus and pulmonary embolism. About half of patients with a subarachnoid hemorrhage die immediately. However, new and better treatment has improved the prognosis.

CAUSES
Cerebral aneurysms may result from a congenital defect, a degenerative process, or a combination. For example, hypertension and atherosclerosis may disrupt blood flow and exert pressure against a congenitally weak arterial wall, stretching it and making it likely to rupture.

SIGNS AND SYMPTOMS
Usually, cerebral aneurysm rupture occurs abruptly and without warning, causing a sudden severe headache, nausea, vomiting and, depending on the severity and location of bleeding, altered level of consciousness, possibly including a deep coma.

Bleeding may lead to nuchal rigidity, back and leg pain, fever, restlessness, irritability, occasional seizures, and blurred vision. Bleeding into the brain tissues causes hemiparesis, hemisensory defects, dysphagia, and visual defects. (See *Danger signs in cerebral aneurysm,* page 52.)

DIAGNOSTIC TESTS
Diagnosis is based on the patient's history and a neurologic examina-

Danger signs in cerebral aneurysm

The health care team must monitor a patient with a cerebral aneurysm for an enlarging aneurysm, rebleeding, intracranial clot, vasospasm, or other complications. These complications may be preceded by:
• a decreased level of consciousness
• a unilateral enlarged pupil
• onset or worsening of hemiparesis or motor deficit
• increased blood pressure
• slowed pulse
• worsening of headache or sudden onset of a headache
• renewed or worsened nuchal rigidity
• renewed or persistent vomiting.
Intermittent signs, such as restlessness, extremity weakness, and speech alterations, can also indicate increasing intracranial pressure.

tion; a computed tomography scan revealing blood in the brain; and magnetic resonance imaging or magnetic resonant angiography, which can identify a brain aneurysm as a "flow void" or by computer reconstruction of the involved blood vessels. However, cerebral angiography is the diagnostic procedure of choice.

TREATMENT
Typically, the aneurysm is repaired to reduce the risk of vasospasm and cerebral infarction. Usually, surgical repair (by clipping, ligation, or wrapping the aneurysm neck with muscle) takes place 7 to 10 days after the initial hemorrhage.

When surgical correction is risky, supportive measures may include bed rest in a quiet, darkened room; avoidance of coffee, other stimulants, and aspirin; and various drugs (analgesics, antihypertensives, calcium channel blockers, corticosteroids, anticonvulsants, sedatives, and possibly the fibrinolytic inhibitor aminocaproic acid).

SPECIAL CONSIDERATIONS
• To minimize the risk of rebleeding and increased ICP, the head of the patient's bed is kept flat or under 30 degrees; visitors are limited; the patient is instructed to avoid caffeine, other stimulants, and strenuous physical activity; and fluid intake is restricted.
• Rectal temperature measurement must be avoided because vagus nerve stimulation may cause cardiac arrest.
• A patient who can eat should receive a high-bulk diet to prevent straining during defecation, which can increase ICP. A stool softener or mild laxative may be needed but fluids shouldn't be forced. A bowel elimination program based on previous habits should be instituted.
• Side rails may be raised to help protect the patient from injury. However, restraints can cause agitation and raise ICP.
• If the patient can't speak, using cards or a slate can permit some communication. Limit conversation to topics that won't further frustrate him. Encourage his family to speak to him in a normal tone, even if he doesn't seem to respond.

Cerebral contusion

Cerebral contusion refers to bruising of brain tissue. More serious than a concussion, a contusion disrupts normal nerve functions in the bruised area and may cause loss of consciousness, hemorrhage, edema, and even death.

CAUSES
Cerebral contusion results from acceleration-deceleration or coup-contrecoup injuries. Such injuries can occur directly beneath the site of impact when the brain rebounds against the skull from the force of a blow (a beat-

ing with a blunt instrument, for example), when the blow drives the brain against the opposite side of the skull, or when the head is hurled forward and stopped abruptly.

In these injuries, the brain continues to move and slaps against the skull (acceleration), then rebounds (deceleration). The brain may also strike against bony prominences inside the skull, causing intracranial hemorrhage or hematoma.

SIGNS AND SYMPTOMS
The patient may have severe scalp wounds and labored respirations. He may lose consciousness for a few minutes or longer. If conscious, he may be drowsy, confused, disoriented, agitated, or even violent. He may display hemiparesis, decorticate or decerebrate posturing, and unequal pupillary response.

Eventually, he should return to a relatively alert state, perhaps with temporary aphasia, slight hemiparesis, or unilateral numbness. A lucid period followed by rapid deterioration suggests epidural hematoma.

DIAGNOSTIC TESTS
An accurate history of the injury and a neurologic examination are the primary diagnostic tools. A computed tomography scan shows damaged tissue, hematomas, and fractures.

TREATMENT
A patent airway must be established and maintained. The patient may need a tracheotomy or endotracheal intubation. A patient with a suspected intracerebral hemorrhage may receive a blood transfusion and undergo a craniotomy to control bleeding and aspirate blood. Fluid intake is restricted to 1,200 to 1,500 ml/day to reduce volume and intracerebral swelling.

SPECIAL CONSIDERATIONS
• If the patient's intubated, hyperventilation should achieve a partial pressure of arterial carbon dioxide of 26 to 28 mm Hg.

• Vital signs are monitored regularly (usually every 15 minutes). Abnormal respirations could indicate a critical neurologic emergency.
• If spinal injury is ruled out, the head of the bed can be elevated to 30 degrees; however, the patient must stay in bed.
• Cerebrospinal fluid (CSF) may leak from the nares and ear canals. If this happens, raising the head of the bed 30 degrees promotes patient comfort. If CSF leaks from the nose, a gauze pad can be placed under the nostrils. If CSF leaks from the ear, position the patient so the ear drains naturally. Neither the ear nor the nose should be packed.

Cerebral palsy
The most common cause of crippling in children, cerebral palsy comprises a group of neuromuscular disorders resulting from prenatal, perinatal, or postnatal central nervous system (CNS) damage. These disorders may become more obvious as the infant grows older.

Three major types of cerebral palsy — *spastic, athetoid,* and *ataxic* — occur, sometimes in mixed forms. Motor impairment may be minimal or severely disabling. Associated defects, such as seizures, speech disorders, and mental retardation, are common.

CAUSES
Conditions that result in cerebral anoxia, hemorrhage, or other CNS damage are probably responsible for cerebral palsy. Prenatal causes include maternal infection or diabetes, radiation, anoxia, toxemia, abnormal placental attachment, malnutrition, and isoimmunization. Perinatal and birth difficulties that can lead to cerebral palsy include forceps delivery, breech presentation, placenta previa, abruptio placentae, and prolapsed cord with delay in delivery of the head. Premature birth, prolonged or unusually rapid labor, and multiple birth are other possible causes.

Diagnostic features of cerebral palsy

Cerebral palsy is suspected whenever an infant:
● has difficulty sucking or keeping the nipple or food in his mouth
● seldom moves voluntarily or has arm or leg tremors with voluntary movement
● crosses the legs when lifted from behind
● has hard-to-separate legs, making diaper changing difficult
● persistently uses only one hand or, as he gets older, uses the hands well but not the legs.

All infants should have a screening test for cerebral palsy as a regular part of their 6-month checkup.

SIGNS AND SYMPTOMS

Spastic cerebral palsy causes hyperactive deep tendon reflexes, increased stretch reflexes, rapid alternating muscle contraction and relaxation, muscle weakness, underdevelopment of affected limbs, and a tendency toward contractures. Typically, the child walks on his toes with a scissors gait, crossing one foot in front of the other.

Athetoid cerebral palsy may cause involuntary grimacing, wormlike writhing, and sharp jerks that impair voluntary movement. Involuntary facial movements may make speech difficult.

Ataxic cerebral palsy may lead to disturbed balance, incoordination, hypoactive reflexes, nystagmus, muscle weakness, tremor, lack of leg movement during infancy, and a wide gait as the child begins to walk.

DIAGNOSTIC TESTS

Early diagnosis requires careful clinical observation during infancy and precise neurologic assessment. (See *Diagnostic features of cerebral palsy*.)

TREATMENT

Cerebral palsy can't be cured, but proper therapy can help the child reach full potential. Treatment involves doctors, nurses, teachers, psychologists, the child's family, and occupational, physical, and speech therapists and may include:
● braces or splints and special appliances to help the child perform activities independently
● range-of-motion exercises to minimize contractures
● orthopedic surgery to correct contractures
● anticonvulsant therapy to control seizures
● muscle relaxants or neurosurgery to decrease spasticity
● artificial urinary sphincter for the incontinent child who can use the hand controls.

SPECIAL CONSIDERATIONS

● The diet must accommodate the child's high energy needs. He may need special utensils and a chair with a solid footrest. Placing food far back in the mouth eases swallowing.
● The child should be encouraged to wash, perform dental care, and dress independently, with assistance only as needed.
● Give all care in an unhurried manner; otherwise, muscle spasticity may increase.

 TEACHING TIP: Encourage the child and family to participate in care so they can continue it properly at home.
● Supportive organizations can provide education and resources. For more information, advise parents to contact the United Cerebral Palsy Association or their local cerebral palsy agency.

Cerebrovascular accident

Commonly called a stroke, cerebrovascular accident (CVA) is a sudden impairment of circulation in one or more of the blood vessels supplying the brain. CVA interrupts or di-

What happens in transient ischemic attack

A transient ischemic attack (TIA) is a recurrent episode of neurologic deficit, lasting from seconds to hours, that clears within 12 to 24 hours. It's usually considered a warning sign of an impending thrombotic cerebrovascular accident. The most distinctive features of TIAs are the short duration of neurologic deficits and complete return of normal function.

Causes of TIA

Microemboli released from a thrombus probably temporarily interrupt blood flow. Small spasms in those arterioles may impair blood flow and also precede TIA.

Clinical findings

Signs and symptoms vary with the location of the affected artery. They include double vision, speech deficits, unilateral blindness, staggering or uncoordinated gait, unilateral weakness or numbness, falling due to weakness in the legs, and dizziness.

Treatment of TIA

During an active TIA, the treatment goal is to prevent a completed stroke. Typically, the patient receives aspirin or anticoagulants to minimize the risk of thrombosis. After or between attacks, preventive treatment includes surgery (carotid endarterectomy or cerebral microvascular bypass).

minishes oxygen supply and often causes serious damage or necrosis in brain tissue.

About half of those who survive a CVA are disabled and experience a recurrence within weeks, months, or years. CVA is the third most common cause of death in the United States. It strikes 500,000 people each year; half of them die as a result.

CVAs are classified according to their course of progression. The least severe is the *transient ischemic attack* (TIA), or "little stroke," caused by a temporary interruption of blood flow. (See *What happens in transient ischemic attack.*) A *progressive stroke,* or stroke-in-evolution, starts with slight neurologic deficit and worsens in a day or two. In a *completed stroke,* neurologic deficits are maximal at onset.

CAUSES

Major immediate causes of CVA are thrombosis, embolism, and hemorrhage. Factors that increase the risk of CVA include a history of TIAs, atherosclerosis, hypertension, arrhythmias, rheumatic heart disease, diabetes mellitus, gout, postural hypotension, cardiac enlargement, high serum triglyceride levels, cigarette smoking, and a family history of CVA.

SIGNS AND SYMPTOMS

Signs and symptoms vary with the artery affected, severity of damage, and extent of secondary circulation that develops to help compensate for decreased blood supply. If CVA occurs in the left hemisphere, signs and symptoms appear on the right side; if it occurs in the right hemisphere, signs and symptoms appear on the left. Stroke signs and symptoms include aphasia, dysphasia, partial paralysis, weakness, numbness, sensory changes, visual disturbances, ataxia, confusion, incontinence, loss of coordination, personality changes, and coma.

Generalized signs and symptoms of CVA include headache, vomiting, mental impairment, seizures, coma, rigidity at the nape of the neck, fever, and disorientation.

DIAGNOSTIC TESTS
Diagnosis is based on physical examination, history of risk factors, and various diagnostic tests. A computed tomography scan shows signs of hemorrhagic stroke immediately. Magnetic resonance imaging or a brain scan may help identify damaged and swollen brain areas. Other tests may include lumbar puncture, ophthalmoscopy, angiography, electroencephalography, and laboratory tests (urinalysis, blood clotting studies, and a complete blood count).

TREATMENT
Surgery may improve cerebral circulation in patients with thrombotic or embolic CVAs. Medications used to treat CVAs include ticlopidine, an antiplatelet drug; tissue plasminogen activator, used experimentally to dissolve clots; anticonvulsants to treat or prevent seizures; corticosteroids to minimize cerebral edema; and analgesics to relieve headache.

SPECIAL CONSIDERATIONS
• If the patient vomits, position him on his side to prevent aspiration.
• High-topped sneakers can help prevent footdrop and contractures. Eggcrate, flotation, or pulsating mattresses or sheepskin can help prevent pressure ulcers.
• Encourage the patient to exercise as much as possible. Range-of-motion exercises should be done for both the affected and unaffected sides.
• Simplify your language if needed but avoid correcting the patient's speech or treating him like a child. If he has aphasia, provide a simple method for him to convey basic needs.
• Never give too much fluid too fast, because this can increase intracranial pressure. Also, before offering food,

the patient's gag reflex should be assessed.
• Physical and occupational therapists can assist in obtaining assistive devices as needed.
• Speech therapy, if indicated, should begin as soon as possible.

 TEACHING TIP: Explain the patient's expected deficits and strengths to family members. Involve them in rehabilitation. Stress that the patient must not substitute acetaminophen for aspirin (if prescribed) and that they must seek immediate help if the patient develops signs or symptoms of an impending CVA (sudden rise in blood pressure, rapid and bounding pulse, headache).

Cervical cancer

The third most common cancer of the female reproductive system, cervical cancer is classified as either preinvasive or invasive.
Preinvasive carcinoma ranges from minimal cervical dysplasia, in which the lower third of the epithelium contains abnormal cells, to carcinoma in situ, in which the full thickness of epithelium contains abnormally proliferating cells. Preinvasive cancer is curable 75% to 90% of the time with early detection and proper treatment. If untreated, it may progress to invasive cervical cancer.

In *invasive carcinoma,* cancer cells penetrate the basement membrane and may spread directly to contiguous pelvic structures or disseminate to distant sites by lymphatic routes.

CAUSES
Although the cause of cervical cancer is unknown, several predisposing factors have been related to its development: sexual intercourse at a young age (under age 16), multiple sexual partners, multiple pregnancies, and human herpesvirus 2 and other bacterial or viral venereal infections.

SIGNS AND SYMPTOMS
Preinvasive cervical cancer produces

no symptoms or other clinically apparent changes. Early invasive cervical cancer causes abnormal vaginal bleeding, persistent vaginal discharge, and postcoital pain and bleeding. In advanced stages, it can cause pelvic pain, vaginal leakage of urine and feces from a fistula, anorexia, weight loss, and anemia.

DIAGNOSTIC TESTS
Papanicolaou (Pap) tests can detect cervical cancer before the disease causes signs and symptoms. An abnormal Pap test routinely calls for colposcopy. Other studies can detect cancer spread.

TREATMENT
Preinvasive lesions may be treated with a total excisional biopsy, cryosurgery, laser destruction, conization, or, rarely, hysterectomy. Therapy for invasive squamous cell carcinoma may include radical hysterectomy and radiation therapy. (See *Radiation implant precautions.*)

SPECIAL CONSIDERATIONS
• After an excisional biopsy, cryosurgery, and laser therapy, the patient can expect vaginal discharge or spotting for about 1 week. She should not douche, use tampons, or have sexual intercourse during this time.

 TEACHING TIP: Because radiation therapy may increase susceptibility to infection, the patient should avoid persons with obvious infections during therapy. Teach her how to recognize signs of infection. Emphasize the need for a follow-up Pap test and a pelvic examination within 3 to 4 months after excisional biopsy, cryosurgery, or laser therapy, and periodically thereafter.

Chalazion
A common eye disorder, a chalazion is a granulomatous inflammation of a meibomian gland in the upper or lower eyelid. Characterized by local-

Radiation implant precautions

If your patient has an internal radiation implant, remember that safety precautions — time, distance, and shielding — begin as soon as the implant is in place.

Protecting the patient
While the implant is in place, the patient should avoid movement and lie flat. (If she prefers, the head of the bed can be elevated slightly.) Leg exercises and other body movements could dislodge the implant.

Protecting yourself and others
Staff should organize time spent with the patient to minimize each person's exposure to radiation.

Be sure to inform all visitors of safety precautions. Hang a sign listing these precautions on the patient's door.

ized swelling, the disorder usually develops slowly over several weeks.

A chalazion may become large enough to press on the eyeball, producing astigmatism; a large chalazion seldom subsides spontaneously. It's generally benign and chronic and can occur at any age; in some patients, it's apt to recur.

CAUSES
Obstruction of the meibomian (sebaceous) gland duct causes a chalazion.

SIGNS AND SYMPTOMS
A chalazion occurs as a painless, hard lump that usually points toward the conjunctival side of the eyelid. Eversion of the lid reveals a red or red-yellow elevated area on the conjunctival surface.

DIAGNOSTIC TESTS

Visual examination and palpation of the eyelid reveal a small bump or nodule. Persistently recurrent chalazions, especially in an adult, necessitate a biopsy to rule out meibomian cancer.

TREATMENT

Initial treatment consists of applying warm compresses to open the lumen of the gland and, occasionally, instilling sulfonamide eye drops. If such therapy fails, or if the chalazion presses on the eyeball or causes a severe cosmetic problem, steroid injection or incision and curettage under local anesthetic may be necessary.

After such surgery, a pressure eye patch applied for 8 to 24 hours controls bleeding and swelling. After patch removal, treatment consists of warm compresses applied for 10 to 15 minutes, two to four times daily, and antimicrobial eye drops or ointment to prevent secondary infection.

SPECIAL CONSIDERATIONS

 TEACHING TIP: Teach proper lid hygiene (water and mild baby shampoo applied with a cotton applicator) to the patient who's disposed to chalazions. Instruct him how to properly apply warm compresses. Tell him to take special care to avoid burning the skin, to always use a clean cloth, and to discard used compresses. Advise him to start applying warm compres-ses at the first sign of lid irritation.

Chancroid

Painful genital ulcers and inguinal adenitis characterize chancroid, or soft chancre. This sexually transmitted disease (STD) occurs worldwide but is particularly common in tropical countries. It affects men more often than women. A high rate of human immunodeficiency virus (HIV) infection has been reported among patients with chancroid.

Chancroidal lesions may heal spontaneously. Usually they respond well to treatment in the absence of secondary infections.

CAUSES

Chancroid results from *Haemophilus ducreyi,* a gram-negative streptobacillus, and is transmitted through sexual contact. Poor hygiene may predispose men — especially those who are uncircumcised — to this disease.

SIGNS AND SYMPTOMS

After a 3- to 5-day incubation period, a small papule appears at the entry site, usually the groin or inner thigh. In men, it may appear on the penis; in women, on the vulva, vagina, or cervix. Occasionally, this papule may erupt on the tongue, lip, breast, or navel.

The papule rapidly ulcerates, becoming painful, soft, and malodorous. Gray and shallow, it bleeds easily and produces pus. It has irregular edges and measures up to 1" (2.5 cm) in diameter. Within 2 to 3 weeks, inguinal adenitis develops, creating suppurated, inflamed nodes that may rupture into large ulcers or buboes. Headache and malaise occur in 50% of patients. During the healing stage, phimosis may develop.

DIAGNOSTIC TESTS

Gram stain smears of ulcer exudate or bubo aspirate are 50% reliable; blood agar cultures are 75% reliable. A biopsy confirms the diagnosis but is reserved for resistant cases or when cancer is suspected. Dark-field examination and serologic testing rule out other STDs that cause similar ulcers. Testing for HIV infection should be done at the time of the diagnosis.

TREATMENT

Drug therapy consists of azithromycin, erythromycin, or ceftriaxone. Aspiration of fluid-filled nodes helps prevent the infection from spreading.

SPECIAL CONSIDERATIONS

• Practice universal precautions when providing care.

Teaching tip: Instruct the patient not to apply lotions, creams, or oils on or near the genitalia or on other lesion sites. Tell him to abstain from sexual contact until healing is complete (usually about 2 weeks after treatment begins) and to wash the genitalia daily with soap and water. Instruct uncircumcised men to retract the foreskin for thorough cleaning.

• To avoid chancroid, persons should avoid sexual contact with infected persons, use condoms during sexual activity, and wash the genitalia with soap and water after sexual activity.

Chlamydial infections

Urethritis in men and urethritis and cervicitis in women compose a group of infections linked to one organism: *Chlamydia trachomatis*. These infections are the most common sexually transmitted diseases in the United States, affecting an estimated 4 million Americans each year. Trachoma inclusion conjunctivitis is a leading cause of blindness in Third World countries.

Untreated, chlamydial infections can lead to such complications as acute epididymitis, salpingitis, pelvic inflammatory disease and, eventually, sterility.

CAUSES

Transmission of *C. trachomatis* primarily follows vaginal or rectal intercourse or oral-genital contact with an infected person. Children born of mothers with chlamydial infections may contract associated conjunctivitis, otitis media, and pneumonia during passage through the birth canal.

SIGNS AND SYMPTOMS

Patients with chlamydial infections may be asymptomatic or may show signs of infection. Signs and symptoms vary with the specific type of chlamydial infection. (See *Clinical features of chlamydial infection.*)

Clinical features of chlamydial infection

Chlamydial infection may cause the following signs and symptoms.

In women

• *Cervicitis* may cause cervical erosion, mucopurulent discharge, pelvic pain, and dyspareunia.

• *Endometritis* or *salpingitis* may lead to signs and symptoms of pelvic inflammatory disease, such as pain and tenderness of the abdomen, cervix, uterus, and lymph nodes; chills; fever; breakthrough bleeding; bleeding after intercourse; and vaginal discharge.

• *Urethral syndrome* may bring on dysuria, pyuria, and urinary frequency.

In men

• *Urethritis* may cause dysuria, erythema, tenderness of the urethral meatus, urinary frequency, pruritus, and urethral discharge.

• *Epididymitis* may cause painful scrotal swelling and urethral discharge.

• *Prostatitis* may cause low back pain, urinary frequency, dysuria, nocturia, and painful ejaculation.

• *Proctitis* may manifest as diarrhea, tenesmus, pruritus, bloody or mucopurulent discharge, and diffuse or discrete ulceration in the rectosigmoid colon.

DIAGNOSTIC TESTS

Laboratory tests provide a definite diagnosis. A swab culture from the infection site establishes a diagnosis of urethritis, cervicitis, salpingitis, endometritis, or proctitis.

TREATMENT

The first-line treatment for adults and adolescents is oral doxycycline for 7

Common sites of calculi formation

Gallstones are most likely to develop at the sites shown here. Keep in mind that small stones may travel.

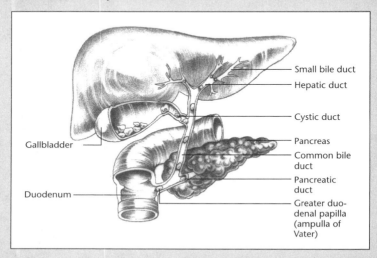

- Small bile duct
- Hepatic duct
- Cystic duct
- Pancreas
- Common bile duct
- Pancreatic duct
- Greater duodenal papilla (ampulla of Vater)
- Gallbladder
- Duodenum

days or oral azithromycin in a single dose. For pregnant women, erythromycin (stearate base) is preferred.

SPECIAL CONSIDERATIONS
- Practice universal precautions when caring for this patient.
- Some states require that all cases of chlamydial infection be reported to local public health authorities.

TEACHING TIP: Make sure the patient understands proper use of prescribed medications. Stress the importance of completing drug therapy, even after symptoms subside; practicing meticulous personal hygiene; avoiding touching the discharge; washing and drying hands before touching the eyes; abstaining from intercourse until both the patient and partner are cured; and informing sexual contacts of the infection.

Cholelithiasis

Cholelithiasis, or gallbladder inflammation, can be painful and is sometimes life-threatening. Usually, it requires surgery to remove grainy deposits in the gallbladder and relieve inflammation.

Cholelithiasis is often associated with deposits of calculi (stones) and inflammation. (See *Common sites of calculi formation*.) The condition may lead to any of the disorders associated with gallstone formation: cholangitis, cholecystitis, choledocholithiasis, or gallstone ileus.

The fifth leading cause of hospitalization among adults, cholelithiasis accounts for 90% of all gallbladder and duct diseases. The prognosis is usually good with treatment. If infection occurs, prognosis depends on its severity and response to antibiotics.

CAUSES

Cholelithiasis results from changes in bile components. Made of cholesterol, calcium bilirubinate, or a mixture of cholesterol and bilirubin pigment, gallstones arise during periods of sluggishness in the gallbladder (such as from pregnancy, oral contraceptives, diabetes mellitus, celiac disease, cirrhosis, or pancreatitis).

SIGNS AND SYMPTOMS

Acute cholelithiasis causes symptoms of a classic gallbladder attack. Such attacks often follow meals rich in fats, or they may occur at night, awakening the patient. They begin with acute abdominal pain in the right upper quadrant that may radiate to the back, between the shoulders, or to the front of the chest. The pain may be so severe that the patient seeks emergency care.

Other features may include recurring fat intolerance, biliary colic, belching, flatulence, indigestion, diaphoresis, nausea, vomiting, chills, low-grade fever, and jaundice.

DIAGNOSTIC TESTS

Ultrasound detects stones in the gallbladder with 96% accuracy. Other tests may include fluoroscopy, endoscopy, computed tomography scans, an injected radioisotope (HIDA) scan of the gallbladder, abdominal X-rays, and blood tests (to help distinguish this disease from others with similar signs).

TREATMENT

Surgery, usually elective, is the treatment of choice. Surgery may include open or laparoscopic cholecystectomy, cholecystectomy with operative cholangiography and, possibly, exploration of the common bile duct. Chenodiol, which dissolves radiolucent stones, is an alternative for patients who are poor surgical risks or who refuse surgery.

Other treatment includes a low-fat diet to prevent attacks and vitamin K for itching, jaundice, and bleeding, which may result from vitamin K deficiency. During an acute attack, the patient may need a nasogastric tube, an I.V. line and, possibly, antibiotics.

SPECIAL CONSIDERATIONS

 TEACHING TIP: At discharge, advise the patient to walk daily but to avoid heavy lifting or straining for 6 weeks. Food restrictions are unnecessary unless he is intolerant to a specific food or has an underlying condition (such as diabetes) that requires restriction.

Chronic fatigue and immune dysfunction syndrome

This recently recognized illness goes by several names, including chronic fatigue syndrome, chronic Epstein-Barr virus, myalgic encephalomyelitis, and "yuppie flu." Typically, chronic fatigue and immune dysfunction syndrome (CFIDS) is marked by debilitating fatigue, neurologic abnormalities, and persistent symptoms that suggest chronic mononucleosis. It commonly affects adults under age 45.

CAUSES

Although the cause of CFIDS is unknown, researchers suspect it may be found in human herpesvirus 6 or in other herpesviruses, enteroviruses, or retroviruses. CFIDS may be associated with a reaction to viral illness that's complicated by dysfunctional immune response and by other factors, such as gender, age, genetic disposition, prior illness, stress, and environment.

SIGNS AND SYMPTOMS

The hallmark of CFIDS is prolonged, often overwhelming fatigue that's commonly associated with a varying complex of other symptoms. To aid disease identification, the Centers for Disease Control and Prevention (CDC) uses a working case definition to group symptoms and severity.

DIAGNOSTIC TESTS

No single test clearly confirms CFIDS.

Diagnosis hinges on the patient's history and the CDC criteria. However, diagnosis is difficult and uncertain because these criteria may not include all forms of the disease and are based on symptoms that can result from other diseases.

TREATMENT
No therapy is known to cure CFIDS. Experimental treatments include the antiviral drug acyclovir and selected immunomodulating agents, such as I.V. gamma globulin, ampligen, and transfer factor.

Symptomatic treatment may include tricyclic antidepressants, histamine$_2$-blocking agents, and antianxiety agents. In some patients, avoiding environmental irritants and certain foods may ease symptoms.

SPECIAL CONSIDERATIONS

TEACHING TIP: Inform the patient that the CFIDS Association and local support groups can provide information and contact with others who share this disease.

Chronic granulomatous disease

In this disease, abnormal neutrophil metabolism impairs phagocytosis, one of the body's chief defense mechanisms. This leads to increased susceptibility to low-virulent or nonpathogenic organisms, such as *Staphylococcus epidermidis, Escherichia coli, Aspergillus,* and *Nocardia.* Patients with chronic granulomatous disease (CGD) may develop granulomatous inflammation, resulting in ischemic tissue damage.

CAUSES
CGD is usually inherited as an X-linked trait, although a variant form also exists. The genetic defect may be associated with an enzyme deficiency.

SIGNS AND SYMPTOMS
Usually, the patient displays signs and symptoms by age 2, associated with infections of the skin, lymph nodes, lung, liver, and bone. Skin infection is characterized by small, well-localized areas of tenderness. Seborrheic dermatitis of the scalp and axilla is also common. Lymph node infection typically causes marked lymphadenopathy with draining lymph nodes and hepatosplenomegaly.

Many patients develop liver abscess, suggested by abdominal tenderness, fever, anorexia, and nausea. Other common infections include osteomyelitis, which causes localized pain and fever; pneumonia; and gingivitis with severe periodontal disease.

DIAGNOSTIC TESTS
Clinical features of osteomyelitis, pneumonia, liver abscess, or chronic lymphadenopathy in a young child provide the first clues to a diagnosis of CGD. An important tool for confirming this diagnosis is the nitroblue tetrazolium (NBT) test, which shows impaired NBT reduction in CGD. Another test measures the rate of intracellular killing by neutrophils; in CGD, killing is delayed or absent.

Other laboratory values may support the diagnosis or help monitor disease activity.

TREATMENT
Early, aggressive treatment of infection is the chief goal. Areas of suspected infection should be biopsied or cultured, with broad-spectrum antibiotics usually started immediately, without waiting for culture results. Confirmed abscesses may be drained or surgically removed.

Many patients receive a combination of I.V. antibiotics, often extended beyond the usual 10- to 14-day course. However, for fungal infections with *Aspergillus* or *Nocardia,* treatment involves amphotericin B.

To treat life-threatening or antibiotic-resistant infection or to help localize infection, the patient may receive granulocyte transfusions. Interferon is an experimental but promising treatment in CGD.

SPECIAL CONSIDERATIONS
● During hospitalization, encourage the patient to continue activities of daily living to the extent possible. A tutor can help the child keep up with schoolwork.

 TEACHING TIP: If the doctor orders prophylactic antibiotics, teach the patient and family how to administer them and how to recognize adverse reactions. Tell them to promptly report signs and symptoms of infection. Encourage good nutrition and hygiene.

Chronic obstructive pulmonary disease

Chronic obstructive pulmonary disease (COPD) is a chronic airway obstruction that results from emphysema, chronic bronchitis, asthma, or any combination of these disorders. The most common chronic lung disease, COPD affects an estimated 17 million Americans. Although it doesn't always produce signs or symptoms and may cause only minimal disability, it tends to worsen with time.

CAUSES
Predisposing factors include cigarette smoking, recurrent or chronic respiratory infections, air pollution, and allergies. Familial and hereditary factors also predispose a person to COPD. Smoking is by far the most important predisposing factor.

SIGNS AND SYMPTOMS
The typical patient, a long-term cigarette smoker, has no signs or symptoms until middle age, when his capacity for exercise or strenuous work gradually starts to decline and a productive cough develops. Subtle at first, these signs and symptoms become more pronounced as the patient ages and the disease progresses.

Eventually, the patient develops dyspnea on minimal exertion, frequent respiratory infections, intermittent or continuous hypoxemia, and grossly abnormal pulmonary function studies. Advanced COPD may cause thoracic deformities, overwhelming disability, cor pulmonale, severe respiratory failure, and death.

DIAGNOSTIC TESTS
A history of cigarette smoking along with results of arterial blood testing and pulmonary function studies help confirm COPD. The patient with emphysema, for instance, typically has increases in residual volume, total lung capacity, and lung compliance and decreases in vital capacity, diffusing capacity, and expiratory volumes.

TREATMENT
Bronchodilators can alleviate bronchospasm and enhance pulmonary secretion clearance. Effective coughing, postural drainage, and chest physiotherapy can help mobilize secretions. Low oxygen concentrations ease symptoms. Antibiotics are given to treat respiratory infections.

SPECIAL CONSIDERATIONS
● Excessive oxygen therapy may eliminate the COPD patient's hypoxic respiratory drive, causing confusion and drowsiness. (See *Helping the patient cope with COPD,* page 64.)

Cirrhosis

This chronic liver disease is characterized by diffuse destruction and fibrotic regeneration of hepatic cells. As necrotic tissue yields to fibrosis, cirrhosis alters liver structure and normal vasculature, impairs blood and lymph flow, and ultimately causes hepatic insufficiency.

Cirrhosis is especially prevalent among malnourished chronic alcoholics over age 50. Mortality is high; many patients die within 5 years of onset.

CAUSES
Liver damage from malnutrition and chronic alcohol ingestion causes *portal* (Laënnec's) cirrhosis (also called

Helping the patient cope with COPD

Most patients with chronic obstructive pulmonary disease (COPD) receive outpatient treatment and need comprehensive instruction to help them comply with therapy. If patient teaching is one of your job responsibilities, provide the following instructions.

Improving respiratory capacity
● Enroll in a pulmonary rehabilitation program if one is available.
● Take slow, deep breaths and exhale through pursed lips to strengthen respiratory muscles.
● Perform deep-breathing exercises and effective coughing techniques as prescribed.

Using medication properly
● Take bronchodilators and other medications exactly as prescribed. Be sure to complete the entire course of prescribed antibiotics.
● If you're using oxygen therapy at home, keep the oxygen flow rate within prescribed limits.
● Quit smoking and avoid other respiratory irritants. If possible, install an air conditioner with an air filter at home.
● To reduce thick secretions, drink 12 to 15 8-oz (237-ml) glasses of water daily. A home humidifier may be beneficial, especially in the winter.

Avoiding infections
● Stay away from persons with respiratory infections.
● Get pneumococcal vaccination and annual influenza vaccinations.
● Practice good oral hygiene to help prevent infection.
● Learn how to recognize early signs of infection.

Other instructions
Maintain a balanced diet. To reduce fatigue when eating, eat small, frequent meals.

nutritional or alcoholic cirrhosis). This form of cirrhosis is the most common. Bile duct diseases, which suppress bile flow, cause *biliary cirrhosis*. Various types of hepatitis cause *postnecrotic cirrhosis*. *Pigment cirrhosis* may stem from disorders such as hemochromatosis. *Cardiac cirrhosis* results from liver damage caused by right-sided heart failure.

SIGNS AND SYMPTOMS
Early indications of cirrhosis usually include GI symptoms (anorexia, indigestion, nausea, vomiting, constipation, diarrhea) and dull abdominal ache.

Major and late signs and symptoms include the following:
● respiratory problems, stemming from hypoxia
● central nervous system effects (such as lethargy, mental changes, asterixis,

peripheral neuritis, hallucinations, and coma)
● bleeding tendencies, anemia
● testicular atrophy, menstrual irregularities, and gynecomastia
● severe pruritus, extreme skin dryness, poor tissue turgor, abnormal pigmentation and, possibly, jaundice
● hepatomegaly, ascites, edema of the legs, hepatic encephalopathy, and hepatorenal syndrome.

DIAGNOSTIC TESTS
Liver biopsy confirms cirrhosis, and X-ray scans check the gallbladder and bile duct for gallstones. Laboratory tests of blood, feces, and urine identify disease extent and complications.

TREATMENT
The patient may benefit from a high-calorie and moderate- to high-protein diet, but must restrict protein intake if hepatic encephalopathy develops.

Sodium is usually restricted to 200 to 500 mg/day, fluids to 1,000 to 1,500 ml/day.

If the patient's condition continues to deteriorate, he may need tube feedings or hyperalimentation. Other supportive measures include supplemental vitamins and thiamine.

Drug therapy requires special caution because the cirrhotic liver can't detoxify harmful substances efficiently. Sedatives are avoided or prescribed with great care.

Paracentesis and infusions of salt-poor albumin may relieve ascites. Surgical procedures include ligation of varices, splenectomy, esophagogastric resection, and splenorenal or portacaval anastomosis to relieve portal hypertension.

SPECIAL CONSIDERATIONS

 TEACHING TIP: Instruct the patient to avoid taking aspirin, straining during defecation, and blowing his nose or sneezing too vigorously. Using an electric razor and soft toothbrush also help to reduce the risk of injury. Stress the need to avoid infections and abstain from alcohol.

● Support groups such as Alcoholics Anonymous may provide information and assistance.

Coal worker's pneumoconiosis

A progressive nodular pulmonary disease, coal worker's pneumoconiosis (also called black lung) occurs in two forms. *Simple coal worker's pneumoconiosis* is characterized by small lung opacities. In *complicated coal worker's pneumoconiosis,* masses of fibrous tissue occasionally develop in the lungs of patients with simple coal worker's pneumoconiosis.

CAUSES

Coal worker's pneumoconiosis results from inhalation and prolonged retention of respirable coal dust particles (less than 5 microns in diameter).

> ## Risk factors for coal worker's pneumoconiosis
>
> The risk of developing coal worker's pneumoconiosis depends on the following:
> ● the person's duration of exposure to coal dust (usually 15 years or longer)
> ● intensity of exposure (dust count, particle size)
> ● mine location
> ● silica content of the coal (anthracite coal has the highest silica content)
> ● the person's susceptibility.
>   The incidence of coal worker's pneumoconiosis is highest among anthracite coal miners in the eastern United States.

(See *Risk factors for coal worker's pneumoconiosis.*)

SIGNS AND SYMPTOMS

Simple coal worker's pneumoconiosis is asymptomatic, especially in nonsmokers. Complicated coal worker's pneumoconiosis may lead to exertional dyspnea and a cough that occasionally produces inky-black sputum.

Other clinical features include increasing dyspnea and a cough that produces milky, gray, clear, or coal-flecked sputum. Recurrent bronchial and pulmonary infections produce yellow, green, or thick sputum.

DIAGNOSTIC TESTS

The patient's history reveals exposure to coal dust. A physical examination shows a barrel chest, hyperresonant lungs with diminished breath sounds, wheezes, and other abnormal breath sounds.

Pulmonary function studies help to evaluate the patient's breathing capacity; arterial blood gas studies reveal the amount of oxygen and carbon dioxide in the blood. In simple coal worker's pneumoconiosis, chest X-rays show small opacities; in complicated coal worker's pneumoconiosis, they show one or more large opaque areas.

TREATMENT

Therapy aims to relieve respiratory symptoms, manage hypoxia and cor pulmonale, and avoid respiratory tract irritants and infection. If tuberculosis develops, the patient receives antitubercular therapy.

Respiratory signs and symptoms may be relieved through bronchodilator therapy with theophylline or aminophylline, oral or inhaled sympathomimetic amines, corticosteroids, or cromolyn sodium aerosol. Chest physiotherapy combined with chest percussion and vibration help remove secretions. Other measures include increased fluid intake, aerosol therapy, inhaled mucolytics, and intermittent positive pressure breathing.

In severe cases, oxygen may be given by cannula or mask if the patient has chronic hypoxia or by mechanical ventilation if the partial pressure of arterial oxygen can't be maintained above 40 mm Hg. Respiratory infections warrant prompt antibiotic administration.

SPECIAL CONSIDERATIONS

• Tuberculosis is a risk for the patient with coal worker's pneumoconiosis. The patient, family, and staff should stay alert for signs and symptoms of developing disease.

 PREVENTION: Advise the patient to stay active but to pace activities and practice relaxation techniques to avoid overexertion. To help prevent infections, instruct him to avoid crowds and persons with respiratory infections, and to receive influenza and pneumococcal vaccines.

Colorectal cancer

Colorectal cancer — cancer of the large intestine — is the second most common visceral neoplasm in the United States and Europe. The disease tends to progress slowly and remain localized for a long time. It's potentially curable in 75% of patients if early diagnosis allows resection before nodal involvement.

CAUSES

The exact cause of colorectal cancer is unknown, but studies showing concentration in areas of higher economic development suggest a relationship to diet (excess animal fat and low fiber). Other risk factors include other digestive tract diseases, age (over 40), history of ulcerative colitis, and familial polyposis.

SIGNS AND SYMPTOMS

Early signs and symptoms are typically vague and depend on the location and function of the bowel segment containing the tumor. (See *Assessing colorectal cancer.*) Later signs and symptoms generally include pallor, cachexia, and ascites.

DIAGNOSTIC TESTS

Only a tumor biopsy can verify colon cancer, but other tests help detect it. For instance, a digital examination can detect almost 15% of colon cancers. Hemoccult tests can reveal blood in stools. Proctoscopy or sigmoidoscopy can detect up to 66% of colon cancers. Colonoscopy permits visual inspection of the colon. Computed tomography scan helps detect cancer spread. Barium X-ray can locate tumors that are undetectable on manual or visual examination.

TREATMENT

The most effective treatment is surgery to remove the tumor and adjacent tissues as well as any lymph nodes that may contain cancer cells. The type of surgery depends on tumor location. Some patients must undergo a colostomy.

Chemotherapy is used to treat metastasis, residual disease, or a recurrent inoperable tumor. Radiation therapy induces tumor regression and may be used before or after

Assessing colorectal cancer

Clinical features of colorectal cancer depend on the location of the tumor.

Cancer on the right side
The patient may have black, tarry stools; anemia; and abdominal aching or pressure or dull cramps. As the disease progresses, he experiences weakness, fatigue, exertional dyspnea, vertigo and, eventually, diarrhea, obstipation, anorexia, weight loss, and vomiting.

Cancer on the left side
The patient may have rectal bleeding, intermittent abdominal fullness or cramping, and rectal pressure. As

the disease progresses, he develops obstipation, diarrhea, or ribbon- or pencil-shaped stools. Typically, passage of stools or flatus relieves the pain. Dark or bright red blood may appear in the feces.

Rectal tumor
The first sign is a change in bowel habits, often starting with an urgent need to defecate on arising or obstipation alternating with diarrhea. The patient may have blood or mucus in stools and a sense of incomplete evacuation. Late in the disease, pain begins as a feeling of rectal fullness that later becomes a dull ache in the rectum or sacral region.

---

surgery or combined with chemotherapy.

SPECIAL CONSIDERATIONS
● The patient should be encouraged to look at and care for the stoma. An enterostomal therapist can help set up a regimen.

 TEACHING TIP: Stress the importance of good hygiene and skin care. To reduce flatus, diarrhea, or constipation, advise the patient to eliminate suspected causative foods from the diet.
● If appropriate, a home health agency can provide follow-up care and counseling.
● Anyone who's had colorectal cancer is at increased risk for another primary cancer. Yearly screening and testing and maintaining a high-fiber diet are important.

Common cold

This acute, usually afebrile viral infection causes inflammation of the upper respiratory tract. It accounts for more time lost from school or work than any other cause and is the most common infectious disease. Although

benign and self-limiting, it can lead to secondary bacterial infections.

CAUSES
About 90% of colds stem from a viral infection of the upper respiratory passages and consequent mucous membrane inflammation. Over a hundred viruses can cause the common cold. Major offenders include rhinoviruses, coronaviruses, myxoviruses, adenoviruses, coxsackieviruses, and echoviruses.

Transmission occurs through airborne respiratory droplets, contact with contaminated objects, and hand-to-hand transmission.

SIGNS AND SYMPTOMS
After a 1- to 4-day incubation period, the common cold produces pharyngitis, nasal congestion, rhinitis, headache, and burning, watery eyes. Other signs and symptoms may include fever (in children), chills, myalgia, arthralgia, malaise, lethargy, and a hacking, nonproductive, or nocturnal cough.

As the cold progresses, signs and symptoms include a feeling of fullness with a copious nasal discharge that often irritates the nose. About 3 days after onset, major signs diminish, but the "stuffed-up" feeling may persist for a week.

DIAGNOSTIC TESTS

No explicit diagnostic test isolates the specific organism responsible for the common cold. Consequently, diagnosis rests on typical upper respiratory signs and symptoms.

Diagnosis must rule out allergic rhinitis, measles, rubella, and other disorders that produce similar early signs and symptoms. A fever higher than 100° F (37.8° C), severe malaise, anorexia, tachycardia, exudate on the tonsils or throat, petechiae, and tender lymph glands may point to more serious disorders and require additional diagnostic tests.

TREATMENT

The primary treatment — aspirin or acetaminophen, fluids, and rest — is symptomatic, as the common cold has no cure. Aspirin eases myalgia and headache, fluids loosen accumulated respiratory secretions and maintain hydration, and rest combats fatigue and weakness. Decongestants can relieve congestion. Steam encourages expectoration.

Pure antitussives relieve severe coughs but are contraindicated with productive coughs. The role of vitamin C remains controversial.

SPECIAL CONSIDERATIONS

• Emphasize that antibiotics don't cure the common cold.

 TEACHING TIP: Tell the patient to maintain bed rest during the first few days, increase his fluid intake, and eat light meals. To avoid spreading colds, advise him to wash his hands often, cover coughs and sneezes, and avoid sharing towels and drinking glasses.
• Suggest hot or cold steam vaporizers.
• Overuse of nose drops or sprays may cause rebound congestion.

Common variable immunodeficiency

Also called acquired hypogammaglobulinemia and agammaglobulinemia with immunoglobulin-bearing B cells, common variable immunodeficiency is characterized by progressive deterioration of B-cell (humoral) immunity. This results in increased susceptibility to infection.

The disorder usually causes symptoms between ages 25 and 40. It affects men and women equally and usually doesn't interfere with normal life span or with normal pregnancy and offspring.

CAUSES

Exactly what causes common variable immunodeficiency isn't known. Most patients have a normal circulating B-cell count but defective synthesis or release of immunoglobulins. Many also exhibit progressive deterioration of T cell–mediated (cell-mediated) immunity.

SIGNS AND SYMPTOMS

In common variable immunodeficiency, pyogenic bacterial infections are characteristic but tend to be chronic rather than acute. Recurrent sinopulmonary infections, chronic bacterial conjunctivitis, and malabsorption are usually the first clues to immunodeficiency.

Common variable immunodeficiency may be associated with autoimmune diseases, such as systemic lupus erythematosus, rheumatoid arthritis, hemolytic anemia, and pernicious anemia, as well as with cancers, such as leukemia and lymphoma.

DIAGNOSTIC TESTS

Characteristic diagnostic markers include decreased serum immunoglobulin M (IgM), IgA, and IgG detected by immunoelectrophoresis, along with a normal circulating B-cell count. Antigenic stimulation confirms inability to produce specific antibodies; cell-mediated immunity may be intact or delayed. X-rays usually show signs of chronic lung disease or sinusitis.

TREATMENT
Patients with common variable immunodeficiency need essentially the same treatment as patients with X-linked hypogammaglobulinemia. Injection of immune globulin (usually weekly to monthly) helps maintain immune response. The patient may also need fresh frozen plasma infusions to provide IgA and IgM.

Antibiotics are the mainstay for combating infection. Regular X-rays and pulmonary function studies help monitor lung infection; chest physiotherapy may forestall or help clear such infection.

SPECIAL CONSIDERATIONS
 PREVENTION: To help prevent severe infection, teach the patient and his family how to recognize its early signs and symptoms. Warn the patient to avoid crowds and persons with active infections.

• Stress the importance of good nutrition and regular follow-up care.

Conjunctivitis
Hyperemia of the conjunctiva from infection, allergy, or chemical reactions characterize conjunctivitis. This disorder usually occurs as benign, self-limiting pinkeye; it may also be chronic, possibly indicating degenerative changes or damage from repeated acute attacks. In the Western hemisphere, conjunctivitis is probably the most common eye disorder.

CAUSES
The most common causative organisms are the following:

• *bacterial: Staphylococcus aureus, Streptococcus pneumoniae, Neisseria gonorrhoeae, Neisseria meningitidis*
• *chlamydial: Chlamydia trachomatis* (inclusion conjunctivitis)
• *viral:* adenovirus types 3, 7, and 8; herpes simplex virus, type 1.

Other causes include allergic reactions to pollen, grass, topical medications, air pollutants, and smoke; occupational irritants; rickettsial diseases; parasitic diseases; and, rarely, fungal infections.

Vernal conjunctivitis results from allergy to an unidentified allergen. Idiopathic conjunctivitis may be associated with certain systemic diseases. Conjunctivitis may occur secondary to pneumococcal dacryocystitis or canaliculitis from candidal infection.

SIGNS AND SYMPTOMS
Conjunctivitis usually begins in one eye and rapidly spreads to the other by contamination of towels, washcloths, or the patient's own hand. It commonly produces hyperemia of the conjunctiva, sometimes accompanied by discharge, tearing, pain, and, with corneal involvement, photophobia. (For specific clinical features of acute and viral conjunctivitis, see *Comparing symptoms of bacterial and viral conjunctivitis,* page 70.)

DIAGNOSTIC TESTS
Physical examination usually reveals redness and swelling of blood vessels in the conjunctiva. Monocytes are predominant in stained smears of conjunctival scrapings if conjunctivitis is caused by a virus. Polymorphonuclear cells predominate if conjunctivitis stems from bacteria; eosinophils predominate if it's allergy-related. Culture and sensitivity tests identify the causative bacterial organism and guide antibiotic therapy.

TREATMENT
Bacterial conjunctivitis requires topical application of the appropriate antibiotic or sulfonamide. In viral conjunctivitis, a sulfonamide or broad-spectrum antibiotic eyedrops may prevent secondary infection. Herpes simplex infection generally responds to treatment with trifluridine drops or vidarabine ointment or oral acyclovir.

Comparing symptoms of bacterial and viral conjunctivitis

In *acute bacterial conjunctivitis* (pinkeye), the infection usually lasts only 2 weeks. The patient typically complains of itching, burning, and the sensation of a foreign body in his eye. The eyelids show a crust of sticky, mucopurulent discharge. If the disorder stems from *Neisseria gonorrhoeae,* however, the discharge is profuse and purulent.

Viral conjunctivitis produces copious tearing with minimal exudate, and enlargement of the preauricular lymph node. Some viruses follow a chronic course and produce severe disabling disease. Others last 2 to 3 weeks.

SPECIAL CONSIDERATIONS

• The eye must not be irrigated because this will only spread infection.
• The patient must use proper handwashing technique because some conjunctivitis forms are highly contagious. Also, he must wash his hands before he uses the medication.

 TEACHING TIP: Teach the patient to instill eyedrops and ointments correctly — without touching the bottle tip to his eye or lashes.

Cor pulmonale

Chronic cor pulmonale is hypertrophy of the heart's right ventricle secondary to certain diseases that affect lung function or structure. The disorder accounts for about 25% of all types of heart failure.

Cor pulmonale follows some disorder of the lungs, pulmonary vessels, chest wall, or respiratory control center. For instance, chronic obstructive pulmonary disease (COPD) produces pulmonary hypertension, which leads to right ventricular hypertrophy and right-sided heart failure. Because cor pulmonale generally occurs late during the course of COPD and other irreversible diseases, the prognosis is poor.

CAUSES

Approximately 85% of patients with cor pulmonale have COPD, and 25% of patients with COPD eventually develop cor pulmonale. (See *Other causes of cor pulmonale.*)

SIGNS AND SYMPTOMS

As long as the heart can compensate for increased pulmonary vascular resistance, clinical features are mostly respiratory (chronic productive cough, exertional dyspnea, wheezing respirations, fatigue, and weakness.) Disease progression leads to dyspnea that worsens on exertion, tachypnea, orthopnea, edema, weakness, and right upper quadrant discomfort.

Signs of cor pulmonale and right-sided heart failure include dependent edema; distended neck veins; enlarged, tender liver; and tachycardia.

DIAGNOSTIC TESTS

Pulmonary artery pressure measurements show increased right-sided heart and pulmonary artery pressures. Other useful tests include echocardiography or angiography, chest X-ray, arterial blood gas analysis, electrocardiography, pulmonary function studies, and hematocrit.

TREATMENT

Treatment goals include reducing hypoxemia, increasing the patient's exercise tolerance and, when possible, correcting the underlying condition. Besides bed rest, treatment may include digitalis glycosides, antibiotics (if respiratory infection is present), potent pulmonary artery vasodilators, and oxygen administration. Acute cases may warrant mechanical ventilation.

PATHOPHYSIOLOGY

Other causes of cor pulmonale

Although cor pulmonale most often is associated with chronic obstructive pulmonary disease, it may also result from the following disorders:
• obstructive lung disease (such as bronchiectasis and cystic fibrosis)
• restrictive lung disease (such as pneumoconiosis)
• loss of lung tissue after extensive lung surgery

• pulmonary vascular disease (such as recurrent thromboembolism)
• respiratory insufficiency without pulmonary disease (as in chest wall disorders, such as kyphoscoliosis, and neuromuscular incompetence resulting from muscular dystrophy or amyotrophic lateral sclerosis)
• living at high altitudes (chronic mountain sickness).

Other treatments may include a low-salt diet, restricted fluid intake, diuretics, phlebotomy (to reduce the red blood cell count), and anticoagulation.

SPECIAL CONSIDERATIONS
• A social service agency can help the patient obtain equipment for home suctioning or supplemental oxygen therapy.

TEACHING TIP: Stress the importance of eating a low-salt diet and immediately reporting edema. Urge the patient to promptly report increased sputum production, a change in sputum color, increased coughing or wheezing, chest pain, fever, and chest tightness. Advise him to avoid crowds and persons known to have pulmonary infections.

Coronary artery disease

The dominant effect of coronary artery disease (CAD) is the loss of oxygen and nutrients to myocardial tissue because of diminished coronary blood flow. This disease is near epidemic in the Western world.

CAUSES
Atherosclerosis is the usual cause of CAD. In this form of arteriosclerosis, fatty, fibrous plaques narrow the lumen of the coronary arteries, reduce the volume of blood that can flow through them, and lead to myocardial ischemia. Plaque formation also predisposes the patient to thrombosis, which can provoke myocardial infarction.

Atherosclerosis has been linked to many risk factors: family history, hypertension, obesity, smoking, diabetes mellitus, stress, a sedentary lifestyle, and high serum cholesterol and triglyceride levels.

Coronary artery spasms may also impede blood flow. These spasms result from a spontaneous, sustained contraction of one or more coronary arteries. The spasms cause ischemia and heart muscle dysfunction.

SIGNS AND SYMPTOMS
The classic symptom of CAD is angina, which is usually described as a burning, squeezing, or tight feeling in the substernal or precordial chest. Chest pain may radiate to the left arm, neck, jaw, or shoulder blade and may be accompanied by nausea, vomiting, fainting, sweating, and cool extremities. Anginal episodes most often follow physical exertion.

Relieving occlusions with angioplasty

For a patient with an occluded coronary artery, percutaneous transluminal coronary angioplasty can open the artery without opening the chest — an important advantage over bypass surgery.

First, coronary angiography must confirm the presence and location of the arterial occlusion. Then, a guide catheter is threaded through the patient's femoral artery into the coronary artery under fluoroscopic guidance.

When angiography shows the guide catheter positioned at the occlusion site, a smaller, double lumen balloon catheter is carefully inserted through the guide catheter and the balloon directed through the occlusion (left illustration). A marked pressure gradient will be obvious.

The balloon is alternately inflated and deflated until an angiogram verifies successful arterial dilation (right illustration) and the pressure gradient has decreased.

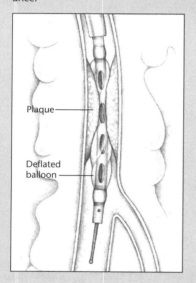

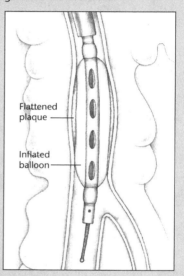

Severe and prolonged anginal pain generally suggests MI, with potentially fatal arrhythmias and mechanical failure.

DIAGNOSTIC TESTS

The patient's history — including the frequency and duration of angina and the presence of associated risk factors — is crucial in evaluating CAD. Diagnostic test results include the following:

• *Electrocardiogram during angina* shows heart damage and, possibly, an irregular heart rhythm.

• *Treadmill or bicycle stress tests* may provoke chest pain and signs of heart damage.

• *Coronary angiography* reveals coronary artery narrowing or blockage.

• *Myocardial perfusion imaging* during treadmill exercise detects damaged heart areas, seen as "cold spots."

TREATMENT

For patients with angina, treatment

aims to either reduce myocardial oxygen demand or increase oxygen supply. Therapy consists mainly of nitrates, beta-adrenergic blockers, or calcium channel blockers. Obstructive lesions may necessitate coronary artery bypass surgery and vein grafting.

Angioplasty may be performed during cardiac catheterization to compress fatty deposits and relieve occlusion in patients with no calcification and partial occlusion. (See *Relieving occlusions with angioplasty.*) Laser angioplasty, a newer procedure, corrects occlusion by melting fatty deposits.

Prevention

Because CAD is so widespread, prevention is crucial. Dietary restrictions aimed at reducing calorie (in obesity), salt, fat, and cholesterol intake can reduce the risk. Stress reduction and abstention from smoking are also beneficial.

Other preventive actions include control of hypertension and high serum cholesterol or triglyceride levels and measures that minimize platelet aggregation and the risk of blood clots.

SPECIAL CONSIDERATIONS

• The patient should be told to call for help immediately if he feels chest, arm, or neck pain.
• After surgery, vigorous chest physiotherapy and guidance in coughing and deep-breathing exercises should be provided.
• The patient must follow the prescribed drug regimen, engage in an exercise program, stop smoking, and monitor his diet.

Crohn's disease

Crohn's disease is an inflammation of any part of the GI tract (usually the terminal ileum). Lacteal blockage in the intestinal wall leads to edema and, eventually, to inflammation, ulceration, stenosis and, possibly, abscesses and fistulas. Inflammation can extend through all layers of the intestinal wall and may involve regional lymph nodes and the mesentery.

Possible complications of Crohn's disease include intestinal obstruction, fistula formation between the small bowel and the bladder, perianal and perirectal abscesses and fistulas, intra-abdominal abscesses, and perforation.

CAUSES

Although the exact cause of Crohn's disease is unknown, possible causes include allergies, a genetic tendency, and other immune disorders and infection.

SIGNS AND SYMPTOMS

Clinical effects vary with the location and extent of the lesion. At first, they may be mild and nonspecific.

The patient with acute disease typically has signs and symptoms that mimic appendicitis — steady, colicky, pain in the right lower quadrant; cramping; tenderness; flatulence; nausea; fever; and diarrhea. Bleeding and bloody stools may occur.

Chronic signs and symptoms (more typical of the disease) are more persistent and less severe. They include diarrhea (four to six stools a day) with pain in the right lower abdominal quadrant, steatorrhea, marked weight loss, weakness, and fatigue.

DIAGNOSTIC TESTS

Laboratory tests show an increase in white blood cells and other imbalances. Barium enema and other X-ray studies may be used to check changes in bowel shape. However, biopsy is the only way to confirm the diagnosis.

TREATMENT

No cure for Crohn's disease exists; treatment is symptomatic. In debilitated patients, therapy includes I.V. hyperalimentation to maintain nutrition while resting the bowel.

Drug therapy may include anti-inflammatory corticosteroids, immunosuppressive agents, and antibacterial agents such as sulfasalazine. Metronidazole is effective in some patients.

The patient must get adequate physical rest, restrict fiber intake (no fruit or vegetables), and eliminate dairy products if he's lactose intolerant.

Surgery may be necessary to correct bowel perforation, massive hemorrhage, fistulas, or acute intestinal obstruction. Extensive disease of the large intestine and rectum may necessitate colectomy with ileostomy.

SPECIAL CONSIDERATIONS
• Good skin care is important after each bowel movement. A clean, covered bedpan should always be within the patient's reach. Ventilating the room helps eliminate odors.
• Before ileostomy, the patient may benefit from a visit by an enterostomal therapist. Meticulous stoma care is important, and the patient and family should learn proper technique.

Croup

This severe inflammation and obstruction of the upper airway can occur as acute laryngotracheobronchitis (most common), laryngitis, or acute spasmodic laryngitis. It must always be distinguished from epiglottitis.

Croup is a childhood disease affecting boys more often than girls (typically between ages 3 months and 3 years) that usually occurs during the winter. Up to 15% of patients have a strong family history of croup. Recovery is usually complete.

CAUSES
Croup usually results from a viral infection. Parainfluenza viruses cause two-thirds of such infections; adenoviruses, respiratory syncytial virus, influenza and measles viruses, and bacteria account for the rest.

SIGNS AND SYMPTOMS
Clinical features include inspiratory stridor, hoarse or muffled vocal sounds, laryngeal obstruction, respiratory distress, and a characteristic sharp, barklike cough.

As croup progresses, it causes inflammatory edema and, possibly, spasm, which can obstruct the upper airway and severely compromise ventilation.

Each form of croup has additional characteristics. Symptoms of *laryngotracheobronchitis* seem to worsen at night. Inflammation causes edema of the bronchi and bronchioles and increasingly difficult expiration, which frightens the child. Other characteristic features include fever, diffusely decreased breath sounds, expiratory rhonchi, and scattered crackles.

Laryngitis usually produces no respiratory distress except in infants. Early signs and symptoms are a sore throat and cough.

Acute spasmodic laryngitis typically begins with mild to moderate hoarseness and nasal discharge, followed by the characteristic cough and noisy inspiration, labored breathing with retractions, rapid pulse, and clammy skin.

DIAGNOSTIC TESTS
When bacterial infection is the cause, throat cultures may identify organisms and rule out diphtheria. A neck X-ray may show areas of upper airway narrowing and swelling. With a child, the doctor looks for foreign body obstruction (a common cause of croupy cough in young children), masses, and cysts.

TREATMENT
For most children with croup, home care with rest, cool humidification during sleep, and antipyretics relieves symptoms. However, respiratory distress that interferes with oral hydration requires hospitalization and parenteral fluid replacement. Bacterial infection calls for antibiotic therapy and possibly supplemental oxygen.

SPECIAL CONSIDERATIONS
• Sore throat can be relieved with soothing, water-based ices, such as fruit sherbet and popsicles.
• Apply petroleum jelly or another

ointment around the nose and lips to soothe irritation.

 TEACHING TIP: When croup doesn't require hospitalization, provide thorough patient and family teaching for home care. Suggest the use of a cool mist humidifier. To relieve croupy spells, tell parents to carry the child into the bathroom, shut the door, and turn on the hot water. Breathing in warm, moist air quickly eases an acute spell of croup.

Cushing's syndrome

Cushing's syndrome is marked by a cluster of clinical abnormalities caused by excessive levels of adrenocortical hormones or related corticosteroids and, to a lesser extent, androgens and aldosterone.

Prognosis depends on the underlying cause. It's poor in untreated persons and in those with untreatable, ectopic, corticotropin-producing carcinoma.

CAUSES

In roughly 70% of patients, Cushing's syndrome results from excess production of corticotropin and consequent hyperplasia of the adrenal cortex. Corticotropin overproduction may stem from pituitary hypersecretion (Cushing's disease), excessive exogenous glucocorticoid use, or a corticotropin-producing tumor in another organ. In the remaining 30% of patients, Cushing's syndrome results from a cortisol-secreting adrenal tumor (usually benign).

SIGNS AND SYMPTOMS

Cushing's syndrome causes rapidly developing adiposity of the face (moon face), neck, and trunk and purple striae on the skin. Typically, the disease induces changes in multiple body systems. (See *Clinical effects of Cushing's syndrome,* page 76.)

DIAGNOSTIC TESTS

Blood hormone levels may indicate the need for further tests. The *dexamethasone suppression test* confirms diagnosis. Another dexamethasone suppression test may be administered to determine if Cushing's syndrome results from Cushing's disease. Ultrasound, computed tomography (CT) scan, or angiography can help localize adrenal tumors. CT scans or magnetic resonance imaging may identify pituitary tumors.

TREATMENT

Radiation, drug therapy, and surgery may be used to restore hormone balance and reverse Cushing's syndrome. For example, pituitary-dependent Cushing's syndrome with adrenal hyperplasia and severe cushingoid signs and symptoms may require hypophysectomy or pituitary irradiation.

Nonendocrine corticotropin-producing tumors must be excised. If signs and symptoms persist, drug therapy follows to decrease cortisol levels.

Aminoglutethimide and ketoconazole decrease cortisol levels. Aminoglutethimide alone, or in combination with metyrapone, may also be useful in metastatic adrenal carcinoma.

Before surgery, the patient with cushingoid signs and symptoms should have special management to control hypertension, edema, diabetes, and cardiovascular manifestations and to prevent infection. Cortisol therapy is essential during and after surgery to help the patient tolerate the physiologic stress caused by pituitary or adrenal removal. Some patients need lifelong steroid replacement therapy.

SPECIAL CONSIDERATIONS

• A diet high in protein and potassium but low in calories, carbohydrates, and sodium can minimize weight gain, edema, and hypertension.

• The patient must watch for and report signs and symptoms of infection — a particular concern in Cushing's syndrome.

 TEACHING TIP: Instruct a patient who needs lifelong steroid replacement to take

Clinical effects of Cushing's syndrome

A patient with Cushing's syndrome may have any of the signs and symptoms below, depending on which body system is affected.

Endocrine and metabolic systems
- Diabetes mellitus, with decreased glucose tolerance, fasting hyperglycemia, and glucosuria

Musculoskeletal system
- Muscle weakness
- Pathologic fractures
- Slender arms and legs
- Skeletal growth retardation in children

Skin
- Purplish striae
- Fat pads above the clavicles, over the upper back, on the face, and throughout the trunk
- Little or no scar formation
- Poor wound healing
- Acne and hirsutism in women

GI system
- Peptic ulcer
- Decreased gastric mucus

Central nervous system
- Irritability
- Emotional lability, ranging from euphoric behavior to depression or psychosis
- Insomnia

Cardiovascular system
- Hypertension
- Left ventricular hypertrophy
- Bleeding, petechiae, and ecchymosis (from capillary weakness)

Immunologic system
- Increased susceptibility to infection
- Decreased resistance to stress
- Suppressed inflammatory response (may mask even a severe infection)

Genitourinary system
- Sodium and fluid retention
- Increased potassium excretion
- Inhibited secretion of antidiuretic hormone
- Ureteral calculi

Reproductive system
- Clitoral hypertrophy, mild virilism, and amenorrhea or oligomenorrhea in women
- Sexual dysfunction

the drug exactly as prescribed, with antacids or meals to minimize gastric irritation; to carry a medical identification card; to immediately report stressful situations such as infections; and to watch closely for fatigue, weakness, and dizziness (symptoms of inadequate steroid dosage) as well as severe swelling and weight gain (signs of overdose). Warn him not to stop taking steroids abruptly because this could trigger a fatal adrenal crisis.

Cystic fibrosis

Cystic fibrosis is a generalized dysfunction of the exocrine glands that affects multiple organ systems. Transmitted as an autosomal recessive trait, it's the most common fatal genetic disease of white children. Cystic fibrosis is fatal by age 16 in about 50% of affected children. Of the rest, some survive to age 30 or beyond. Death typically results from pneumonia, emphysema, or atelectasis.

CAUSES
The recently identified gene responsible for cystic fibrosis encodes a protein that involves chloride transport across epithelial membranes. The immediate causes of signs and symptoms are increased viscosity of bronchial, pancreatic, and other mucous gland secretions and consequent obstruction of glandular ducts.

SIGNS AND SYMPTOMS

Clinical effects may become apparent soon after birth or may take years to develop. They include major aberrations in sweat gland, respiratory, and GI functions.

Sweat gland dysfunction can eventually induce fatal shock and arrhythmias, especially in hot weather. Respiratory symptoms reflect obstructive changes in the lungs. (See *Respiratory features of cystic fibrosis*.) GI symptoms may begin with meconium ileus (failure to excrete meconium) in a newborn; this condition leads to symptoms of intestinal obstruction.

Eventually, obstruction of the pancreatic ducts and resulting enzyme deficiencies lead to bulky, foul-smelling, pale stools with a high fat content. This malabsorption induces poor weight gain, poor growth, ravenous appetite, distended abdomen, thin extremities, and poor turgor. Inability to absorb fats produces deficiency of vitamins A, D, E, and K, leading to clotting problems, retarded bone growth, and delayed sexual development.

The disease also induces changes in the pancreas, causing insufficient insulin production, abnormal glucose tolerance, and glycosuria.

DIAGNOSTIC TESTS

Cystic fibrosis is diagnosed if a person has two clearly positive sweat tests along with one of the following:
• an obstructive lung disease, confirmed pancreatic insufficiency, or failure to thrive and a family history of cystic fibrosis
• chest X-rays showing early signs of obstructive lung disease
• stool specimen lacking the enzyme trypsin.

TREATMENT

Specific treatment depends on the organ systems involved. To combat sweat electrolyte losses, treatment includes generous salting of foods and, during hot weather, sodium supplementation. Oral pancreatic enzymes with meals and snacks are given to

---

Respiratory features of cystic fibrosis

Patients with cystic fibrosis typically experience wheezy respirations; a dry, nonproductive, paroxysmal cough; dyspnea; and tachypnea. These changes eventually lead to severe atelectasis and emphysema.

Other respiratory signs include:
• barrel chest
• cyanosis
• clubbed fingers and toes
• recurring bronchitis and pneumonia.

---

offset pancreatic enzyme deficiencies. The child must eat a diet low in fat but high in protein and calories and must take vitamin supplements.

Management of pulmonary dysfunction includes chest physiotherapy, postural drainage, and breathing exercises several times daily. Aerosol therapy before postural drainage helps to loosen secretions. Dornase alfa, a genetically engineered pulmonary enzyme, helps to thin airway mucus, improving lung function and reducing the risk of pulmonary infection.

In a patient with pulmonary infection, mucopurulent secretions must be loosened and removed. Broad-spectrum antimicrobials help combat infection. Oxygen therapy is used as needed. Clinical trials of aerosol gene therapy show promise in reducing pulmonary symptoms.

SPECIAL CONSIDERATIONS

 TEACHING TIP: Instruct the patient and family about the disease and its treatment.
• Using an air conditioner and humidifier can decrease the patient's vulnerability to respiratory infections.
• The family may wish to undergo ge-

netic counseling. The Cystic Fibrosis Foundation is a good source of information.

Cytomegalovirus infection

Cytomegalovirus (CMV) infection is caused by the cytomegalovirus, an ether-sensitive virus belonging to the herpes family. The disease occurs worldwide and is transmitted by human contact.

About four out of five people over age 35 have been infected with CMV. In most cases, the disease is so mild that it's overlooked. However, CMV infection during pregnancy can harm the fetus, possibly leading to stillbirth, brain damage, and other birth defects or to severe neonatal illness.

CAUSES
CMV has been found in the saliva, urine, semen, breast milk, feces, blood, and vaginal and cervical secretions of infected persons. Transmission usually occurs through contact with infected secretions, which harbor the virus for months or even years.

The virus may be transmitted by sexual contact and can travel across the placenta, causing a congenital infection. Immunosuppressed patients run a 90% chance of contracting CMV infection. Recipients of blood transfusions from donors with positive CMV antibodies are at some risk.

SIGNS AND SYMPTOMS
Most patients have mild, nonspecific complaints or none at all; in these patients, the disease usually runs a self-limiting course. Some patients experience inflammatory reactions in the lungs, liver, GI tract, eyes, and central nervous system. In some adults, CMV may cause CMV mononucleosis, with 3 weeks or more of irregular, high fever.

Immunodeficient patients, such as those with AIDS, and patients receiving immunosuppressives may devel-

op pneumonia or other secondary infections. AIDS patients may also develop disseminated CMV infection, which may cause chorioretinitis (resulting in blindness), colitis, or encephalitis.

Infected infants ages 3 to 6 months usually appear asymptomatic but may develop hepatic dysfunction, hepatosplenomegaly, spider angiomas, pneumonitis, and lymphadenopathy. Congenital CMV infection is seldom apparent at birth, but can lead to brain damage.

DIAGNOSTIC TESTS
Although virus isolation in urine is the most sensitive laboratory method, the diagnosis can also rest on virus isolation from saliva, throat, cervix, white blood cell, and biopsy specimens.

TREATMENT
Because CMV infection is usually self-limiting, treatment aims to relieve signs and symptoms and prevent complications. The immunosuppressed patient may receive acyclovir, ganciclovir, and foscarnet.

SPECIAL CONSIDERATIONS
• Thorough hand washing can reduce the risk of infection in patients with CMV infection.
• Observe universal precautions when handling body secretions.

 PREVENTION: To help prevent CMV infection, warn immunosuppressed patients and pregnant women to avoid exposure to persons with confirmed or suspected CMV infection.

Dermatitis

An inflammation of the skin, dermatitis occurs in several forms: atopic (discussed here), seborrheic, nummular, contact, chronic, localized neurodermatitis, exfoliative, and stasis.

Atopic dermatitis (atopic or infantile eczema) is a chronic inflammatory response often associated with other atopic diseases, such as bronchial asthma and allergic rhinitis. It usually develops in infants between ages 1 month and 1 year, commonly in those with a strong family history of atopic disease.

Typically, this form of dermatitis flares and subsides repeatedly before finally resolving during adolescence. However, it can persist into adulthood.

CAUSES
The cause of atopic dermatitis is unknown, but there is a genetic predisposition exacerbated by factors such as food allergies, infections, irritating chemicals, and temperature and humidity extremes. Approximately 10% of childhood cases are caused by allergy to certain foods, particularly eggs, peanuts, milk, and wheat. Chronic skin irritation usually continues even after exposure to the allergen has ended or after the irritation has been systemically controlled.

SIGNS AND SYMPTOMS
Atopic skin lesions generally begin as erythematous areas on excessively dry skin. In children, lesions typically appear on the forehead, cheeks, and extensor surfaces of the arms and legs; in adults, at flexion points (antecubital fossa, popliteal area, and neck).

During flare-ups, pruritus and scratching cause edema, crusting, and scaling. Eventually, chronic atopic lesions lead to multiple areas of dry, scaly skin, with white dermatographia, blanching, and lichenification.

DIAGNOSTIC TESTS
A family history of allergy and chronic inflammation suggests atopic dermatitis. Serum immunoglobulin E levels are often elevated. Other skin lesions, such as seborrheic dermatitis, are ruled out by examining the distribution of skin lesions.

TREATMENT
The patient must eliminate allergens and avoid irritants and other precipitating factors. Local and systemic measures relieve itching and inflammation. Topical application of a corticosteroid ointment often alleviates inflammation. Between steroid doses, a moisturizing cream can help retain moisture. Systemic corticosteroid therapy should be used only during extreme exacerbations.

SPECIAL CONSIDERATIONS
● An individual schedule and plan for daily skin care can help the patient manage this condition. He should bathe in tepid water and use a nonfatty soap. When lesions are acutely inflamed, bathing may be restricted to plain water.
● Lubricating the skin after bathing may promote comfort. Applying occlusive dressings (such as plastic film) intermittently as necessary can help to clear lichenified skin patches.

 PREVENTION: Advise the patient to keep fingernails short to help reduce the risk of injury and the risk of infection from scratching.

Diabetes insipidus

A disorder of water metabolism, diabetes insipidus results from a defi-

Water deprivation test

This definitive test for diabetes insipidus measures urine osmolality, which reflects renal concentration capacity after a period of water deprivation and after injection of vasopressin, a pituitary hormone.

Test procedure
The evening before and the morning of the test, fluids are withheld to induce dehydration. (In a patient with polyuria exceeding 10 L/day, fluids are withheld only during the morning of the test.) A urine sample is collected hourly in the morning for osmolality measurement. At noon, a blood sample is drawn for osmolality measurement. If serum osmolality exceeds 288 mOsm/kg (the level of adequate hydration), vasopressin is injected subcutaneously. Within an hour, a urine specimen is collected for osmolality measurement.

Precautions
During this test, the patient must be weighed and vital signs monitored every 2 hours. A 2 lb (1-kg) weight loss normally accompanies adequate dehydration. If weight loss exceeds 4½ lb (2 kg), the test is discontinued.

Test results
A rise of more than 9% in urine osmolality after vasopressin injection indicates diabetes insipidus.

ciency of circulating vasopressin (also called antidiuretic hormone). It's characterized by excessive fluid intake and hypotonic polyuria. In uncomplicated diabetes insipidus, the prognosis is good with adequate water replacement, and patients usually lead normal lives.

Normally, the hypothalamus synthesizes vasopressin. The posterior pituitary gland stores vasopressin and releases it into the general circulation, where it causes the kidneys to reabsorb water. In diabetes insipidus, the absence of vasopressin allows the filtered water to be excreted in the urine instead of being reabsorbed.

CAUSES
Diabetes insipidus results from an intracranial neoplastic or metastatic lesion, hypophysectomy or other neurosurgery, skull fracture, or head trauma that damages the neurohypophyseal structures. It can also result from infection, granulomatous disease, and vascular lesions; it may be idiopathic or familial.

SIGNS AND SYMPTOMS
The patient's history typically shows an abrupt onset of extreme polyuria (up to 30 L/day), which causes extreme thirst and ingestion of great quantities of water. Some patients also experience nocturia. A few have extreme fatigue from inadequate rest caused by frequent voiding and excessive thirst.

Other features of diabetes insipidus include signs and symptoms of dehydration, which usually begin abruptly.

DIAGNOSTIC TESTS
Urinalysis reveals almost colorless urine of low osmolality (50 to 200 mOsm/kg) and low specific gravity (less than 1.005). However, confirmation of the diagnosis requires the water deprivation test. (See *Water deprivation test.*)

TREATMENT
Until the cause of diabetes insipidus is identified and eliminated, administration of vasopressin or a vasopressin stimulant can control fluid balance and prevent dehydration.

SPECIAL CONSIDERATIONS
• Fluid intake and output are monitored carefully and maintained at lev-

els adequate to prevent severe dehydration.

• If the patient experiences dizziness or muscle weakness, take safety precautions, such as raising the side rails and assisting him to walk.

 TEACHING TIP: Instruct the patient to administer desmopressin by nasal spray only after the onset of polyuria — not before — to prevent excess fluid retention and water intoxication. Tell him to wear a medical identification bracelet and carry medication at all times.

• Weight gain may mean that the medication dosage is too high and should be reported to the patient's health care provider. Polyuria recurrence indicates that the dosage is too low.

Diabetes mellitus

A chronic disease of absolute or relative insulin deficiency or resistance, diabetes mellitus is characterized by disturbances in carbohydrate, protein, and fat metabolism. The disease occurs in two forms: *type I, insulin-dependent diabetes mellitus,* and the more prevalent *type II, non-insulin-dependent diabetes mellitus.*

Type I usually occurs before age 30; typically, the patient requires exogenous insulin and dietary management to achieve control. Type II usually occurs in obese adults after age 40 and is most often treated with diet and exercise.

A leading cause of death by disease in the United States, diabetes mellitus contributes to about 50% of myocardial infarctions and about 75% of cerebrovascular accidents as well as to renal failure and peripheral vascular disease. It's also the leading cause of new blindness.

CAUSES

The effects of diabetes mellitus result from insulin deficiency, which compromises the body tissue's access to essential nutrients for fuel and storage. The precise cause of both type I and type II diabetes mellitus remains unknown. Genetic factors may play a part in development of all types; autoimmune disease and viral infections may be risk factors in type I. Other risk factors include obesity, physiologic or emotional stress, pregnancy, and some medications.

Pregnancy places special demands on carbohydrate metabolism to increase, even in a healthy woman. Consequently, pregnancy may lead to a prediabetic state, to the conversion of an asymptomatic diabetic state to a symptomatic one, or to complications in a patient with previously stable diabetes. Nonetheless, the maternal and fetal prognoses can be good if maternal blood glucose is well controlled and diabetic complications are prevented. Infant illness and mortality hinge on recognizing and successfully controlling hypoglycemia, which may develop within hours after delivery.

SIGNS AND SYMPTOMS

Diabetes may begin dramatically with ketoacidosis in type I or insidiously. The most common symptom is fatigue. Insulin deficiency causes hyperglycemia, which pulls fluid from body tissues, causing osmotic diuresis, polyuria, dehydration, polydipsia, dry mucous membranes, and poor skin turgor. In ketoacidosis and hyperglycemic hyperosmolar nonketotic coma, dehydration may cause hypovolemia and shock. Type I diabetes mellitus may lead to weight loss and hunger.

Over time, diabetes may cause retinopathy, nephropathy, atherosclerosis, peripheral and autonomic neuropathy, and infections of the skin, urinary tract, and vagina.

DIAGNOSTIC TESTS

In June 1997, the American Diabetes Association (ADA) issued new diagnostic guidelines that broaden the definition of diabetes and may lead to detection of 2 million new cases. A person is now considered to have diabetes if his fasting plasma glucose level equals or exceeds 126 mg/dl on at least two occasions. (Formerly, dia-

What your patient needs to know about diabetes mellitus

The patient with diabetes mellitus needs comprehensive teaching to help him manage the disease. If your job involves patient teaching, tailor your instructions to the patient's needs, abilities, and developmental stage. Make sure to cover the following topics:
● purpose and goals of treatment
● dietary guidelines
● names, dosages, and administration of diabetes medications
● adverse medication reactions to report
● prescribed exercise program
● procedures he should follow to monitor his condition
● importance of meticulous hygiene
● recognizing and immediately reporting symptoms of hypoglycemia and hyperglycemia.

betes was defined as a level of 140 mg/dl or higher). Patients with fasting plasma glucose levels of 110 to 125 mg/dl are in a danger zone of impaired glucose metabolism. The ADA recommends that all healthy persons age 45 and older get tested every 3 years. Federal health authorities have endorsed the new guidelines.

TREATMENT
Effective treatment for both types of diabetes normalizes blood glucose and decreases complications. Treatment for type I diabetes includes insulin replacement, diet, and exercise. Pancreas transplantation is experimental and requires chronic immunosuppression. In type II diabetes, the patient may need oral antidiabetic drugs.

Treatment of both types requires a strict diet planned to meet nutritional needs, control blood glucose levels, and reach and maintain appropriate body weight. For the obese patient with type II diabetes, weight reduction is a goal. In type I, the calorie allotment may be high.

Treatment of long-term diabetic complications may include transplantation or dialysis for renal failure, photocoagulation for retinopathy, and vascular surgery for large-vessel disease.

SPECIAL CONSIDERATIONS

 ACTION STAT: Stay alert for signs and symptoms of acute complications from diabetic therapy — altered mentation, dizziness, weakness, pallor, tachycardia, diaphoresis, seizures, and coma. If the patient is conscious, he must immediately receive carbohydrates in the form of fruit juice, hard candy, or honey; if he's unconscious, he must receive glucagon or dextrose I.V.
● The patient must take an active role in checking for signs of complications and taking steps to prevent problems. For instance, he must know how to care for all injuries, cuts, and blisters; recognize signs of urinary tract infection and renal disease; have regular ophthalmologic examinations; and manage diabetes during minor illness.

 TEACHING TIP: Compliance with the therapeutic regimen is essential. Emphasize the importance of blood glucose control on the patient's long-term health. (See *What your patient needs to know about diabetes mellitus.*)

Disseminated intravascular coagulation

Disseminated intravascular coagulation (DIC) occurs as a complication of diseases and conditions that accelerate clotting, which leads to small blood vessel occlusion, organ necro-

PATHOPHYSIOLOGY

Conditions that can cause DIC

A wide range of diseases, disorders, and other conditions can trigger the chain of events that characterizes disseminated intravascular coagulation (DIC). They include:
- infection
- obstetric complications
- neoplastic disease
- disorders that produce necrosis, such as extensive burns and trauma, brain tissue destruction, transplant rejection, and hepatic necrosis
- heatstroke
- shock
- poisonous snakebite
- cirrhosis

- fat embolism
- incompatible blood transfusion
- cardiac arrest
- surgery necessitating cardiopulmonary bypass
- giant hemangioma
- severe venous thrombosis.

It's not clear why such conditions lead to DIC — nor is it certain that they lead to it through a common mechanism. In many patients, the triggering mechanisms may be the entrance of foreign protein into the circulation and vascular endothelial injury.

sis, depletion of circulating clotting factors and platelets, and activation of the fibrinolytic system. These events, in turn, can provoke severe hemorrhage. Clotting in the microcirculation usually affects the kidneys and extremities but may occur in the brain, lungs, pituitary and adrenal glands, and GI mucosa.

DIC generally is an acute condition but may be chronic in cancer patients. The prognosis depends on early detection and treatment, severity of the hemorrhage, and treatment of the underlying condition.

CAUSES
DIC may result from a wide range of conditions. (See *Conditions that can cause DIC*.)

SIGNS AND SYMPTOMS
The most significant clinical feature of DIC is abnormal bleeding, *without* an accompanying history of a serious hemorrhagic disorder. Signs of such bleeding include cutaneous oozing, petechiae, ecchymoses, and hematomas caused by bleeding into the skin. Bleeding from sites of surgical or invasive procedures and from the

GI tract are equally significant, as are acrocyanosis and signs of acute tubular necrosis.

Related signs and symptoms include nausea, vomiting, dyspnea, oliguria, convulsions, coma, shock, failure of major organ systems, and severe muscle, back, and abdominal pain.

DIAGNOSTIC TESTS
Abnormal bleeding in the absence of a known hematologic disorder suggests DIC. Initial laboratory findings supporting a tentative diagnosis include:
- prolonged prothrombin time (greater than 15 seconds)
- prolonged partial thromboplastin time (greater than 60 seconds)
- decreased fibrinogen levels (less than 150 mg/dl)
- decreased platelets (less than 100,000/mm^3)
- increased fibrin degradation products (often greater than 100 µg/ml).

Final confirmation of DIC may be difficult because many of these test results also occur in other disorders.

TREATMENT

Successful management of DIC necessitates prompt recognition and adequate treatment of the underlying disorder. Treatment may be supportive or highly specific.

If the patient isn't actively bleeding, supportive care alone may reverse DIC. However, active bleeding may require heparin I.V. and administration of blood, fresh-frozen plasma, platelets, or packed red blood cells to support hemostasis.

SPECIAL CONSIDERATIONS

• Protecting the patient from injury may require complete bed rest during bleeding episodes.
• I.V. and venipuncture sites should be checked frequently for bleeding. Alert other personnel to the patient's tendency to hemorrhage.

Diverticular disease

In this disorder, bulging pouches (diverticula) in the GI wall push the mucosal lining through the surrounding muscle. The most common site for diverticula is the sigmoid colon, although they may develop anywhere, from the proximal end of the pharynx to the anus.

Diverticular disease has two clinical forms. In *diverticulosis,* diverticula are present but don't cause signs or symptoms. In *diverticulitis,* diverticula are inflamed and may cause potentially fatal obstruction, infection, or hemorrhage.

CAUSES

Diverticula probably result from high intraluminal pressure on weak areas within the GI wall, where blood vessels enter. Diet may be a contributing factor because lack of roughage reduces fecal residue, narrows the bowel lumen, and leads to higher intra-abdominal pressure during defecation.

In diverticulitis, retained undigested food mixed with bacteria accumulates in the diverticular sac, forming a hard mass (fecalith). This substance cuts off the blood supply to the thin walls of the sac, making them more susceptible to attack by colonic bacteria. Inflammation follows, possibly leading to perforation, abscess, peritonitis, obstruction, or hemorrhage.

SIGNS AND SYMPTOMS

Although *diverticulosis* usually produces no symptoms, it may cause recurrent left lower quadrant pain. Such pain, often accompanied by alternating constipation and diarrhea, is relieved by defecation or passage of flatus.

Mild diverticulitis produces moderate left lower quadrant pain, mild nausea, gas, irregular bowel habits, low-grade fever, and leukocytosis. In *severe diverticulitis,* diverticula may rupture and produce abscesses or peritonitis. Symptoms of rupture include abdominal rigidity and left lower quadrant pain. Peritonitis follows release of fecal material from the rupture site and causes signs and symptoms of sepsis and shock (high fever, chills, hypotension). Rupture of diverticula near a vessel may cause microscopic or massive hemorrhage.

Chronic diverticulitis may cause fibrosis and adhesions that narrow the bowel lumen and lead to bowel obstruction. Signs and symptoms of incomplete obstruction include constipation, ribbonlike stools, intermittent diarrhea, and abdominal distention.

DIAGNOSTIC TESTS

Because it rarely produces signs or symptoms, diverticular disease is often discovered coincidentally during a physical examination that includes an upper GI barium X-ray series.

TREATMENT

The two forms of the disease call for different treatment regimens.

Diverticulosis

Asymptomatic diverticulosis generally doesn't require treatment. Intestinal diverticulosis with pain, mild GI distress, constipation, or difficult defecation may respond to a liquid or bland diet, stool softeners, and occasional doses of mineral oil. After pain subsides, patients also benefit from a high-residue diet and bulk medication such as psyllium.

Diverticulitis

Treatment of mild diverticulitis may include bed rest, a liquid diet, stool softeners, a broad-spectrum antibiotic, meperidine to control pain and relax smooth muscle, and an antispasmodic to control muscle spasms. Diverticulitis that doesn't respond to medical treatment requires colonic resection to remove the involved segment. Perforation, peritonitis, obstruction, or a fistula that accompanies diverticulitis may require a temporary colostomy to drain abscesses and rest the colon, followed by anastomosis.

SPECIAL CONSIDERATIONS

● The patient should take bulk-forming cathartics (if prescribed) with plenty of water.

 TEACHING TIP: Explain that the recommended high-fiber diet may cause temporary flatulence and discomfort.

Dysmenorrhea

The most common gynecologic complaint, dysmenorrhea — painful menstruation — is a leading cause of absenteeism from school and work. Dysmenorrhea can be a primary disorder or occur secondary to an underlying disease.

Because dysmenorrhea almost always follows an ovulatory cycle, both the primary and secondary forms are rare during the anovulatory cycles of menses. After age 20, dysmenorrhea is generally secondary.

CAUSES

Although primary dysmenorrhea is unrelated to any identifiable cause, possible contributing factors include hormonal imbalances and psychogenic factors. The pain of dysmenorrhea probably results from increased prostaglandin secretion.

Treatments for dysmenorrhea

In *primary dysmenorrhea,* administration of sex steroids is an alternative to treatment with antiprostaglandins or analgesics. In such therapy, oral contraceptives relieve pain by suppressing ovulation. Because persistently severe dysmenorrhea may have a psychogenic cause, psychological evaluation and appropriate counseling may be helpful.

Secondary dysmenorrhea may necessitate surgery to correct an underlying disorder, such as endometriosis or uterine leiomyoma. However, surgical treatment is used only if conservative therapy fails.

Dysmenorrhea may also arise secondary to such gynecologic disorders as endometriosis, cervical stenosis, uterine leiomyomas, uterine malposition, pelvic inflammatory disease, pelvic tumors, or adenomyosis.

SIGNS AND SYMPTOMS

Dysmenorrhea produces sharp, intermittent, cramping lower abdominal pain, which usually radiates to the back, thighs, groin, and vulva. Such pain starts with or immediately before menstrual flow and peaks within 24 hours.

Dysmenorrhea also may be associated with signs and symptoms of premenstrual syndrome (urinary frequency, nausea, vomiting, diarrhea, headache, chills, abdominal bloating, painful breasts, depression, irritability).

DIAGNOSTIC TESTS

Pelvic examination and a detailed patient history may suggest the cause of dysmenorrhea. Primary dysmenorrhea is diagnosed when secondary causes are ruled out. Appropriate tests (laparoscopy, dilation and curettage, X-rays) are used to diagnose underlying disorders in secondary dysmenorrhea.

TREATMENT
Initial treatment aims to relieve pain. Pain-relief measures may include analgesics, narcotics (rarely used), prostaglandin inhibitors, and heat applied to the lower abdomen (not recommended in young adolescents). Other treatment depends on whether the condition is primary or secondary. (See *Treatments for dysmenorrhea*.)

SPECIAL CONSIDERATIONS

 TEACHING TIP: Instruct the patient to keep a diary of menstrual symptoms; this may provide valuable information that aids diagnosis and treatment.

Ear canal tumors, benign

Benign tumors may develop anywhere in the ear canal. Common types include keloids, osteomas, and sebaceous cysts. These tumors rarely become malignant. With proper treatment, the prognosis is excellent.

CAUSES

Keloids may result from surgery or trauma, such as ear piercing. Osteomas have no known cause; however, a predisposing factor is swimming in cold water. Sebaceous cysts result from obstruction of a sebaceous gland.

SIGNS AND SYMPTOMS

A benign ear tumor is usually asymptomatic. If it becomes infected, the patient may experience pain, fever, or inflammation. (Pain is often a symptom of cancer.) If the tumor grows large enough to obstruct the ear canal by itself or through accumulated cerumen and debris, it may cause hearing loss and a sensation of pressure.

DIAGNOSTIC TESTS

Clinical features and the patient history suggest a benign tumor of the ear canal; otoscopy confirms it. A biopsy rules out cancer.

TREATMENT

Generally, a benign tumor requires surgical excision if it obstructs the ear canal, is cosmetically undesirable, or becomes malignant.

Treatment of keloids may include surgery followed by repeated injections of long-acting steroids into the suture line. Excision must be complete, but even this may not prevent recurrence.

Surgical excision of an osteoma consists of elevating the skin from the surface of the bony growth and shaving the osteoma with a mechanical burr or drill.

Before surgery, a sebaceous cyst requires preliminary treatment with antibiotics to reduce inflammation. To prevent recurrence, excision must be complete, including the sac or capsule of the cyst.

SPECIAL CONSIDERATIONS

● Good aural hygiene is vital after surgery. Until the ear completely heals, the patient should not insert anything into the ear or allow water to enter the ear. Covering the ears with a cap when showering can prevent problems.

Eardrum perforation

Perforation of the eardrum is a rupture of the tympanic membrane. Such injury may lead to otitis media and hearing loss.

CAUSES

The usual cause of perforated eardrum is trauma — deliberate or accidental insertion of sharp objects (cotton swabs, bobby pins) or sudden excessive changes in pressure (as from an explosion, a blow to the head, flying, or diving). The injury may also result from untreated otitis media and, in children, from acute otitis media.

SIGNS AND SYMPTOMS

Sudden onset of severe earache and bleeding from the ear are the first sign and symptom of a perforated eardrum. Other clinical features include hearing loss, tinnitus, and vertigo. Purulent otorrhea within 48 hours of injury signals infection.

DIAGNOSTIC TESTS

Severe earache and bleeding from the

ear in a patient with a history of traumatic injury strongly suggest a perforated eardrum. Direct visualization of the perforated tympanic membrane with an otoscope confirms it.

TREATMENT

If the ear is bleeding, a sterile, cotton-tipped applicator is used to absorb the blood, and the patient is checked for purulent drainage or evidence of cerebrospinal fluid leakage. A specimen culture may be ordered. A sterile dressing is applied over the outer ear, and the patient is referred to an ear specialist.

A large perforation with uncontrolled bleeding may require immediate surgery to approximate the ruptured edges. Treatment may include a mild analgesic, a sedative to decrease anxiety, and an oral antibiotic.

SPECIAL CONSIDERATIONS

• *Irrigation of the ear is absolutely contraindicated.*

 PREVENTION: Instruct the patient not to blow his nose or get water in his ear canal until the perforation heals.

• Stay alert for signs of child abuse and report it if it's suspected.

Ebola virus infection

One of the most frightening viruses to come out of the African subcontinent, the Ebola virus first appeared in 1976. More than 400 people in Zaire and neighboring Sudan were killed by the hemorrhagic fever that the virus caused. Since then, *Ebola* virus has been responsible for several outbreaks.

Ebola is morphologically similar to the Marburg virus. Both viruses cause headache, malaise, myalgia, and high fever, progressing to severe diarrhea, vomiting, and internal and external hemorrhage.

As the infection progresses, severe complications, including liver and kidney dysfunction, dehydration, and hemorrhage, may develop. In pregnant women, Ebola virus leads to abortion and massive hemorrhage.

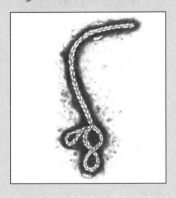

Ebola Zaire

This illustration shows Ebola Zaire, one of three strains of the Ebola virus that cause hemorrhagic illness in humans.

The prognosis for Ebola virus infection is extremely poor, with a mortality as high as 90%. Death usually results during the second week of illness from organ failure or hemorrhage.

Four strains of the Ebola virus are know to exist: Ebola Zaire, Ebola Sudan, Ebola Tai, and Ebola Reston. (See *Ebola Zaire.*) Ebola Reston causes illness only in monkeys, not in humans as do the other three.

CAUSES

Ebola virus infection is caused by an unclassified ribonucleic acid virus that passes from person to person by direct contact with infected blood, body secretions, or organs. Nosocomial and community-acquired transmission can occur. Contaminated needles can also cause the infection. Transmission through semen may occur up to 7 weeks after clinical recovery. The virus remains contagious even after the patient has died.

SIGNS AND SYMPTOMS

The patient usually complains of flu-like signs and symptoms (headache,

Preventing the spread of Ebola virus

When caring for a patient in the early stages of Ebola virus infection, practicing universal precautions generally prevents its transmission. As the disease progresses, though, the patient develops diarrhea and begins vomiting and hemorrhaging, greatly increasing the risk that the disease will spread through contact with infected blood and body fluids.

The Centers for Disease Control and Prevention recommends the following guidelines to help prevent the spread of this deadly disease:
- Keep the patient in isolation throughout the course of the disease.
- If possible, place the patient in a negative-pressure room at the beginning of hospitalization to avoid the need for transfer as the disease progresses.
- Restrict nonessential staff members from entering the patient's room.

- Make sure anyone who enters the patient's room wears gloves and a gown to prevent contact with any surface in the room that may have been soiled.
- Use barrier precautions to prevent skin or mucous membrane exposure to blood or other body fluids, secretions, or excretions when caring for the patient.
- If you must come within 3' (1 m) of the patient, also wear a face shield or surgical mask and goggles or eyeglasses with side shields.
- *Don't* reuse gloves or gowns unless they have been completely disinfected.

Postdeath measures

Any patient who dies of the disease should be promptly buried or cremated. Continue to use precautions to prevent contact with the patient's body fluids and secretions even after the patient's death.

---

malaise, myalgia, fever, cough, and sore throat), which first appear within 3 days of infection. As the virus spreads through the body, inspection reveals bruising as capillaries rupture and dead blood cells infiltrate the skin. A maculopapular eruption appears after the fifth day of infection. The patient may also display melena, hematemesis, epistaxis, and bleeding gums. In the final disease stages, the skin blisters and sloughs off, blood seeps from all orifices, and the patient begins vomiting his liquefied internal organs.

DIAGNOSTIC TESTS
The patient's history usually reveals contact with an infected person. Specialized laboratory tests reveal specific antigens or antibodies and may show the isolated virus. Tests also demonstrate neutrophil leukocytosis, hypofibrinogenemia, thrombocy-

topenia, and microangiopathic hemolytic anemia.

TREATMENT
No cure exists for Ebola virus infection; treatment consists mainly of intensive supportive care. I.V. fluids help offset the effects of severe dehydration. Before the onset of clinical shock, the patient may receive replacement of plasma. He may also receive heparin to prevent disseminated intravascular coagulation. Administration of plasma that contains Ebola virus-specific antibodies is experimental.

SPECIAL CONSIDERATIONS
- Throughout treatment, the patient should remain in isolation.
- Take appropriate precautions when caring for a patient who may have Ebola virus infection. (See *Preventing the spread of Ebola virus.*)

Encephalitis

A severe inflammation of the brain, encephalitis is characterized by intense lymphocytic infiltration of brain tissues and the leptomeninges. Such infiltration causes cerebral edema, degeneration of the brain's ganglion cells, and diffuse nerve cell destruction.

Encephalitis is usually caused by a mosquito-borne or, in some areas, a tick-borne virus. However, transmission by means other than arthropod bites may occur through ingestion of infected goat's milk and accidental injection or inhalation of the virus.

CAUSES

Encephalitis generally results from infection with arboviruses specific to rural areas. However, in urban areas, it's most commonly caused by enteroviruses (coxsackievirus, poliovirus, and echovirus). Other causes include herpesvirus, mumps virus, human immunodeficiency virus, adenoviruses, and demyelinating diseases following measles, varicella, rubella, or vaccination.

SIGNS AND SYMPTOMS

Usually, the acute illness begins with sudden onset of fever, headache, and vomiting and progresses to include signs and symptoms of meningeal irritation (stiff neck and back) and neuronal damage (drowsiness, coma, paralysis, convulsions, ataxia, organic psychoses). After the acute phase, coma may persist for days or weeks.

The severity of arbovirus encephalitis may range from subclinical to rapidly fatal necrotizing disease. Herpes encephalitis also produces signs and symptoms that vary from subclinical to acute and often fatal disease. Associated effects include disturbances of taste or smell.

DIAGNOSTIC TESTS

During an encephalitis epidemic, diagnosis hinges on the patient's health history and clinical findings. Sporadic cases make it difficult to distinguish encephalitis from other illnesses that produce fever. When possible, identification of the virus in cerebrospinal fluid (CSF) or blood confirms this diagnosis.

In all forms of encephalitis, CSF pressure is elevated, and the fluid is often clear. White blood cell and protein levels in CSF are slightly elevated. Electroencephalography reveals abnormalities.

TREATMENT

The antiviral agent acyclovir is effective only against herpes encephalitis. Treatment of all other forms of encephalitis is entirely supportive.

Drug therapy includes an anticonvulsant, glucocorticoids to reduce cerebral inflammation and edema, furosemide or mannitol to reduce cerebral swelling, sedatives for restlessness, and aspirin or acetaminophen to relieve headache and reduce fever. Fluids and electrolytes are given to prevent dehydration, and antibiotics are used for an associated infection such as pneumonia. Isolation is unnecessary.

SPECIAL CONSIDERATIONS

• Fluid overload must be avoided because it may increase cerebral edema.
• The patient must be positioned carefully to prevent joint stiffness and neck pain, and should be turned often. Range-of-motion exercises can help prevent contractures.
• Darkening the room may ease photophobia and headache.
• Reassure the patient and his family that behavior changes caused by encephalitis usually disappear.

Endocarditis

Also called infective endocarditis or bacterial endocarditis, endocarditis is an infection of the endocardium, heart valves, or a cardiac prosthesis, resulting from bacterial or fungal invasion. This invasion produces vegetative growths on the heart valves, endocardial lining of a heart chamber, or the endothelium of a blood vessel that may embolize to the spleen, kidneys, central nervous system, and lungs. (See *Infecting organisms in endocarditis*.)

In endocarditis, fibrin and platelets aggregate on the valve tissue and engulf circulating bacteria or fungi that flourish and produce friable verrucous vegetations. Such vegetations may cover the valve surfaces, causing ulceration and necrosis; they may also extend to the chordae tendineae, leading to their rupture and subsequent valvular insufficiency.

Untreated endocarditis is usually fatal, but with proper treatment, about 70% of patients recover.

CAUSES

Most cases of endocarditis occur in I.V. drug abusers, patients with prosthetic heart valves, and those with mitral valve prolapse. These conditions have surpassed rheumatic heart disease as the leading risk factors.

SIGNS AND SYMPTOMS

Early clinical features may include malaise, weakness, fatigue, weight loss, anorexia, arthralgia, night sweats, chills, valvular insufficiency and, in 90% of patients, an intermittent fever that may recur for weeks. A more acute onset is associated with highly pathogenic organisms such as *Staphylococcus aureus*.

Endocarditis often causes a loud, regurgitant murmur typical of the underlying heart lesion. A sudden change in a murmur or discovery of a new murmur in the presence of fever is a classic sign of endocarditis.

In about 30% of patients, embolization from vegetating lesions or diseased valvular tissue may produce typical features of splenic, renal, cerebral, or pulmonary infarction or of peripheral vascular occlusion.

Other signs may include splenomegaly; petechiae of the skin and the buccal, pharyngeal, or conjunctival mucosa; and splinter hemorrhages under the nails.

DIAGNOSTIC TESTS

Three or more blood cultures in a

Infecting organisms in endocarditis

In patients with native valve endocarditis who aren't I.V. drug abusers, causative organisms usually include streptococci, staphylococci, or enterococci. Although many other bacteria occasionally cause the disorder, fungal causes are rare in this group. The mitral valve is involved most commonly, followed by the aortic valve.

In endocarditis patients who are I.V. drug abusers, *Staphylococcus aureus* is the most common infecting organism. Less commonly, streptococci, enterococci, gram-negative bacilli, or fungi cause the disorder. In most cases, the tricuspid valve is involved, followed by the aortic and then the mitral valve.

In patients with prosthetic valve endocarditis, "early" cases (those that develop within 60 days of valve insertion) are usually due to staphylococcal infection. However, gram-negative aerobic organisms, fungi, streptococci, enterococci, or diphtheroids may also cause the disorder. The course is often severe and is associated with a high mortality rate. "Late" cases (occurring after 60 days) present similarly to native valve endocarditis.

24- to 48-hour period identify the causative organism in up to 90% of patients. The remaining 10% may have negative blood cultures, possibly suggesting fungal infection or infections that are hard to diagnose.

Echocardiography may identify valvular damage; an electrocardiogram may show atrial fibrillation and other irregular heart rhythms that accompany valvular disease.

TREATMENT

Therapy aims to eradicate the infecting organism. Antimicrobial therapy should start promptly and continue over 4 to 6 weeks. Supportive treatment includes bed rest, aspirin for fever and aches, and sufficient fluid intake. Severe valvular damage may require corrective surgery.

SPECIAL CONSIDERATIONS

 ACTION STAT: Embolization is common during the first 3 months of treatment. Notify the doctor immediately if the patient experiences such signs and symptoms as hematuria, pleuritic chest pain, left upper quadrant pain, and paresis.

• Susceptible patients may need prophylactic antibiotics before, during, and after dental work, childbirth, and genitourinary, GI, or gynecologic procedures.

Endometriosis

Endometriosis refers to the presence of endometrial tissue outside the lining of the uterine cavity. Such ectopic tissue is generally confined to the pelvic area, but it can appear anywhere in the body.

Ectopic endometrial tissue responds to normal stimulation in the same way that the endometrium does. During menstruation, ectopic tissue bleeds, causing inflammation of surrounding tissues. This inflammation results in fibrosis, leading to adhesions that produce pain and infertility.

Active endometriosis usually occurs between ages 30 and 40, especially in women who postpone childbearing. Severe symptoms of endometriosis may have an abrupt onset or may develop over many years. Infertility is the primary complication of endometriosis.

CAUSES

The mechanisms by which endometriosis causes symptoms are unknown. The main theories to explain this disorder are:

• transtubal regurgitation of endometrial cells and implantation at ectopic sites

• coelomic metaplasia (repeated inflammation may induce metaplasia of mesothelial cells to the endometrial epithelium)

• lymphatic or hematogenous spread (to explain extraperitoneal disease).

SIGNS AND SYMPTOMS

The classic symptom is acquired dysmenorrhea, which may produce constant pain in the lower abdomen, vagina, posterior pelvis, and back. This pain usually begins 5 to 7 days before menses reaches its peak and lasts 2 to 3 days. It differs from primary dysmenorrheal pain, which is more cramplike and concentrated in the abdominal midline. Other clinical features depend on the location of the ectopic tissue.

DIAGNOSTIC TESTS

Palpation during a pelvic examination may detect multiple tender nodules on uterosacral ligaments or between the rectum and vagina. These nodules enlarge and become more tender during menses.

Palpation may also uncover ovarian enlargement in the presence of endometrial cysts on the ovaries or thickened, nodular adnexa. Laparoscopy must confirm the diagnosis and determine the disease stage before treatment begins.

TREATMENT

Therapy varies with the disease stage and the patient's age and desire to have children. Conservative therapy for young women who want to have children includes androgens such as danazol. Progestins and oral contraceptives also relieve symptoms. Gonadotropin-releasing hormone agonists have induced disease remission.

When ovarian masses are present, surgery must rule out cancer. The treatment of choice for women who don't want to bear children and for those with extensive disease is a total abdominal hysterectomy with bilateral salpingo-oophorectomy.

SPECIAL CONSIDERATIONS

• Because infertility is a possible complication, the patient should be advised not to postpone childbearing.

 PREVENTION: To help prevent retrograde flow in a patient with a narrow vagina or small introitus, instruct her to use sanitary napkins instead of tampons.

Enterobiasis

Also called pinworm, seatworm, or threadworm infection, enterobiasis is a benign intestinal disease caused by the nematode *Enterobius vermicularis.* Found worldwide, it's common even in temperate regions with good sanitation. It's the most prevalent helminthic infection in the United States.

CAUSES

Adult pinworms live in the intestine; female worms migrate to the perianal region to deposit their ova. Direct transmission occurs when the patient's hands transfer infective eggs from the anus to the mouth. Indirect transmission occurs through contact with contaminated articles, such as linens and clothing.

Enterobiasis infection and reinfection are most common in children between ages 5 and 14 and in certain institutionalized groups because of poor hygiene and frequent hand-to-mouth activity. Crowded living conditions often lead to its spread to other family members. (See *Preventing enterobiasis.*)

SIGNS AND SYMPTOMS

Asymptomatic enterobiasis is often overlooked. However, intense perianal pruritus may occur, especially at night. Pruritus disturbs sleep and causes irritability, scratching, skin irritation and, sometimes, vaginitis.

DIAGNOSTIC TESTS

A history of anal itching suggests pinworm; microscopic identification of *Enterobius* eggs recovered from the perianal area with a cellophane tape swab confirms it. A stool sample is

---

Preventing enterobiasis

To help prevent enterobiasis, parents should bathe children daily (showers are preferable to tub baths) and change underwear and bed linens daily.

Children should be instructed in proper personal hygiene, with emphasis on hand washing after defecation and before handling food. Nail biting should be discouraged; if the child can't stop, he should wear gloves until the infection clears.

---

generally egg- and worm-free because these worms deposit their eggs outside the intestine and die after migrating to the anus.

TREATMENT

Drug therapy with pyrantel, piperazine, or mebendazole destroys these parasites. Effective eradication requires simultaneous treatment of family members and, in institutions, other patients.

SPECIAL CONSIDERATIONS

• Patients should be informed that pyrantel colors stools and vomitus bright red.
• *All* outbreaks of enterobiasis should be reported to school authorities.

Epididymitis

This infection of the epididymis, the testicle's cordlike excretory duct, is one of the most common infections of the male reproductive tract. Usually affecting adults, it's rare before puberty. Epididymitis may spread to the testicle itself, causing orchitis; bilateral epididymitis may cause sterility.

CAUSES

Epididymitis usually results from pyogenic organisms, such as staphylococci, *Escherichia coli,* and streptococci. Generally, such organisms result from established urinary tract infection or prostatitis and reach the epididymis through the lumen of the vas deferens.

Other causes include trauma, gonorrhea, syphilis, or a chlamydial infection. Trauma may reactivate a dormant infection or initiate a new one. Epididymitis can be a complication of prostatectomy; it may also result from chemical irritation by extravasation of urine through the vas deferens.

SIGNS AND SYMPTOMS
The key signs and symptoms are pain, extreme tenderness, and swelling in the groin and scrotum. Other clinical effects include high fever, malaise, and a characteristic waddle — an attempt to protect the groin and scrotum during walking. An acute hydrocele may result from inflammation.

DIAGNOSTIC TESTS
A tentative diagnosis can be made based on the patient's history, physical findings, and description of signs and symptoms. Tests that confirm the diagnosis include a white blood cell count, urinalysis, urine culture and sensitivity tests, urethral discharge and prostatic secretion cultures and, possibly, segmented bacteriologic localization cultures. Scrotal ultrasonography may help differentiate acute epididymitis from other conditions.

TREATMENT
The goal of treatment is to reduce pain and swelling and combat infection. Therapy must begin immediately, particularly in the patient with bilateral epididymitis, because sterility is always a threat.

During the acute phase, treatment consists of bed rest, scrotal elevation with towel rolls or adhesive strapping, broad-spectrum antibiotics, and analgesics. Ice application may reduce swelling and relieve pain. (Heat is contraindicated because it may damage germinal cells.) When pain

and swelling subside to allow walking, an athletic supporter may prevent pain. The use of corticosteroids to help combat inflammation is controversial.

In the older patient undergoing open prostatectomy, bilateral vasectomy may be necessary to prevent epididymitis as a postoperative complication; however, antibiotic therapy alone may prevent it. When epididymitis is refractory to antibiotic therapy, epididymectomy under local anesthetic is necessary.

SPECIAL CONSIDERATIONS
 TEACHING TIP: Instruct the patient to complete prescribed antibiotic therapy even after signs and symptoms subside.

Epiglottitis
Acute epiglottitis is an inflammation of the epiglottis that tends to cause airway obstruction. It typically strikes children between ages 2 and 8. A critical emergency, epiglottitis can prove fatal in 8% to 12% of victims unless it's recognized and treated promptly.

CAUSES
Epiglottitis usually results from infection with the bacterium *Haemophilus influenzae* type B. Occasionally, it results from pneumococci and group A streptococci.

SIGNS AND SYMPTOMS
Sometimes preceded by an upper respiratory infection, epiglottitis may rapidly progress to complete upper airway obstruction within 2 to 5 hours. Laryngeal obstruction results from inflammation and edema of the epiglottis. Accompanying signs and symptoms include high fever, stridor, sore throat, dysphagia, irritability, restlessness, and drooling.

To relieve severe respiratory distress, the child with epiglottitis may hyperextend his neck, sit up, and lean forward with his mouth open, tongue protruding, and nostrils flaring as he tries to breathe. He may develop inspiratory retractions and rhonchi.

DIAGNOSTIC TESTS

In acute epiglottitis, throat examination reveals a large, edematous, bright red epiglottis. Such examination should follow lateral neck X-rays and, generally, should *not* be performed if the suspected obstruction is large.

During throat examination, a laryngoscope and endotracheal (ET) tubes should be available because a tongue depressor can cause sudden complete airway obstruction. Trained personnel, such as an anesthesiologist, should be on hand to secure an emergency airway.

TREATMENT

A child with acute epiglottitis and airway obstruction requires emergency hospitalization; he may need emergency ET intubation or a tracheotomy and should be monitored in an intensive care unit. Respiratory distress that interferes with swallowing necessitates parenteral fluid administration.

A patient with acute epiglottitis should receive a 10-day course of parenteral antibiotics — usually a second- or third-generation cephalosporin. Oxygen therapy and arterial blood gas monitoring may be desirable.

SPECIAL CONSIDERATIONS

• Emergency equipment should be kept on hand at all times. (See *Staying prepared for airway obstruction.*)

Epilepsy

Epilepsy, or seizure disorder, is a condition of the brain characterized by susceptibility to recurrent seizures (paroxysmal events associated with abnormal electrical discharges of neurons in the brain). Epilepsy is believed to affect 1% to 2% of the population. The prognosis is good if the patient adheres strictly to prescribed treatment.

Staying prepared for airway obstruction

If a child has epiglottitis, the following equipment should be available in case of sudden complete airway obstruction:
• a tracheotomy tray
• endotracheal tubes
• a handheld resuscitation bag
• oxygen equipment
• a laryngoscope with blades of various sizes.

Increasing restlessness, increasing pulse, fever, dyspnea, and retractions may indicate the need for emergency tracheotomy.

CAUSES

In about half of epilepsy cases, the cause is unknown. However, some possible causes include:
• birth trauma (inadequate oxygen supply to the brain, blood incompatibility, or hemorrhage)
• perinatal infection
• anoxia
• infectious diseases (meningitis, encephalitis, brain abscess)
• head injury or trauma.

SIGNS AND SYMPTOMS

The hallmarks of epilepsy are recurring seizures, which can be classified as partial or generalized. Some patients may be affected by more than one type.

Partial seizures

Arising from a localized area of the brain, partial seizures cause specific symptoms. In some patients, partial seizure activity may spread to the entire brain, causing a generalized seizure. Partial seizures include jacksonian and complex partial seizures (psychomotor or temporal lobe).

Jacksonian seizures begin as localized motor seizures characterized by a spread of abnormal activity to adjacent brain areas. They typically produce a stiffening or jerking in one ex-

First aid for seizures

Generalized tonic-clonic seizures may necessitate first aid. Cover the following points when teaching the patient's family how to give first aid correctly.

During the seizure

• Don't restrain the person. Instead, help him to a lying position, loosen any tight clothing, and place something flat and soft, such as a pillow, jacket, or hand, under his head. Clear the area of hard objects.
• If the person's teeth are clenched, don't force anything into his mouth. This could lacerate his mouth and lips or displace teeth, causing respiratory distress.
• If the person's mouth is open, protect his tongue by placing a soft object (such as a folded cloth) between his teeth.
• Turn his head to provide an open airway.
• If the person has a complex partial seizure, protect him from injury by gently calling his name and directing him away from the source of danger.

After the seizure

Once the seizure subsides, reassure the person that he's all right, orient him to time and place, and inform him that he's had a seizure.

tremity, accompanied by a tingling sensation in the same area. The patient seldom loses consciousness.

Simple partial sensory seizures involve perceptual distortion, which can include hallucinations.

Signs of *complex partial seizures* vary but usually include purposeless behavior. These seizures may begin with an aura, which represents the beginning of abnormal electrical discharges within a focal area of the brain. The aura may include a pungent smell, GI distress (nausea, indigestion), a rising or sinking feeling in the stomach, a dreamy feeling, an unusual taste, or a visual disturbance. Overt signs of complex partial seizures include a glassy stare, picking at one's clothes, aimless wandering, lip-smacking or chewing motions, and unintelligible speech.

Generalized seizures

These seizures are marked by a generalized electrical abnormality within the brain. They include several distinct types.

Absence seizures are most common in children. They usually begin with a brief change in level of consciousness, indicated by blinking or rolling of the eyes. The patient retains his posture and continues preseizure activity. Typically, each seizure lasts from 1 to 10 seconds.

Myoclonic (bilateral massive epileptic myoclonus) seizures are characterized by brief, involuntary muscle movements.

Generalized tonic-clonic seizures typically begin with a loud cry. The patient then falls to the ground, losing consciousness. The body stiffens (tonic phase), then alternates between episodes of muscular spasm and relaxation (clonic phase). Tongue-biting, incontinence, labored breathing, apnea, and cyanosis may occur. The seizure stops in 2 to 5 minutes.

Akinetic seizures are characterized by a general loss of postural tone and a temporary loss of consciousness. They occur in young children and are sometimes called "drop attacks" because they cause the child to fall.

Status epilepticus is a continuous seizure state that can occur in all seizure types. The most life-threatening example is generalized tonic-clonic status epilepticus, a continuous seizure without intervening return of consciousness. Status epilepticus is accompanied by respiratory distress.

DIAGNOSTIC TESTS

The patient's personal and family history, a description of seizure activity, and physical and neurologic findings may suggest epilepsy. Computed tomography scans or magnetic resonance imaging may indicate abnormalities in internal brain structures.

Diagnosis is confirmed when electroencephalography provides evidence of the continuing tendency to have seizures. Other tests may include serum glucose and calcium studies, skull X-rays, lumbar puncture, brain scan, and cerebral angiography.

TREATMENT

Generally, treatment consists of drug therapy specific to the type of seizure. The most commonly prescribed drugs are phenytoin, carbamazepine, phenobarbital, and primidone administered individually for generalized tonic-clonic seizures and complex partial seizures. Valproic acid, clonazepam, and ethosuximide are commonly prescribed for absence seizures. Gabapentin and felbamate are newer anticonvulsant drugs.

If drug therapy fails, treatment may include surgical removal of a demonstrated focal lesion to attempt to stop seizures. Emergency treatment of status epilepticus usually consists of diazepam, phenytoin, and phenobarbital; dextrose 50% I.V.; and thiamine I.V. (in chronic alcoholism or withdrawal).

 TEACHING TIP: Teach family members and other caregivers how to administer first aid in case a seizure occurs. (See *First aid for seizures.*)

Epistaxis (nosebleed)

Epistaxis, or nosebleed, may be a primary disorder or may occur secondary to another condition. Such bleeding in children generally originates in the anterior nasal septum and tends to be mild. In adults, it's most likely to originate in the posterior septum and can be severe.

CAUSES

Epistaxis usually follows trauma from external or internal causes: a blow to the nose, nose picking, or insertion of a foreign body. Less commonly, it follows polyps; acute or chronic infections, such as sinusitis or rhinitis; or inhalation of chemicals that irritate the nasal mucosa.

SIGNS AND SYMPTOMS

Blood oozing from the nostrils usually originates in the anterior nose and is bright red. Blood from the back of the throat originates in the posterior area and may be dark or bright red.

In severe epistaxis, blood may seep behind the nasal septum; it may also appear in the middle ear and in the corners of the eyes.

Associated effects depend on the severity of bleeding. Moderate blood loss may produce light-headedness, dizziness, and slight respiratory difficulty. Severe hemorrhage causes hypotension, rapid and bounding pulse, dyspnea, and pallor. Bleeding is considered severe if it persists longer than 10 minutes after pressure is applied.

DIAGNOSTIC TESTS

Although simple observation confirms epistaxis, inspection with a bright light and nasal speculum is necessary to locate the bleeding site. Blood tests used to evaluate a patient with epistaxis include hemoglobin and hematocrit, platelet count, prothrombin time, and partial thromboplastin time. Diagnosis must rule out underlying systemic causes of epistaxis.

TREATMENT

For anterior bleeding, a cotton ball saturated with epinephrine is held at the bleeding site and external pressure is applied. This is followed by cauterization with electrocautery or silver nitrate stick. If these measures don't control bleeding, petrolatum gauze nasal packing may be needed.

For posterior bleeding, treatment includes gauze packing inserted through the nose or postnasal pack-

E. coli incidence

The incidence of *Escherichia coli* infection is highest among travelers returning from other countries, particularly Mexico, Southeast Asia, and South America. *E. coli* infection also induces other diseases, especially in people whose resistance is low.

A new strain, *E. coli* 0157:H7, has been reported. It's associated with undercooked hamburger.

Escherichia coli and other Enterobacteriaceae infections

Enterobacteriaceae — a group of mostly aerobic, gram-negative bacilli — cause local and systemic infections, including an invasive diarrhea resembling shigella and, more often, a noninvasive, toxin-mediated diarrhea resembling cholera.

Escherichia coli and other Enterobacteriaceae cause most nosocomial infections. Noninvasive, enterotoxin-producing *E. coli* infections may be a major cause of diarrheal illness in children in the United States. (See E. coli *incidence*.)

CAUSES
Although some strains of *E. coli* exist as part of the normal GI flora, infection usually results from certain non-indigenous strains. For example, non-invasive diarrhea results from two toxins produced by strains called enterotoxic or enteropathogenic *E. coli*. These toxins interact with intestinal juices and promote excessive loss of chloride and water.

In the invasive form, *E. coli* directly invades the intestinal mucosa without producing enterotoxins, thereby causing local irritation, inflammation, and diarrhea. Normal strains can cause infection in immunocompromised patients.

Transmission can occur directly from an infected person or indirectly by ingestion of contaminated food or water or contact with contaminated utensils. Incubation takes 12 to 72 hours.

SIGNS AND SYMPTOMS
Noninvasive diarrhea may cause abrupt onset of watery diarrhea with cramping abdominal pain and, in severe illness, acidosis. Invasive infection produces chills, abdominal cramps, and diarrheal stools containing blood and pus.

Infantile diarrhea from an *E. coli* infection is usually noninvasive; it be-

ing inserted through the mouth, depending on the bleeding site. The nasal balloon catheter also controls bleeding effectively.

Other measures
Antibiotics may be appropriate if packing must remain in place longer than 24 hours. If local measures fail to control bleeding, additional treatment may include supplemental vitamin K and, for severe bleeding, blood transfusions and surgical ligation or embolization of a bleeding artery.

SPECIAL CONSIDERATIONS
● To control epistaxis, the patient should remain seated in an upright position while the soft portion of the nostril is compressed against the septum continuously for 5 to 10 minutes. Then an ice collar or cold, wet compresses are applied to the nose. Bleeding should stop after 10 minutes.

 PREVENTION: Instruct the patient to avoid picking the nose or inserting foreign objects in it, and to avoid bending or lifting. Also mention that sneezing with the mouth open can reduce the risk of epistaxis.

gins with loose, watery stools that change from yellow to green and contain little mucus or blood. Vomiting, listlessness, irritability, and anorexia often precede diarrhea. This condition can progress to fever, severe dehydration, acidosis, and shock.

DIAGNOSTIC TESTS
A working diagnosis of *E. coli* infection depends on clinical observation alone. A firm diagnosis requires sophisticated procedures such as bioassays that are expensive and time-consuming. Diagnosis must rule out salmonellosis and shigellosis, common infections that produce similar signs and symptoms.

TREATMENT
Effective treatment consists of isolation, correction of fluid and electrolyte imbalance and, in an infant, I.V. antibiotics. For cramping and diarrhea, bismuth subsalicylate may be given.

SPECIAL CONSIDERATIONS
 PREVENTION: To help prevent spread of this infection, all hospital personnel and visitors should be screened for diarrhea and avoid direct patient contact during epidemics. Other preventive measures include proper hand washing technique and enteric precautions (private room, gown and gloves while handling feces, hand washing before entering and after leaving the patient's room).
• *E. coli* cases should be reported to local public health authorities.

Esophageal cancer
Nearly always fatal, esophageal cancer usually develops in men over age 60. The disease occurs worldwide, but incidence varies geographically. It's most common in Japan, China, the Middle East, and parts of South Africa.

CAUSES
The cause of esophageal cancer is unknown, but predisposing factors include chronic irritation caused by heavy smoking and excessive use of alcohol, stasis-induced inflammation, and nutritional deficiency. Most esophageal tumors arise in squamous cell epithelium; a few are adenocarcinomas; fewer still are melanomas and sarcomas.

SIGNS AND SYMPTOMS
Dysphagia and weight loss are the most common presenting signs and symptoms. Dysphagia is mild and intermittent at first but soon becomes constant. Pain, hoarseness, coughing, and esophageal obstruction follow. Cachexia usually develops.

DIAGNOSTIC TESTS
Esophageal X-rays, with barium swallow and motility studies, reveal structural and filling defects and reduced peristalsis. Endoscopic examination of the esophagus, biopsies, and cytologic tests confirm esophageal tumors.

TREATMENT
Whenever possible, treatment includes resection to maintain a passageway for food. This may require such radical surgery as esophagogastrectomy with jejunal or colonic bypass grafts. Palliative surgery may include a feeding gastrostomy. Other therapies may include radiation, chemotherapy, or insertion of prosthetic tubes to bridge the tumor and relieve dysphagia.

SPECIAL CONSIDERATIONS
• Offering the patient something to chew before each feeding promotes gastric secretions and provides a semblance of normal eating.
• The patient's family or other caregivers may need instruction in gastrostomy tube care.

Esophageal diverticula
Hollow outpouchings of one or more layers of the esophageal wall, esophageal diverticula occur in three main areas: just above the upper

esophageal sphincter (Zenker's diverticulum, the most common type), near the midpoint of the esophagus (traction), and just above the lower esophageal sphincter (epiphrenic).

CAUSES

Esophageal diverticula result from primary muscular abnormalities that may be congenital or from inflammatory processes adjacent to the esophagus.

When the pouch results from increased intraesophageal pressure, *Zenker's diverticulum* occurs. It's caused by developmental muscular weakness of the posterior pharynx above the border of the cricopharyngeal muscle.

When the pouch is pulled out by adjacent inflamed tissue or lymph nodes, a *midesophageal (traction) diverticulum* occurs. This is a response to scarring and pulling on esophageal walls by an external inflammatory process such as tuberculosis.

A rare condition, *epiphrenic diverticulum* usually accompanies an esophageal motor disturbance such as esophageal spasm. It's thought to result from traction and pulsation.

SIGNS AND SYMPTOMS

Midesophageal and epiphrenic diverticula with an associated motor disturbance (achalasia or spasm) seldom produce signs or symptoms. Zenker's diverticulum produces distinctly staged signs and symptoms: initially, throat irritation and, later, dysphagia and near-complete obstruction.

In early stages, regurgitation occurs soon after eating; in later stages, regurgitation is delayed and may even occur during sleep. Other signs and symptoms include noise when liquids are swallowed, chronic cough, hoarseness, and a bad taste in the mouth or foul breath.

DIAGNOSTIC TESTS

X-rays taken after a barium swallow usually confirm the diagnosis. Esophagoscopy can rule out other lesions;

however, the procedure risks rupturing the diverticulum.

TREATMENT

Zenker's diverticulum usually calls for palliative treatment, such as a bland diet, thorough chewing, and drinking water after eating to flush out the sac. Severe symptoms or a large diverticulum necessitate surgery to remove the sac or promote drainage. An esophagomyotomy may be needed to prevent recurrence.

A midesophageal diverticulum seldom requires therapy except when esophagitis aggravates the risk of rupture. In that case, treatment includes antacids and an antireflux regimen: keeping the head elevated, staying upright for 2 hours after eating, eating small meals, controlling chronic coughing, and avoiding constrictive clothing.

Epiphrenic diverticulum requires treatment of accompanying motor disorders by repeated dilatations of the esophagus, of acute spasm by anticholinergic administration and diverticulum excision, and of dysphagia or severe pain by surgical excision or suspending the diverticulum to promote drainage.

SPECIAL CONSIDERATIONS

• If the patient regurgitates food and mucus, he should be positioned carefully with his head elevated or turned to one side to prevent aspiration. Also, he should empty any visible outpouching in the neck by massage or postural drainage before retiring.

Esophagitis, corrosive

Inflammation and damage to the esophagus after ingestion of a caustic chemical is called corrosive esophagitis. This injury may be temporary or may lead to permanent stricture (narrowing or stenosis) of the esophagus that's correctable only through surgery.

Severe injury can quickly lead to esophageal perforation, mediastinitis,

Helping patients with corrosive esophagitis

Because the adult who has ingested a corrosive agent has usually done so with suicidal intent, encourage and assist him and his family to seek psychological counseling.

If a child has ingested a chemical, provide emotional support for the parents. They'll be distraught and may feel guilty about the accident. After the emergency and without emphasizing blame, discuss appropriate preventive measures, such as locking accessible cabinets and keeping all corrosive agents out of a child's reach.

and death from infection, shock, and massive hemorrhage.

CAUSES
The most common chemical injury to the esophagus follows ingestion of lye or other strong alkalies and, less often, ingestion of strong acids. The type and amount of chemical ingested determines the severity and location of damage.

In children, household chemical ingestion is accidental; in adults, it's usually deliberate. (See *Helping patients with corrosive esophagitis.*)

SIGNS AND SYMPTOMS
Effects vary from none to intense pain in the mouth and chest, marked salivation, inability to swallow, and tachypnea. Bloody vomitus containing pieces of esophageal tissue signals severe damage. Signs and symptoms of esophageal perforation and mediastinitis indicate destruction of the entire esophagus. Inability to speak suggests laryngeal damage.

The acute phase subsides in 3 to 4 days, enabling the patient to eat again. Signs and symptoms of dysphagia return if stricture develops.

DIAGNOSTIC TESTS
A history of chemical ingestion and physical examination revealing oropharyngeal burns usually confirm the diagnosis. The type and amount of chemical ingested must be identified by such methods as examining empty containers of the ingested material.

To delineate the extent and location of the esophageal injury and assess burn depth, the patient may undergo endoscopy. *Barium swallow* may identify segmental spasm or fistula.

TREATMENT
The usual treatment includes monitoring the patient's condition, administering corticosteroids to control inflammation and inhibit fibrosis, giving a broad-spectrum antibiotic to protect the corticosteroid-immunosuppressed patient against infection by his own mouth flora, and performing endoscopy early.

Bougienage
This procedure involves passing a bougie — a slender, flexible, cylindrical instrument — into the esophagus to dilate it and minimize stricture. Some doctors begin bougienage immediately and continue it regularly; others delay it for a week to avoid the risk of esophageal perforation.

Surgery
Immediate surgery may be necessary for esophageal perforation; it may also be done later to correct stricture untreatable with bougienage.

Supportive treatment
Other treatment includes I.V. therapy to replace fluids or total parenteral nutrition while the patient can't swallow, gradually progressing to clear liquids and a soft diet.

SPECIAL CONSIDERATIONS
• Induced vomiting and gastric lavage *must not be done* in a patient who has ingested a corrosive chemical. These procedures can cause further damage to the GI mucosa.

Exophthalmos

Exophthalmos is the unilateral or bilateral bulging or protrusion of the eyeballs or their apparent forward displacement (with lid retraction).

CAUSES
Exophthalmos commonly results from ophthalmic Graves' disease, in which the eyeballs are displaced forward and the lids retract. Unilateral exophthalmos may also result from trauma (such as fracture of the ethmoid bone). Other conditions that can lead to exophthalmos include hemorrhage, varicosities, thrombosis, and edema — all of which similarly displace one or both eyeballs.

Other systemic and ocular causes of exophthalmos include infection such as orbital cellulitis, tumors and neoplastic diseases, parasitic cysts in surrounding tissue, and pseudoexophthalmos paralysis of extraocular muscles.

SIGNS AND SYMPTOMS
The obvious sign is a bulging eyeball, commonly with diplopia if extraocular muscle edema causes misalignment. A rim of the sclera may be visible around the limbus, and the patient may blink infrequently.

Other signs and symptoms depend on the cause. Pain may accompany traumatic exophthalmos, a tumor may produce conjunctival hyperemia or chemosis, and retraction of the upper lid predisposes the patient to exposure keratitis.

DIAGNOSTIC TESTS
This disorder is usually obvious on physical examination. Exophthalmometer readings showing the degree of eyeball projection and misalignment between the eyes can confirm the diagnosis.

TREATMENT
Effective treatment varies with the cause. Eye trauma may require cold compresses for the first 24 hours, followed by warm compresses, and prophylactic antibiotic therapy. After edema subsides, surgery may be necessary.

Eye infection warrants treatment with broad-spectrum antibiotics during the 24 hours preceding positive identification of the organism, followed by specific antibiotics.

A patient with exophthalmos resulting from an orbital tumor may initially benefit from antibiotic or corticosteroid therapy. Eventually, surgical exploration of the orbit and excision of the tumor, enucleation, or exenteration may be necessary. When primary orbital tumors can't be fully excised as encapsulated lesions, radiation and chemotherapy may be used.

Treatment of Graves' disease may include antithyroid drugs or partial or total thyroidectomy to control hyperthyroidism, initial high doses of systemic corticosteroids for optic neuropathy, and protective lubricants.

Surgery may involve lateral tarsorrhaphy (suturing the lateral sections of the eyelids together) to correct lid retraction or orbital decompression (removal of the superior and lateral orbital walls) if vision is threatened.

SPECIAL CONSIDERATIONS
• The exposed cornea can be protected with lubricants and patching when appropriate.

Fallopian tube cancer

Primary fallopian tube cancer is extremely rare, accounting for fewer than 0.5% of all gynecologic cancers. It usually strikes postmenopausal women in their 50s and 60s. Because this disease is generally well advanced at the time of diagnosis, the prognosis is poor.

CAUSES

The causes of fallopian tube cancer aren't clear, but the disease appears to be linked with nulliparity: Over one-half of the women with this disease have never had children.

SIGNS AND SYMPTOMS

Generally, early-stage fallopian tube cancer produces no symptoms. In late-stage disease, signs and symptoms include an enlarged abdomen with a palpable mass, amber-colored vaginal discharge, and excessive bleeding during menstruation.

Other features are abdominal cramps, frequent urination, persistent constipation, weight loss, and unilateral colicky pain.

Metastasis occurs by local extension or by lymphatic spread to the abdominal organs or to the pelvic, aortic, and inguinal lymph nodes. Metastasis beyond the abdominal area is rare.

DIAGNOSTIC TESTS

Unexplained postmenopausal bleeding and an abnormal Papanicolaou test suggest this diagnosis, but laparotomy is usually necessary to confirm it. When such cancer involves both the ovary and fallopian tube, the primary site is hard to identify.

The preoperative workup includes routine blood studies, an electrocardiogram, ultrasound or plain film of the abdomen to help delineate tumor mass, and excretory urography to assess renal function and to show urinary tract anomalies and ureteral obstruction. A chest X-ray can rule out metastasis.

TREATMENT

Fallopian tube cancer is treated with surgery, chemotherapy, external radiation, or a combination of these. Even when surgery has removed all evidence of disease, all patients should receive some form of adjunctive therapy (radiation or chemotherapy).

SPECIAL CONSIDERATIONS

• Psychological support can greatly reduce the patient's anxiety. If she seems worried about the effect of surgery on her sexual activity, reassure her that this surgery won't inhibit sexual intimacy.
• After surgery, the patient should be turned often and helped to reposition herself, using pillows for support. She should be encouraged to walk within 24 hours.
• Radiation may cause a skin reaction, bladder irritation, bone marrow suppression, and other systemic reactions. During and after treatment, adverse effects of radiation and chemotherapy are treated as required.
• To minimize adverse effects of radiation and chemotherapy, the patient should eat a high-carbohydrate, high-protein, low-fat, low-bulk diet designed to maintain caloric intake but reduce bulk. Several small meals a day instead of three large ones helps ensure adequate nutrition.

 PREVENTION TIP: To help detect fallopian tube and other gynecologic cancers early, stress the importance of a regular pelvic examination for all female patients. Tell them to contact a doctor promptly about any gynecologic symptom.

Reversing fatty liver

Patients with fatty liver may be able to reverse the disease by following appropriate guidelines. Here's what patients should know about self-care.

Eliminating the underlying cause

- Alcoholics should get counseling.
- Diabetics should learn about proper care, including insulin administration, diet, and exercise as well as the need for long-term medical supervision.
- Obese patients should learn about proper diet and exercise. Patients who are more than 20% overweight should be under medical supervision.
- Patients receiving liver-toxic drugs and those who risk occupational exposure to DDT should watch for and immediately report signs of toxicity.

Complying with therapy

Inform patients that fatty liver is reversible only if they strictly follow the therapeutic program. Otherwise, they risk permanent liver damage.

Fatty liver

Fatty liver (steatosis) is a common disorder in which triglycerides and other fats accumulate in liver cells. In severe fatty liver, fat constitutes as much as 40% of the liver's weight (as opposed to 5% in a normal liver) and the liver's weight may increase from 3.3 lb (1.5 kg) to as much as 11 lb (5 kg).

Minimal fatty changes are temporary and asymptomatic; severe or persistent changes may cause liver dysfunction. Fatty liver usually can be reversed simply by eliminating the cause. (See *Reversing fatty liver*.) However, this disorder can result in recurrent infection or sudden death from fat emboli in the lungs.

CAUSES

The most common cause of fatty liver in the United States and Europe is chronic alcoholism, with the severity of hepatic disease directly related to the amount of alcohol consumed.

Other causes include malnutrition (especially protein deficiency), obesity, diabetes mellitus, jejunoileal bypass surgery, Cushing's syndrome, Reye's syndrome, pregnancy, large doses of hepatotoxins (such as I.V. tetracycline), carbon tetrachloride intoxication, prolonged I.V. hyperalimentation, and DDT poisoning.

Whatever the underlying cause, fatty liver probably results from mobilization of fatty acids from adipose tissues or altered fat metabolism.

SIGNS AND SYMPTOMS

Clinical features vary with the degree of fat infiltration. Many patients are asymptomatic.

The most typical sign is a large, tender liver (hepatomegaly). Other common features are right upper quadrant pain (with massive or rapid infiltration), ascites, edema, jaundice, and fever.

Nausea, vomiting, and anorexia occur in fewer cases. Spleen enlargement usually accompanies cirrhosis. Rarer changes are spider angiomas, varices, transient gynecomastia, and menstrual disorders.

DIAGNOSTIC TESTS

Typical clinical features suggest fatty liver — especially in patients who are alcoholic, obese, malnourished, or severely diabetic. A biopsy is used to confirm the disease. Diagnosis is supported by the liver function tests, such as:

- albumin — somewhat low
- globulin — usually elevated
- cholesterol — usually elevated
- total bilirubin — increased
- alkaline phosphatase — elevated
- transaminase — usually low (less than 300 U)
- prothrombin time — possibly prolonged.

TREATMENT

Essentially supportive, treatment consists of correcting the underlying condition or eliminating its cause. For instance, when fatty liver results from I.V. hyperalimentation, decreasing the rate of carbohydrate infusion may correct the disease.

In alcoholic fatty liver, abstinence from alcohol and a proper diet can begin to correct liver changes within 4 to 8 weeks. The patient requires comprehensive teaching.

SPECIAL CONSIDERATIONS

• Because malnutrition is a concern in patients with chronic illness, an adequate diet is important.
• If the patient is obese, weight loss is crucial. All members of the health care team should provide positive reinforcement for losing weight.

Femoral or popliteal aneurysm

These forms of aneurysm occur in the walls of the major peripheral arteries. Aneurysmal formations may be *fusiform* (spindle-shaped) or *saccular* (pouchlike). They may be singular or multiple segmental lesions, commonly affecting both legs, and may accompany other arterial aneurysms located in the abdominal aorta or iliac arteries.

These aneurysms occur most commonly in men over age 50. The clinical course is usually progressive, eventually ending in thrombosis, embolization, and gangrene. Elective surgery before complications arise greatly improves the prognosis.

CAUSES

Femoral and popliteal aneurysms typically result from atherosclerosis. Rarely, they stem from congenital weakness in the arterial wall. Other causes include trauma, bacterial infection, and peripheral vascular reconstructive surgery.

SIGNS AND SYMPTOMS

Popliteal aneurysms may cause pain in the popliteal space if they're large enough to compress the medial popliteal nerve as well as edema and venous distention if the vein is compressed. Femoral and popliteal aneurysms can produce signs and symptoms of severe ischemia in the leg or foot.

Signs and symptoms of acute aneurysmal thrombosis include severe pain, loss of pulse and color, coldness in the affected leg or foot, and gangrene. Distal petechial hemorrhages may arise from aneurysmal emboli.

DIAGNOSTIC TESTS

In femoral aneurysm, the diagnosis is usually confirmed by bilateral palpation of a pulsating mass above or below the inguinal ligament. When thrombosis has occurred, palpation detects a firm, nonpulsating mass.

Arteriography or ultrasonography may be indicated in doubtful situations. Arteriography also may detect associated aneurysms. Ultrasound may help determine the size of the popliteal or femoral artery.

TREATMENT

Femoral and popliteal aneurysms require surgical bypass and reconstruction of the artery, usually with an autogenous saphenous vein graft replacement. Arterial occlusion that causes severe ischemia and gangrene may necessitate leg amputation.

SPECIAL CONSIDERATIONS

• After arterial surgery, the patient is monitored for early signs and symptoms of thrombosis or graft occlusion (loss of pulse, decreased skin temperature and sensation, severe pain) and infection (fever).
• To prevent venostasis and thrombus formation, urge the patient to walk as soon as possible after surgery.

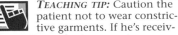 *TEACHING TIP:* Caution the patient not to wear constrictive garments. If he's receiving anticoagulants, suggest measures to prevent bleeding such as using an electric shaver instead of a razor. Also tell him to avoid trauma, tobacco,

and aspirin and to report immediately signs of bleeding: bleeding gums, easy bruising, and black, tarry stools. Emphasize the importance of having follow-up blood studies to monitor anticoagulant therapy. Because the saphenous vein graft replacement can fail or another aneurysm may develop, instruct the patient to immediately report recurrence of symptoms.

Folic acid deficiency anemia

Folic acid deficiency anemia is a common, slowly progressive, megaloblastic anemia. It most commonly strikes infants, adolescents, pregnant and breast-feeding females, alcoholics, the elderly, and patients with malignant or intestinal diseases.

CAUSES
Folic acid deficiency anemia may result from:
• alcohol abuse
• poor diet
• impaired absorption (due to intestinal dysfunction from such disorders as celiac disease, tropical sprue, regional jejunitis, or bowel resection)
• bacteria competing for available folic acid
• overcooking, which can destroy much of the folic acid in foods
• limited storage capacity in infants
• prolonged drug therapy (anticonvulsants, estrogens)
• increased folic acid requirements, such as from pregnancy, rapid growth periods, and neoplastic diseases.

SIGNS AND SYMPTOMS
Folic acid deficiency anemia gradually produces clinical features that resemble those of other megaloblastic anemias, but without the neurologic manifestations: progressive fatigue, shortness of breath, palpitations, weakness, tongue inflammation (glossitis), nausea, anorexia, headache, fainting, irritability, forgetfulness, pallor, and slight jaundice.

DIAGNOSTIC TESTS
Laboratory findings such as an abnormally low serum folate level are the keys to diagnosis. The Schilling test and a therapeutic trial of vitamin B_{12} injections distinguish between folic acid deficiency anemia and pernicious anemia (which is more likely to affect the nervous system).

TREATMENT
Folic acid supplements and elimination of contributing causes are the primary treatments. Supplements may be given orally (usually 1 to 5 mg/day) or parenterally (to patients who are severely ill, have malabsorption, or are unable to take oral medication). Many patients respond favorably to a well-balanced diet.

If the patient has combined B_{12} and folate deficiencies, folic acid replenishment alone may aggravate neurologic dysfunction.

SPECIAL CONSIDERATIONS
 TEACHING TIP: Urge the patient to comply with the prescribed course of therapy and to continue taking supplements even after he begins to feel better.
• Good oral hygiene helps ease tongue inflammation. The patient should use a mild or diluted mouthwash and a soft toothbrush regularly.
• Scheduling regular rest periods until the patient is able to resume normal activity can reduce fatigue caused by anemia. Take the patient's need for rest into account when performing care activities.

 PREVENTION TIP: To help prevent folic acid deficiency anemia, stress the importance of a well-balanced diet high in folic acid. Daily folic acid requirements can be met by including a food from each food group in every meal. Advise mothers who aren't breast-feeding to give their infants commercially prepared formulas.

Gallbladder and bile duct cancers

Cancer of the gallbladder is rare, accounting for fewer than 1% of all cancers. It's usually found coincidentally in patients with cholecystitis (gallbladder inflammation).

Adenocarcinoma accounts for 85% to 95% of all cases of gallbladder cancer; squamous cell, 5% to 15%. Mixed-tissue types are rare.

Gallbladder cancer is rapidly progressive and usually fatal; patients seldom live a year after diagnosis. The disease usually isn't diagnosed until after cholecystectomy, when it's typically in an advanced, metastatic stage.

Extrahepatic bile duct cancer causes approximately 3% of cancer deaths in the United States. It occurs in both males and females between ages 60 and 70. The usual site is the bifurcation in the common duct.

CAUSES

Many clinicians view gallbladder cancer as a complication of gallstones. However, this theory is controversial.

The cause of extrahepatic bile duct cancer isn't known. However, statistics show an unexplained increased incidence in patients with ulcerative colitis. This association may stem from a common cause — perhaps an immune mechanism — or chronic use of certain drugs by the colitis patient.

SIGNS AND SYMPTOMS

Clinically, gallbladder cancer closely resembles cholecystitis: pain in the epigastrium or right upper quadrant, weight loss, anorexia, nausea, vomiting, and jaundice. However, chronic, progressively severe pain in an afebrile patient suggests cancer; in contrast, simple gallstones cause sporadic pain.

Another clue to cancer is a palpable gallbladder with obstructive jaundice.

Some patients also have an enlarged liver and spleen.

Features of bile duct cancer

Progressive profound jaundice is commonly the first sign of obstruction caused by extrahepatic bile duct cancer. Jaundice usually is accompanied by chronic pain in the epigastrium or right upper quadrant, radiating to the back.

DIAGNOSTIC TESTS

No single test can diagnose gallbladder cancer. However, laboratory tests support this diagnosis when they suggest liver dysfunction and extrahepatic biliary obstruction. The following tests are used to confirm gallbladder cancer:
• complete blood count, routine urinalysis, electrolyte studies, enzymes
• liver function tests (which typically reveal elevated serum bilirubin, urine bile and bilirubin, and urobilinogen levels as well as elevated serum alkaline phosphatase levels)
• occult blood in stools
• cholecystography (which may show stones or calcification)
• cholangiography (which may pinpoint the site of common duct obstruction)
• magnetic resonance imaging (which may detect tumors).

To confirm extrahepatic bile duct cancer, the doctor usually orders liver function studies and endoscopic retrograde cannulization of the pancreas. This study identifies the tumor site and allows access for obtaining a biopsy specimen.

TREATMENT

Surgical treatment of gallbladder cancer is essentially palliative. If the cancer invades gallbladder muscles, the survival rate is less than 5%, even with massive resection. Although some cases of long-term survival (4 to 5 years) have been reported, few patients survive longer than 6 months after surgery for gallbladder cancer.

Surgery is usually indicated to relieve the obstruction and jaundice that result from extrahepatic bile duct cancer.

Other palliative measures for both types of cancer include radiation, radiation implants (mostly used for local and incisional recurrences), and chemotherapy. However, all of these treatments have had limited effects.

SPECIAL CONSIDERATIONS
After biliary resection:
• The patient usually is placed in low Fowler's position. Encouraging deep breathing and coughing can help prevent postoperative respiratory problems.
• The high incision makes the patient want to take shallow breaths. Using analgesics and splinting the abdomen with a pillow or an abdominal binder may ease breathing.
• A nasogastric tube and a T tube will be in place for 24 to 72 hours postoperatively to relieve distention. Securing the T tube to minimize tension on it prevents it from being pulled out.

Gastric cancer

Common throughout the world, gastric cancer can affect various parts of the stomach. (See *Sites of gastric cancer.*)

The disease occurs in all races, but with unexplained differences in geographic and cultural incidence. For example, mortality is high in Japan, Iceland, Chile, and Austria. In the United States, incidence has decreased 50% during the past 25 years, and the death rate is one-third that of 30 years ago. This decrease has been attributed, without proof, to the well-balanced American diet and to refrigeration, which reduces nitrate-producing bacteria in food.

Gastric cancer metastasizes rapidly to the regional lymph nodes, omentum, liver, and lungs. Prognosis depends on the disease stage at the time

of diagnosis. Overall, the 5-year survival rate is approximately 15%.

CAUSES
The cause of gastric cancer is unknown. This cancer commonly is associated with gastritis and gastric atrophy. Predisposing factors include smoking and high alcohol intake. Genetic factors also may play a role. Suggested dietary factors include certain types of food preparation, physical properties of some foods, and certain methods of food preservation (especially smoking, pickling, or salting).

SIGNS AND SYMPTOMS
Early clues to gastric cancer are chronic dyspepsia and epigastric discomfort, followed in later stages by weight loss, anorexia, a feeling of fullness after eating, anemia, and fatigue. If the cancer is in the cardia, the first sign may be dysphagia and, later, vomiting. Some patients also have bloody stools.

DIAGNOSTIC TESTS
Diagnosis rests primarily on evaluation of any persistent or recurring GI changes and complaints. To rule out other conditions producing similar symptoms, evaluation includes testing of blood, stools, and stomach fluid specimens. Additional tests typically include barium X-rays of the GI tract, which reveal changes in the stomach's shape, loss of flexibility and of ability to enlarge, and abnormalities in the gastric mucosa. Gastroscopy helps rule out other abnormalities of the mucosa.

Studies that help determine if the cancer has spread to other organs include computed tomography scans, chest X-rays, liver and bone scans, and liver biopsy.

TREATMENT
Surgery is often the treatment of choice. Even in patients whose disease isn't considered surgically curable, resection offers palliation and improves potential benefits from chemotherapy and radiation.

PATHOPHYSIOLOGY

Sites of gastric cancer

In order of decreasing frequency, gastric cancer affects the pylorus and antrum, lesser curvature, cardia, body of the stomach, and greater curvature.

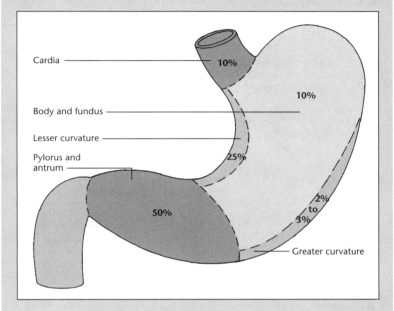

The nature and extent of the tumor determine appropriate surgery. Common procedures include subtotal gastrectomy and total gastrectomy. If gastric cancer has spread to other regions, more extensive surgery is necessary.

Other treatments

Chemotherapy for gastric cancer may help control symptoms and prolong survival. Antiemetics minimize nausea, which increases as the cancer advances. Antispasmodic drugs and antacids may help relieve GI distress.

In more advanced stages, sedatives and tranquilizers may be necessary to control overwhelming anxiety. Narcotics may be necessary to relieve severe and unremitting pain.

Radiation has been particularly useful when combined with chemotherapy in patients who have nonresectable or partially resectable disease.

SPECIAL CONSIDERATIONS

● High-calorie, well-balanced meals minimize the effects of radiation therapy. Fluids such as ginger ale minimize nausea and vomiting.
● After a total gastrectomy, the patient must eat small meals for the rest of his life. Some patients need pancreatin and sodium bicarbonate after meals to prevent or control steatorrhea and dyspepsia.

Identifying the causes of acute gastritis

The following conditions may cause an attack of acute gastritis:

• chronic ingestion of irritating foods such as hot peppers (or an allergic reaction to them) or alcohol

• drugs such as aspirin and other nonsteroidal anti-inflammatory agents (in large doses), cytotoxic agents, caffeine, corticosteroids, antimetabolites, phenylbutazone, and indomethacin

• ingestion of poisons, especially DDT, ammonia, mercury, carbon tetrachloride, and corrosive substances

• endotoxins released from infecting bacteria, such as staphylococci, *Escherichia coli,* or *Salmonella.*

• acute illnesses, especially when the patient has had major traumatic injuries, burns, severe infection, major surgery, or hepatic, renal, or respiratory failure.

 PREVENTION TIP: After gastrectomy, the patient may experience dumping syndrome and malabsorption of vitamin B_{12}. To help prevent vitamin B_{12} deficiency, advise him to follow the doctor's recommendations for taking lifelong vitamin and iron supplements.

• The doctor may recommend steroids, antidepressants, wine, or brandy to boost the appetite.

• If all treatments fail, patient care centers on keeping the patient comfortable and free from pain and providing psychological support.

Gastritis

An inflammation of the gastric mucosa, gastritis may be acute or chronic. It can occur at any age. *Acute gastritis* produces mucosal reddening, edema, hemorrhage, and erosion.

Chronic gastritis is common among elderly people and patients with pernicious anemia. Often it's present as chronic atrophic gastritis, in which all gastric mucosal layers are inflamed, with reduced numbers of chief and parietal cells.

CAUSES

Acute gastritis has many causes, ranging from consumption of irritating foods to acute illness. (See *Identifying the causes of acute gastritis*.)

Chronic gastritis may be associated with peptic ulcer disease or gastrostomy; both conditions cause chronic reflux of pancreatic secretions, bile, and bile acids from the duodenum into the stomach.

Recurring exposure to irritating substances, such as drugs, alcohol, cigarette smoke, or environmental agents, also may lead to chronic gastritis. Sometimes chronic gastritis accompanies pernicious anemia, renal disease, or diabetes mellitus. Infection with *Helicobacter pylori* is a common cause of nonerosive chronic gastritis.

SIGNS AND SYMPTOMS

After exposure to the offending substance, the patient with *acute gastritis* typically reports rapid such symptoms as epigastric discomfort, indigestion, cramping, anorexia, nausea, vomiting, and hematemesis. These symptoms last from a few hours to a few days.

The patient with *chronic gastritis* may describe similar symptoms or may have only mild epigastric discomfort. Or his complaints may be vague, such as an intolerance for spicy or fatty foods or slight pain relieved by eating. The patient with chronic atrophic gastritis may have no symptoms.

DIAGNOSTIC TESTS

Laboratory tests can detect traces of blood in vomitus or stools (or both) if gastric bleeding is suspected. Also, blood tests may help distinguish anemia from bleeding. Gastroscopy (with a biopsy) confirms gastritis when done before lesions heal.

TREATMENT
Bacterial gastritis is treated with antibiotics and ingested poisons are neutralized with the appropriate antidote. Histamine$_2$-receptor antagonists such as cimetidine may block gastric secretions. Antacids may be used as buffers.

For critically ill patients, antacids given hourly, with or without histamine antagonists, may reduce the frequency of gastritis attacks. Some patients also require analgesics. Until healing occurs, oxygen needs, blood volume, and fluid and electrolyte balance must be monitored.

When gastritis causes massive bleeding, treatment involves blood replacement, iced saline lavage, angiography with vasopressin infused in normal saline solution and, sometimes, surgery.

Vagotomy and pyloroplasty have achieved limited success when conservative treatments fail. Rarely, partial or total gastrectomy is required.

Simply avoiding aspirin and spicy foods may relieve chronic gastritis. If symptoms persist, the doctor may recommend antacids. If pernicious anemia is the underlying cause of gastritis, vitamin B$_{12}$ may be given parenterally. A combination of bismuth and an antibiotic such as amoxicillin may relieve *H. pylori* infection; however, eradication is difficult.

SPECIAL CONSIDERATIONS
• As foods are reintroduced to normalize the diet, note the patient's reactions to each food.
• A bland diet of smaller, more frequent meals may reduce irritating gastric secretions. Avoiding alcohol, caffeine, and aspirin-containing compounds also may minimize problems.
• If pain or nausea decreases the patient's appetite, analgesics or antiemetics given 1 hour before meals may be helpful.

 TEACHING TIP: Advise the patient to seek immediate attention for recurring symptoms, such as hematemesis, nausea, or vomiting.

Gastroenteritis
Also called intestinal flu, traveler's diarrhea, viral enteritis, and food poisoning, gastroenteritis is a self-limiting disorder characterized by diarrhea, nausea, vomiting, and abdominal cramping. Occurring in persons of all ages, it is a major cause of illness and death in underdeveloped nations.

In the United States, gastroenteritis is the second leading cause of lost work time and the fifth cause of death among young children. In elderly and debilitated people, the condition can be life-threatening.

CAUSES
Gastroenteritis has many possible causes, including the following:
• bacteria (responsible for acute food poisoning) — *Staphylococcus aureus, Salmonella, Shigella, Clostridium botulinum, Escherichia coli, Clostridium perfringens*
• amoebae — especially *Entamoeba histolytica*
• parasites — *Ascaris, Enterobius,* and *Trichinella spiralis*
• viruses (may be responsible for traveler's diarrhea) — adenoviruses, echoviruses, or coxsackieviruses
• ingestion of toxins — plants or toadstools
• drug reactions — antibiotics
• enzyme deficiencies
• food allergens.

The bowel reacts to any of these enterotoxins with hypermotility, producing severe diarrhea and causing depletion of intracellular fluid.

SIGNS AND SYMPTOMS
Clinical features vary with the pathologic organism and the level of GI tract involved. Adults typically experience diarrhea, abdominal discomfort, nausea, and vomiting. Other possible features include fever,

malaise, and loud bowel sounds caused by intestinal hyperactivity.

In children and elderly and debilitated people, gastroenteritis produces the same symptoms, but inability to tolerate electrolyte and fluid losses leads to a higher mortality.

DIAGNOSTIC TESTS
Diagnosis rests on the patient history and stool specimens or blood samples showing bacteria or parasites that can cause gastroenteritis.

TREATMENT
Usually supportive, treatment involves bed rest, nutritional support, and increased fluid intake. A young child, an elderly or debilitated person, or someone with severe gastroenteritis may need to be hospitalized. Treatment also may involve specific antimicrobials, I.V. fluid and electrolyte replacement, bismuth-containing compounds, and antiemetics.

SPECIAL CONSIDERATIONS
● Giving broth, ginger ale, or lemonade as tolerated can offset fluid and electrolyte losses in the patient who can eat. A varied diet may improve compliance. The patient should avoid milk and milk products, which may provoke recurrence.
● Anal irritation can be eased with warm sitz baths or witch hazel compresses.
● If food poisoning is probable, public health authorities should be notified.

 PREVENTION TIP: Good hygiene may prevent gastritis from recurring. Advise patients to cook foods thoroughly, especially pork; to refrigerate perishable foods, such as milk, mayonnaise, potato salad, and cream-filled pastry; to wash their hands with warm water and soap before handling food, especially after using the bathroom; to clean utensils thoroughly; and to avoid tap water and raw fruits or vegetables in foreign countries.

Gastroesophageal reflux

In this disorder, gastric or duodenal contents, or both, flow backward into the esophagus and past the lower esophageal sphincter (LES). Reflux may or may not cause symptoms or pathologic changes. Persistent reflux may lead to reflux esophagitis (inflammation of the esophageal mucosa). The prognosis varies with the underlying cause.

CAUSES
The function of the LES — a high-pressure area in the lower esophagus, just above the stomach — is to prevent gastric contents from backing up into the esophagus. Normally, the LES creates pressure, closing the lower end of the esophagus, but relaxes after each swallow to allow food into the stomach.

Gastroesophageal reflux occurs when LES pressure is deficient or when pressure within the stomach exceeds LES pressure. Predisposing factors include:
● pyloric surgery (alteration or removal of the pylorus), which allows reflux of bile or pancreatic juice
● long-term nasogastric intubation (more than 4 to 5 days)
● any agent that lowers LES pressure, such as food, alcohol, cigarettes, anticholinergics (atropine, belladonna, propantheline), and other drugs (morphine, diazepam, and meperidine)
● hiatal hernia
● any condition or position that increases intra-abdominal pressure.

SIGNS AND SYMPTOMS
Gastroesophageal reflux doesn't always cause symptoms. Its most common feature is heartburn, which may grow more severe with vigorous exercise, bending, or lying down and may be relieved by antacids or sitting upright.

Some patients have pain from esophageal spasm; it tends to be chronic and may mimic angina pectoris, spreading to the neck, jaws, and arms.

Other signs and symptoms of reflux include:
• severe burning, squeezing pain while swallowing, which may be followed by a dull substernal ache
• dysphagia stemming from esophageal spasm, stricture, or esophagitis
• bleeding (bright red or dark brown).

Pulmonary problems may occur if gastric contents flow into the throat and cause aspiration. These include chronic pulmonary disease or nocturnal wheezing, bronchitis, asthma, morning hoarseness, and cough.

In children, other signs of reflux include failure to thrive and forceful vomiting from esophageal irritation. Such vomiting may cause aspiration pneumonia.

DIAGNOSTIC TESTS
After a careful history and physical examination, visual inspection of the throat lining identifies the problem. To evaluate the condition further, the doctor may order a barium swallow X-ray. In children, X-rays can detect the backup.

TREATMENT
Effective management relieves symptoms by reducing intra-abdominal pressure and reflux through gravity, neutralizing gastric contents, and strengthening the LES with drug therapy. Severe cases may warrant surgery.

Positional therapy
To reduce intra-abdominal pressure and reflux, the patient should sleep in a reverse Trendelenburg position (with the head of the bed elevated) and avoid lying down after meals and late-night snacks.

Drug therapy
Antacids given 1 hour and 3 hours after meals and at bedtime are effective for intermittent reflux. For intensive therapy, antacids are given hourly. A nondiarrheal, nonmagnesium antacid (aluminum carbonate, aluminum hydroxide) may be preferred.

Bethanechol, which increases LES pressure, stimulates smooth-muscle contraction and decreases esophageal

Do's and don'ts for patients with reflux

Thorough teaching can help patients cope better with gastroesophageal reflux. Besides telling the patient about the causes of reflux, review ways to prevent reflux with an antireflux regimen (medication, diet, and positional therapy). Also make sure he knows which symptoms to watch for and report.

Some do's
• Advise the patient to sit upright, particularly after meals.
• Tell the patient to eat small, frequent meals — at least 2 to 3 hours before lying down.
• Urge him to take antacids, as prescribed.

Some don'ts
• Caution the patient to avoid any circumstance that increases intra-abdominal pressure, such as bending, coughing, vigorous exercise, tight clothing, constipation, and obesity.
• Tell him to avoid substances that reduce sphincter control. These include cigarettes, alcohol, fatty foods, and certain drugs.
• Instruct him to avoid highly seasoned food, acidic juices, alcoholic drinks, bedtime snacks, and foods high in fat or carbohydrates.

acidity after meals. Metoclopramide and cimetidine also have been effective.

Surgery
Surgical intervention may be necessary to control severe and refractory symptoms, such as pulmonary aspiration, hemorrhage, obstruction, severe pain, perforation, incompetent LES, or associated hiatal hernia.

Surgical procedures create an artificial closure at the gastroesophageal junction. Also, vagotomy or pyloroplasty may be combined with an antireflux regimen to modify gastric contents.

SPECIAL CONSIDERATIONS
● Before diagnostic studies, the patient should receive special instructions — for example, he shouldn't eat for 6 to 8 hours before a barium X-ray or endoscopy.
● Patient teaching should include ways to avoid and treat reflux. (See *Do's and don'ts for patients with reflux,* page 113.)

Genital herpes

An acute inflammatory disease of the genitalia, primary genital herpes usually is self-limiting but may cause painful local or systemic disease. Prognosis varies with the patient's age, strength of his immune defenses, and infection site.

In neonates and immunocompromised patients such as those with acquired immunodeficiency syndrome, genital herpes commonly is severe, leading to complications and high mortality.

CAUSES
Genital herpes usually results from infection with herpes simplex virus Type 2, although some studies report increasing incidence of infection with herpes simplex virus Type 1. The disease typically is transmitted through sexual intercourse, orogenital sexual activity, kissing, and hand-to-body contact.

Pregnant women may transmit the infection to neonates during vaginal delivery. Such transmitted infection may be localized (for instance, in the eyes) or disseminated and may be associated with central nervous system involvement.

SIGNS AND SYMPTOMS
After a 3- to 7-day incubation period, fluid-filled vesicles appear, usually on the cervix (the primary infection site) and possibly on the labia, perianal skin, vulva, or vagina of the female and on the glans penis, foreskin, or penile shaft of the male. Lesions may also form on the mouth or anus.

In both males and females, the vesicles (usually painless at first) rupture and become extensive, shallow, painful ulcers, with redness, edema, tender inguinal lymph nodes, and yellow oozing centers.

DIAGNOSTIC TESTS
Diagnosis requires a physical examination and patient history. Laboratory results may show characteristic antibody and cell findings. Diagnosis is confirmed if the virus appears in fluid from blisters or is implicated in tests that identify specific antigens.

TREATMENT
Acyclovir has proved to be an effective treatment for genital herpes. The drug may be given I.V. to hospitalized patients with severe genital herpes or to those who are immunocompromised and have a potentially life-threatening herpes infection.

Oral acyclovir may be prescribed for patients with first-time infections or recurrent outbreaks. Daily prophylaxis with acyclovir reduces the frequency of recurrences.

SPECIAL CONSIDERATIONS
 TEACHING TIP: Instruct the patient to get adequate rest and nutrition and to keep the lesions dry. Caution him to avoid sexual activity while lesions are present and to use condoms during all sexual exposures. Urge the patient to have all sexual partners seek medical examination.
● The female patient should have a Papanicolaou test every 6 months.
● Newborns are at risk from vaginal delivery. Pregnant patients with herpes should consider cesarean delivery.
● The Herpes Resource Center, an American Social Health Association group, is a support resource.

Genital warts

Also called venereal warts or condylomata acuminata, genital warts consist of papillomas with fibrous tissue overgrowth from the dermis and thickened epithelial coverings. They're uncommon before puberty or after menopause.

Certain types of human papillomavirus (HPV) infections have been strongly associated with genital dysplasia and, over a period of years, with cervical neoplasia.

CAUSES

Infection with one of the more than 60 known strains of HPV causes genital warts, which are transmitted through sexual contact. Warts grow rapidly in the presence of heavy perspiration, poor hygiene, or pregnancy and commonly accompany other genital infections.

SIGNS AND SYMPTOMS

After a 1- to 6-month incubation period (usually 2 months), genital warts develop on moist surfaces. For instance, in males, they form within the urethral meatus and, less commonly, on the penile shaft; in females, on the vulva and on vaginal and cervical walls.

In both sexes, papillomas spread to the perineum and perianal area. These painless warts start as tiny red or pink swellings that grow (sometimes to 4" [10 cm]) and become pedunculated. Typically, multiple swellings give them a cauliflower-like appearance. If infected, these warts become malodorous.

Most patients report no symptoms; a few complain of itching or pain.

DIAGNOSTIC TESTS

Microscopic examination of scrapings from wart cells helps to distinguish genital warts. Applying 5% acetic acid (white vinegar) to the warts turns them white.

TREATMENT

The initial treatment goal is to eradicate associated genital infections. Warts commonly resolve spontaneously. Topical drug therapy (10% to 25% podophyllum in tincture of benzoin, trichloroacetic acid, or bichloroacetic acid) removes small warts.

Warts larger than 1" (2.5 cm) usually are removed by carbon dioxide laser treatment, cryosurgery, or electrocautery.

The goal of treatment is to remove exophytic warts and to ease signs and symptoms. No therapy has proved effective in eradicating HPV. Relapse commonly occurs.

SPECIAL CONSIDERATIONS

● If the patient has been treated with topical drug therapy as described above, the medication should be washed off with soap and water 4 to 6 hours after applying it.
● Women with genital warts should have annual Papanicolaou tests.

 TEACHING TIP: Advise the patient to encourage sexual partners to seek examination for HPV, human immunodeficiency virus, and other sexually transmitted diseases.

Giardiasis

Also known as *Giardia* enteritis and lambliasis, giardiasis is an infection of the small bowel caused by the symmetrical flagellate protozoan *Giardia lamblia*. A mild infection may not produce intestinal symptoms. In untreated giardiasis, symptoms wax and wane; with treatment, recovery is complete.

Giardiasis occurs worldwide but is most common in developing countries and other areas with poor sanitation and hygiene. In the United States, giardiasis is most common in travelers who have recently returned from endemic areas and in campers who drink unpurified water from contaminated streams.

CAUSES

G. lamblia has two stages: the cystic stage and the trophozoite stage. Giardiasis results from ingesting *G. lamblia* cysts in fecally contaminated water or from fecal-oral transfer of cysts in an infected person.

When cysts enter the small bowel, they become trophozoites and attach themselves with their sucking disks

Preventing giardiasis

To help prevent the spread of giardiasis, follow these guidelines:
● Use good personal hygiene, particularly proper hand-washing technique. Teach patients about proper hygiene, too.
● Warn travelers to endemic areas not to drink water or eat uncooked and unpeeled fruits or vegetables because they may have been rinsed in contaminated water. (Prophylactic drug therapy isn't recommended.)
● Advise campers to purify all stream water before drinking it.

to the bowel's epithelial surface. Then the trophozoites encyst again, travel down the colon, and are excreted. Unformed feces that pass quickly through the intestine may contain trophozoites as well as cysts.

Probably because of frequent hand-to-mouth activity, children are more likely to become infected with *G. lamblia* than adults. Giardiasis does not confer immunity, so reinfections may occur. (See *Preventing giardiasis*.)

SIGNS AND SYMPTOMS
Attachment of *G. lamblia* to the intestinal lumen causes superficial mucosal invasion and destruction, inflammation, and irritation. These effects decrease food transit time through the small intestine and result in malabsorption.

Such malabsorption leads to chronic GI complaints (such as abdominal cramps); pale, loose, greasy, malodorous, and frequent stools (from 2 to 10 daily); and nausea. Stools may contain mucus but not pus or blood. Chronic giardiasis may produce fatigue and weight loss in addition to these typical findings.

DIAGNOSTIC TESTS
Giardiasis should be suspected when travelers who have visited endemic ar-

eas or campers who may have drunk unpurified water develop symptoms.

Diagnosis requires laboratory examination of fresh stool specimens. A barium X-ray of the small bowel may show mucous membrane swelling and barium segmentation.

TREATMENT
Giardiasis responds readily to a 10-day course of metronidazole or a 7-day course of quinacrine and oral furazolidone. Severe diarrhea may necessitate parenteral fluid replacement to prevent dehydration if oral fluid intake is inadequate.

SPECIAL CONSIDERATIONS
● If the patient requires hospitalization, enteric precautions are needed. When caring for such a patient, pay strict attention to hand washing, particularly after handling feces. Quickly dispose of fecal material. (Normal sewage systems can remove and process infected feces adequately.)
● Patients should not drink alcoholic beverages while taking metronidazole because they may provoke a disulfiram-like reaction.
● Epidemic situations should be reported to public health authorities.

Glaucoma

Glaucoma refers to a group of disorders in which intraocular pressure rises dangerously high. Glaucoma can damage the optic nerve. If untreated, it can lead to gradual vision loss and, ultimately, blindness.

Glaucoma occurs in several forms: chronic open-angle (primary), acute angle-closure, congenital (inherited as an autosomal recessive trait), and secondary to other causes.

Glaucoma affects 2% of the U.S. population over age 40 and accounts for 12% of all cases of new blindness in the United States. With early treatment, the prognosis is good.

CAUSES
Chronic open-angle glaucoma results from overproduction of aqueous humor or obstructed outflow of aqueous

humor through the trabecular mesh-work or Schlemm's canal. This form, which accounts for 90% of glaucoma cases, commonly runs in families.

Acute angle-closure (narrow-angle) glaucoma results from obstructed outflow of aqueous humor due to anatomically narrow angles between the anterior iris and posterior corneal surface, shallow anterior chambers, a thickened iris that causes angle closure on pupil dilation, or a bulging iris that presses on the trabeculae, closing the angle.

Secondary glaucoma may result from uveitis, trauma, or drugs (such as steroids.) Vein occlusion or diabetes may lead to new vessel formation (neovascularization) in the angle.

SIGNS AND SYMPTOMS
Clinical features vary with the form of glaucoma.

Chronic open-angle glaucoma
Usually bilateral, chronic open-angle glaucoma has a gradual onset and a slowly progressive course. Signs and symptoms appear late in the disease and include mild aching in the eyes, peripheral vision loss, seeing halos around lights, and reduced visual acuity that's uncorrectable with glasses.

Acute angle-closure glaucoma
Acute angle-closure glaucoma typically has a rapid onset. Signs and symptoms may include unilateral inflammation and pain, pressure over the eye, a moderately dilated pupil that's nonreactive to light, a cloudy cornea, blurring, decreased visual acuity, photophobia, and seeing halos around lights. Increased intraocular pressure (IOP) may result in nausea and vomiting, causing glaucoma to be misinterpreted as GI distress.

Unless treated promptly, acute angle-closure glaucoma leads to blindness in 3 to 5 days.

DIAGNOSTIC TESTS
Loss of peripheral vision and changes in the optic disk confirm glaucoma. Special examinations aid diagnosis.

- Tonometry measures IOP and provides a baseline for later comparison.
- Slit-lamp examination allows examination of the cornea, iris, and lens.
- Gonioscopy determines the angle of the anterior chamber to distinguish between chronic open-angle and acute angle-closure glaucoma.
- Ophthalmoscopy provides a look at the fundus, where cupping and shrinkage of the optic disk are visible in chronic open-angle glaucoma. These changes appear later in chronic angle-closure glaucoma if the disease isn't brought under control. In acute angle-closure glaucoma, the optic disk looks pale.
- Perimetry or visual field tests reveal peripheral vision loss, pinpointing the extent of chronic open-angle deterioration.

TREATMENT
Treatment varies with the form of glaucoma.

Therapy for chronic open-angle glaucoma
Drug therapy is the treatment of choice for chronic open-angle glaucoma. Treatment initially decreases aqueous humor production through beta blockers, epinephrine, or diuretics.

Drug treatment also may involve miotic eyedrops such as pilocarpine to promote aqueous humor outflow. Patients who don't respond to drug therapy may be candidates for an iridectomy, argon laser trabeculoplasty (ALT), or trabeculectomy. (See *Understanding trabeculectomy,* page 118.)

Iridectomy is a surgical filtering procedure that creates an opening for aqueous outflow. In ALT, an argon laser beam produces a thermal burn that changes the surface of the trabecular meshwork and increases aqueous outflow.

Therapy for acute angle-closure glaucoma
Acute angle-closure glaucoma requires immediate treatment to lower IOP. If drug therapy fails to lower IOP, laser iridotomy or surgical pe-

Understanding trabeculectomy

In trabeculectomy, used to treat open-angle glaucoma, a flap of sclera is dissected free to expose the trabecular meshwork. Then this discrete tissue block is removed and a peripheral iridectomy is performed. This produces an opening for aqueous outflow under the conjunctiva.

ripheral iridectomy must be performed promptly to save the patient's vision.

Preoperatively, drug therapy (acetazolamide, pilocarpine, and I.V. mannitol or oral glycerin) is used to lower IOP. Severe pain may necessitate narcotic analgesics.

SPECIAL CONSIDERATIONS

● The patient must comply with prescribed drug therapy to avoid optic disk changes, vision loss, and an increase in IOP.
● After peripheral iridectomy, cycloplegic eyedrops are instilled in the affected eye. (Using them in the normal eye may trigger acute angle-closure glaucoma in this eye.)

 PREVENTION TIP: Glaucoma screening is vital for early detection and prevention. Urge everyone over age 35 to have an annual tonometric examination.

Glomerulonephritis, acute poststreptococcal

Also called acute glomerulonephritis, acute poststreptococcal glomerulonephritis (APSGN) is a relatively common bilateral inflammation of the renal glomeruli. It follows a streptococcal infection of the respiratory tract or, less commonly, a skin infection such as impetigo.

APSGN is most common in boys ages 3 to 7 but can occur at any age. Up to 95% of children and up to 70% of adults with APSGN recover fully; the rest may progress to chronic renal failure within months.

CAUSES

APSGN results from entrapment and collection of antigen-antibody in the glomerular capillary membranes (the antibody is produced as an immunologic mechanism in response to streptococcus). Such entrapment causes inflammatory damage and impedes glomerular function.

Sometimes, the immune complement further damages the glomerular membrane. The damaged and inflamed glomerulus is no longer selectively permeable, allowing red blood cells and proteins to filter through as the glomerular filtration rate falls. Uremic poisoning may ensue.

SIGNS AND SYMPTOMS

APSGN commonly begins within 1 to 3 weeks after untreated pharyngitis. Signs and symptoms include mild to moderate edema, oliguria (urine output of less than 400 ml/24 hours), proteinuria, azotemia, hematuria, and fatigue.

Mild to severe hypertension may result from either sodium or water retention or inappropriate renin release. Heart failure from hypervolemia leads to pulmonary edema.

DIAGNOSTIC TESTS

A detailed patient history and physical examination are followed by laboratory tests, including urinalysis to assess kidney filtration, a throat culture to check for *Streptococcus*, renal ultrasound to check for kidney enlargement, and kidney biopsy to confirm the diagnosis or to assess renal status.

TREATMENT

The goals of treatment are to relieve symptoms and prevent complications. Vigorous supportive care in cludes bed rest, fluid restrictions, dietary sodium restrictions, and correction of electrolyte imbalances (rarely, dialysis is necessary).

Therapy may include diuretics (such as metolazone or furosemide) to reduce extracellular fluid overload and an antihypertensive (such as hydralazine). Use of antibiotics to prevent secondary infection or transmission to others is controversial.

SPECIAL CONSIDERATIONS
• The patient benefits from a diet high in calories and low in protein, sodium, potassium, and fluids.
• Bed rest is necessary during the acute phase. As symptoms subside, the patient can gradually resume normal activities.
• Providing good nutrition, using meticulous hygiene, and preventing contact with infected persons can help prevent secondary infection in a debilitated patient.
• The patient must have follow-up examinations during the convalescent months to detect chronic renal failure. These examinations include blood pressure checks, urinary protein, and renal function assessments.
• Pregnant women with a history of APSGN should have frequent medical evaluations because pregnancy further stresses the kidneys and increases the risk of chronic renal failure.

 PREVENTION TIP: To help prevent APSGN, instruct the patient with a history of chronic upper respiratory tract infections to immediately report signs of infection (fever, sore throat).

Glomerulonephritis, chronic

A slowly progressive disease, chronic glomerulonephritis is characterized by inflammation of the renal glomeruli, which results in sclerosis, scarring, and eventual renal failure.

The condition usually goes undetected until the progressive phase begins, marked by proteinuria, cylindruria (granular tube casts in urine), and hematuria. By the time it produces symptoms, it is usually irreversible.

CAUSES
Chronic glomerulonephritis may result from primary renal disorders or certain systemic conditions. (See *Causes of chronic glomerulonephritis,* page 120.)

SIGNS AND SYMPTOMS
Chronic glomerulonephritis usually develops gradually without symptoms — commonly over many years. However, at any time, it may suddenly become progressive, producing nephrotic syndrome, hypertension, proteinuria, and hematuria.

In late stages, the patient may experience uremic symptoms, such as azotemia, nausea, vomiting, pruritus, dyspnea, malaise, and fatigue. Mild to severe edema and anemia may accompany these symptoms.

Severe hypertension may cause heart enlargement, leading to heart failure. It also may hasten the onset of advanced renal failure, eventually necessitating dialysis or transplantation.

DIAGNOSTIC TESTS
Patient history and physical findings seldom suggest glomerulonephritis. Suspicion develops from:
• urinalysis revealing proteinuria, hematuria, cylindruria, and red blood cell casts
• rising blood urea nitrogen and serum creatinine levels showing advanced renal insufficiency
• X-rays or ultrasonography revealing smaller kidneys
• kidney biopsy that identifies underlying disease.

TREATMENT
Effective treatment aims to:
• control hypertension with antihypertensives and a sodium-restricted diet
• correct fluid and electrolyte imbalances through restrictions and replacement

---

Causes of chronic glomerulonephritis

Renal conditions that can bring on chronic glomerulonephritis include:
- membranoproliferative glomerulonephritis
- membranous glomerulopathy
- focal glomerulosclerosis
- rapidly progressive glomerulonephritis
- poststreptococcal glomerulonephritis (less common).

Systemic causes of this disease include:
- lupus erythematosus
- Goodpasture's syndrome
- hemolytic-uremic syndrome.

- reduce edema with diuretics such as furosemide
- prevent heart failure.

For some patients, treatment also includes antibiotics (for symptomatic urinary tract infections), dialysis, or transplantation.

SPECIAL CONSIDERATIONS
- The patient should consume a low-sodium, high-calorie diet with adequate protein.
- Good skin care helps to reduce pruritus and edema.

 TEACHING TIP: Instruct the patient to continue prescribed antihypertensives as scheduled, even if he is feeling better, and to report any adverse effects. If he's receiving diuretics, advise him to take them in the morning to avoid sleep disruption caused by the need to void. Instruct him to report signs and symptoms of infection, and to avoid contact with people who have infections.

Gonorrhea

A common venereal disease, gonorrhea is an infection of the genitourinary tract and, occasionally, the rectum, pharynx, and eyes. In females, untreated gonorrhea can lead to chronic pelvic inflammatory disease (PID) and sterility. After adequate treatment, prognosis is excellent.

CAUSES
Transmission of *Neisseria gonorrhoeae*, the organism that causes gonorrhea, almost exclusively follows sexual contact with an infected person. Children born of infected mothers may contract gonococcal ophthalmia neonatorum during passage through the birth canal. Children and adults with gonorrhea can contract gonococcal conjunctivitis by touching their eyes with contaminated hands.

SIGNS AND SYMPTOMS
Although many infected males may be asymptomatic, after a 3- to 6-day incubation period some develop symptoms of urethritis, including painful urination and purulent urethral discharge, with redness and swelling at the infection site. Most infected females are asymptomatic but may develop inflammation and a greenish yellow cervical discharge.

Other clinical features vary with the site involved:
- urethra: dysuria, urinary frequency and incontinence, purulent discharge, itching, and red and edematous meatus
- vulva: occasional itching, burning, and pain due to exudate from an adjacent infected area
- vagina: engorgement, redness, swelling, and profuse purulent discharge
- pelvis: severe pelvic and lower abdominal pain, muscular rigidity, tenderness, and abdominal distention. As the infection spreads, nausea, vomiting, fever, and tachycardia may develop in patients with salpingitis or PID.

Untreated gonorrhea can spread through the blood to the joints, tendons, meninges, and heart lining, causing gonococcal septicemia. (See *Clinical features of gonococcal septicemia.*)

Eye involvement

Signs of gonococcal ophthalmia neonatorum include lid edema, bilateral conjunctival infection, and abundant purulent discharge 2 to 3 days after birth. Adult conjunctivitis causes unilateral conjunctival redness and swelling. Unless treated, gonococcal conjunctivitis can progress to corneal ulceration and blindness.

DIAGNOSTIC TESTS

A culture from the infected body part usually establishes the diagnosis by isolating the organism. A Gram stain supports the diagnosis and may be sufficient to confirm gonorrhea in men. A culture of eye scrapings confirms gonococcal conjunctivitis.

TREATMENT

For adults and adolescents, the recommended treatment for uncomplicated gonorrhea caused by susceptible non-penicillinase-producing *N. gonorrhoeae* is a single 125-mg dose of ceftriaxone I.M.; for presumptive treatment of concurrent *Chlamydia trachomatis* infection, 100 mg doxycycline orally twice daily for 7 days.

A single dose of ceftriaxone and erythromycin for 7 days is recommended for pregnant patients and those allergic to penicillin.

All regimens should be continued for 24 to 48 hours after improvement begins; then therapy may be switched to a different regimen to complete a full week of antimicrobial therapy.

SPECIAL CONSIDERATIONS

• Administration of two drops of 1% silver nitrate or erythromycin in the eyes of all neonates immediately after birth is a routine precaution. Newborn infants of infected mothers should be checked for signs and symptoms of infection.

 TEACHING TIP: Until cultures prove negative, the patient is still infectious and can transmit gonococcal infection. Urge him to inform sexual contacts of the infection so they can seek treatment.

• In the patient with gonococcal

Clinical features of gonococcal septicemia

Gonococcal septicemia, which can occur if gonorrhea goes untreated, affects both sexes but is more common in females. Typical signs and symptoms include:

• tender papillary skin lesions on the hands and feet (which may be pustular, hemorrhagic, or necrotic)

• migratory polyarthralgia

• polyarthritis and tenosynovitis of the wrists, fingers, knees, or ankles.

Untreated septic arthritis leads to progressive joint destruction.

---

arthritis, moist heat can ease pain in affected joints.

• All cases of gonorrhea should be reported to local public health authorities for follow-up on sexual contacts. All cases of gonorrhea in children should be reported to child abuse authorities.

 PREVENTION TIP: To help prevent gonorrhea, advise all patients to avoid anyone suspected of being infected, to use condoms during intercourse, to wash genitalia before and after intercourse, and to avoid sharing washcloths or douche equipment.

Gout

Also called gouty arthritis, gout is a metabolic disease in which urate deposits develop in the joints, which may cause painful arthritis. Gout can strike any joint but favors those in the feet and legs.

Hyperuricemia results from the breakdown of nucleic acid. Increased concentration of uric acid leads to urate deposits, called tophi, in joints or tissues, causing local necrosis or fibrosis.

Primary gout usually strikes men older than age 30 and postmenopausal women. *Secondary gout* occurs in older people.

Gout follows an intermittent course and leaves many patients free from symptoms for years between attacks. However, the disease sometimes leads to chronic disability or incapacitation and, rarely, to severe hypertension and progressive renal disease. With treatment, the prognosis is good.

CAUSES

Although the exact cause of primary gout remains unknown, it seems to be linked to a genetic defect in purine metabolism, which causes overproduction of uric acid (hyperuricemia), retention of uric acid, or both.

Secondary gout develops during the course of another disease, such as obesity, diabetes mellitus, hypertension, sickle cell anemia, or renal disease.

Pseudogout occurs when calcium pyrophosphate crystals collect in the periarticular joint structures. (See *All about pseudogout.*)

SIGNS AND SYMPTOMS

Gout develops in four stages: asymptomatic, acute, intercritical, and chronic. In *asymptomatic gout,* serum urate levels rise but produce no symptoms.

Acute stage

As gout progresses, it may cause hypertension or nephrolithiasis, with severe back pain. The first acute attack strikes suddenly and peaks quickly. Extremely painful, this attack commonly involves the metatarsophalangeal joint of the great toe. Affected joints appear hot, tender, inflamed, dusky red, or cyanotic.

Intercritical stage

Symptom-free intervals between gout attacks are called intercritical periods. Most patients have a second attack within 6 months to 2 years, but in some the second attack is delayed for 5 to 10 years.

Chronic stage

Eventually, chronic polyarticular gout sets in. This final, unremitting disease (called chronic or tophaceous gout) is marked by persistent painful polyarthritis with large, subcutaneous tophi in cartilage, synovial membranes, tendons, and soft tissue.

Chronic inflammation and tophaceous deposits trigger secondary joint degeneration, with eventual deformity and disability. Kidney involvement leads to chronic renal dysfunction.

DIAGNOSTIC TESTS

Evidence of gout can be found in fluid taken from an inflamed joint or a deposit and by checking the blood uric acid level. In chronic gout, X-rays show damage to cartilage and bones.

TREATMENT

The goal of therapy is to terminate an acute attack, reduce hyperuricemia, and prevent recurrences, complications, and kidney stones.

Therapy for acute gout

Treatment for an acute attack consists of bed rest; immobilization and protection of the inflamed, painful joints; and local heat or cold application. Analgesics such as acetaminophen relieve the pain of mild attacks, but acute inflammation usually requires colchicine administration every hour for 8 hours until pain subsides.

Therapy for chronic gout

A continuing maintenance dosage of allopurinol may be given to suppress uric acid formation or control uric acid levels, preventing further attacks. Colchicine may be given to prevent recurrent acute attacks until the uric acid level returns to normal. Uricosuric agents (probenecid and sulfinpyrazone) promote uric acid excretion and inhibit accumulation of uric acid.

In some cases, the patient must undergo surgery to improve joint function or correct deformities. Tophi must be excised and drained if they become infected or ulcerated. Or they

All about pseudogout

Pseudogout (also called chondro-calcinosis) is an arthritic disease marked by calcium pyrophosphate deposits in the peripheral joints. It often strikes patients over age 50 who have diabetes mellitus or osteoarthritis. Without treatment, pseudogout leads to permanent joint damage in about one-half of the patients it affects.

Clinical features

Like gout, pseudogout causes abrupt joint pain and swelling. These recurrent, self-limiting attacks may be triggered by stress, trauma, surgery, severe dieting, thiazide therapy, and alcohol abuse. Associated symptoms are similar to those of rheumatoid arthritis.

Diagnosis and treatment

Diagnosis hinges on joint aspiration and a synovial biopsy to detect calcium pyrophosphate crystals. X-rays reveal calcific densities in the fibrocartilage and linear markings along bone ends. Blood tests may detect an underlying endocrine or metabolic disorder.

Effective treatment of pseudogout may include joint aspiration to relieve fluid pressure; instillation of steroids; administration of analgesics, phenylbutazone, salicylates, or other nonsteroidal anti-inflammatory drugs; and, if appropriate, treatment of the underlying endocrine or metabolic disorder.

---

may be removed to prevent ulceration, improve the patient's appearance, or make it easier for him to wear shoes or gloves.

SPECIAL CONSIDERATIONS
• Bed rest is encouraged. A bed cradle is used to keep bed covers off extremely sensitive, inflamed joints.
• Hot or cold packs can ease inflamed joints.
• Drinking plenty of fluids helps to prevent kidney stones.

 TEACHING TIP: Advise the patient to avoid high-purine foods, such as anchovies, liver, sardines, kidneys, sweetbreads, lentils, and alcoholic beverages. If the patient is taking probenecid or sulfinpyrazone, instruct him to avoid aspirin and other salicylates; their combined effect causes urate retention. Instruct the patient receiving allopurinol, probenecid, or other drugs to immediately report adverse effects (drowsiness, dizziness, nausea, vomiting, urinary frequency, and dermatitis).
• Long-term colchicine therapy is es-

sential during the first 3 to 6 months of treatment with uricosuric drugs or allopurinol.

Granulocytopenia and lymphocytopenia

In *granulocytopenia (agranulocytosis),* a marked reduction in the number of circulating granulocytes occurs. Although this implies that all granulocytes (neutrophils, basophils, eosinophils) are reduced, granulocytopenia usually refers to decreased neutrophils. This disorder, which can occur at any age, is associated with infections and ulcerative lesions of the throat, GI tract, other mucous membranes, and skin. Its severest form is agranulocytosis.

Lymphocytopenia (lymphopenia) is a rare deficiency of circulating lymphocytes (leukocytes produced mainly in lymph nodes).

In both granulocytopenia and lymphocytopenia, the total white blood cell (WBC) count may fall to dangerously low levels, leaving the body unprotected against infection. The prognosis depends on the underlying cause of the condition and whether or not it can be treated. Untreated, severe granulocytopenia can be fatal in 3 to 6 days.

CAUSES
Granulocytopenia and lymphocytopenia have numerous causes. (See *Understanding the causes of granulocytopenia and lymphocytopenia.*)

SIGNS AND SYMPTOMS
Patients with granulocytopenia typically experience slowly progressive fatigue and weakness, followed by sudden onset of overwhelming infection (fever, chills, tachycardia, anxiety, headache, and extreme prostration); oral or colonic ulceration; pharyngeal ulceration; pneumonia; and septicemia, possibly leading to mild shock.

Patients with lymphocytopenia may exhibit enlarged lymph nodes, spleen, and tonsils as well as signs and symptoms of an associated disease.

DIAGNOSTIC TESTS
Granulocytopenia is diagnosed by a thorough patient history to check for precipitating factors. The doctor also performs a thorough physical examination to check for clinical effects of an underlying disorder and orders various tests. The test results confirm the diagnosis:
• complete blood count revealing a marked reduction in neutrophils and a WBC count lower than 2,000/µl, with few observable granulocytes
• bone marrow examination showing few granulocytic precursor cells beyond the most immature forms.

With lymphocytopenia, the lymphocyte count measures less than 1,500/µl in adults or less than 3,000/µl in children.

TREATMENT
Effective management of granulocytopenia must identify and eliminate the cause and control infection until the bone marrow can generate more

leukocytes. Usually, this means that drug or radiation therapy must be stopped and antibiotic treatment begun immediately, even while awaiting test results. Treatment also may include antifungal preparations.

Administration of granulocyte- or granulocyte-macrophage colony-stimulating factor is a newer treatment used to stimulate bone marrow production of neutrophils. Spontaneous restoration of leukocyte production in bone marrow generally occurs within 1 to 3 weeks.

Treatment of lymphocytopenia includes eliminating the cause and managing any underlying disorders.

SPECIAL CONSIDERATIONS
• The patient requires protective isolation (preferably with laminar air flow).

 TEACHING TIP: Instruct the patient and family in proper hand-washing technique and correct use of gowns and masks.
• Adequate nutrition and hydration are important because malnutrition worsens immunosuppression. The patient with mouth sores should receive a high-calorie liquid diet and use a straw to make drinking less painful.
• Good oral hygiene (warm saline water gargles and rinses, analgesics, and anesthetic lozenges) increases patient comfort and promotes healing.

 PREVENTION TIP: To help detect granulocytopenia and lymphocytopenia in early stages, the WBC count of any patient receiving radiation or chemotherapy should be closely monitored.

Guillain-Barré syndrome

Guillain-Barré syndrome is an acute, rapidly progressive and potentially fatal form of polyneuritis that causes muscle weakness and mild distal sensory loss. The syndrome can occur at any age but is most common between ages 30 and 50. Recovery is spontaneous and complete in about 95% of patients, although mild mo-

Understanding the causes of granulocytopenia and lymphocytopenia

A wide variety of conditions can lead to a deficiency of granulocytes (granulocytopenia) or of lympho-cytes (lymphocytopenia).

Granulocytopenia may result from:
- decreased production of granulo-cytes in the bone marrow, such as from radiation or drug therapy, aplastic anemia, bone marrow can-cers, and some hereditary disorders
- increased peripheral destruction of granulocytes, such as from viral and bacterial infections and certain drugs that carry antigens that attack blood cells and cause acute reactions
- greater utilization of granulocytes, such as from infectious mononucle-osis and other infections.

Causes of lymphocytopenia in-clude:
- decreased lymphocyte production, as from a genetic or a thymic abnor-mality or an immunodeficiency dis-order, such as ataxia-telangiectasia or thymic dysplasia
- increased lymphocyte destruction, such as from radiation or chemo-therapy with alkylating agents
- lymphocyte loss, as with postsurgi-cal thoracic duct drainage or from intestinal lymphangiectasia, or ele-vated plasma corticoid levels (due to stress, corticotropin or steroid treat-ment, or congestive heart failure).

tor or reflex deficits in the feet and legs may persist.

CAUSES

The precise cause of Guillain-Barré syndrome is unknown, but it may be a cell-mediated immune response with an attack on peripheral nerves in response to a virus.

About 50% of patients have a re-cent history of minor febrile illness, usually an upper respiratory tract in-fection (less commonly, gastroenteri-tis). When infection precedes the on-set of Guillain-Barré syndrome, signs and symptoms of infection subside before neurologic features appear.

Other possible precipitating factors include surgery, rabies or swine in-fluenza vaccination, viral illness, Hodgkin's or other malignant disease, and systemic lupus erythematosus.

SIGNS AND SYMPTOMS

Muscle weakness — the major neuro-logic feature — usually affects the legs first, then extends to the arms and facial nerves in 24 to 72 hours. Sometimes, muscle weakness devel-ops in the arms first or in the arms

and legs simultaneously. In milder disease forms, muscle weakness may affect only the cranial nerves or may not occur at all.

Paresthesia, another common neu-rologic symptom, sometimes pre-cedes muscle weakness but tends to vanish quickly. However, some pa-tients never develop this symptom.

Other clinical features may include facial diplegia, dysphagia or dysar-thria and, less commonly, weakness of the muscles supplied by cranial nerve XI.

Muscle weakness develops so quick-ly that muscle atrophy doesn't occur, but hypotonia and areflexia do. Stiff-ness and pain in the form of a severe "charley horse" are common.

The clinical course of Guillain-Barré syndrome is divided into three phas-es. (See *Three phases of Guillain-Barré syndrome,* page 126.)

Complications

Significant complications of Guillain-Barré syndrome include mechanical ventilatory failure, aspiration, pneu-monia, sepsis, joint contractures, and deep vein thrombosis. Unexplained

Three phases of Guillain-Barré syndrome

Signs and symptoms of Guillain-Barré syndrome tend to occur in three distinct phases.

• The *initial phase* begins when the first definitive sign or symptom develops. It ends 1 to 3 weeks later, when no further deterioration is noted.

• The *plateau phase* may last from several days to 2 weeks.

• The *recovery phase* (which presumably coincides with remyelination and regrowth of axonal processes) extends over 4 to 6 months. However, patients with severe disease may take up to 2 years to recover, and recovery may not be complete.

autonomic nervous system involvement may cause sinus tachycardia or bradycardia, hypertension, postural hypotension, or loss of bladder and bowel sphincter control.

DIAGNOSTIC TESTS
A history of recent febrile illness and typical clinical features suggest Guillain-Barré syndrome. Several days after symptom onset, the protein level in cerebrospinal fluid begins to rise, peaking in 4 to 6 weeks. A complete blood count initially shows leukocytosis and a shift to immature cell forms early in the illness, but blood studies soon return to normal. Diagnosis must rule out similar diseases such as acute poliomyelitis.

TREATMENT
Primarily supportive, treatment consists of endotracheal intubation or tracheotomy if the patient has difficulty clearing secretions. A trial dose of prednisone may be tried if the disease takes a relentlessly progressive course. Plasmapheresis is useful during the initial phase but offers no benefit if begun 2 weeks after onset.

SPECIAL CONSIDERATIONS
• Ascending sensory loss precedes motor loss. Stay alert for these signs.

• Respiratory support should begin at the first sign of dyspnea or a decreasing partial pressure of carbon dioxide.

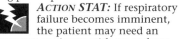 *ACTION STAT:* If respiratory failure becomes imminent, the patient may need an emergency airway with an endotracheal tube.

• After each position change, the patient's circulation should be stimulated through massage of pressure points. Foam, gel, or alternating pressure pads can be used at contact points.

• Passive range-of-motion exercises can be completed, perhaps using a Hubbard tank.

To help prevent aspiration, the patient's gag reflex should be tested and the head of the bed elevated before feedings.

• Postural hypotension is a risk as the patient regains strength and can tolerate a vertical position. If necessary, toe-to-groin elastic bandages or an abdominal binder should be used to prevent postural hypotension.

• Weak abdominal muscles may necessitate manual pressure on the bladder (Credé's method) before urination can occur.

• Prune juice and a high-bulk diet can prevent and relieve constipation. Some patients may need suppositories or Fleet enemas.

 TEACHING TIP: Before discharge, teach the patient and family how to transfer the patient from bed to wheelchair and from wheelchair to toilet or to tub, and how to walk short distances with a walker or a cane. Also provide instruction in helping the patient eat, compensate for facial weakness, and avoid skin breakdown.

Haemophilus influenzae infection

A small, gram-negative, pleomorphic aerobic bacillus, *Haemophilus influenzae* causes disease in many organ systems but most commonly attacks the respiratory system. In exudates, this organism predominantly resembles a coccobacillus.

H. influenzae is a common cause of epiglottitis, laryngotracheobronchitis, pneumonia, bronchiolitis, otitis media, and meningitis. Less often, it leads to bacterial endocarditis, conjunctivitis, facial cellulitis, septic arthritis, and osteomyelitis.

CAUSES

H. influenzae pneumonia is an increasingly common nosocomial infection. It infects about one-half of all children before age 1 and virtually all children by age 3, although a new vaccine given at ages 2, 4, and 6 months has reduced this number.

SIGNS AND SYMPTOMS

H. influenzae provokes a characteristic tissue response — acute suppurative inflammation. When this organism infects the larynx, trachea, and bronchial tree, it leads to mucosal edema and thick exudate; when it invades the lungs, it causes bronchopneumonia.

In the pharynx, *H. influenzae* usually produces no remarkable changes, except when it causes epiglottitis, which generally affects both the laryngeal and pharyngeal surfaces.

The pharyngeal mucosa may be reddened, rarely with soft yellow exudate. More often, it appears normal or shows only slight diffuse redness, even while severe pain makes swallowing difficult or impossible. These infections typically cause high fever and generalized malaise.

DIAGNOSTIC TESTS

Isolation of the organism confirms *H. influenzae* infection, usually with a blood culture. Other laboratory findings typically include a high white blood cell (WBC) count, a low WBC count in young children with severe infection, and *H. influenzae* bacteremia, found in many patients with meningitis.

TREATMENT

H. influenzae infection usually responds to a 2-week course of ampicillin (although resistant strains are becoming more common), cephalosporins, or chloramphenicol.

SPECIAL CONSIDERATIONS

• Proper positioning, humidification (croup tent) in children, and suctioning are used as needed to promote adequate respiratory function.
• For home treatment, the patient can use a room humidifier or breathe moist air from a shower or bath as necessary.

PREVENTION TIP: To help reduce the risk of infection, the *H. influenzae* vaccine should be given to children ages 2 (or younger) to 6. Measures that help prevent spread of this disease include maintaining respiratory isolation, using proper hand-washing technique, properly disposing of respiratory secretions, placing soiled tissues in a plastic bag, and decontaminating all equipment.

Hantavirus pulmonary syndrome

Mainly occurring in the southwestern United States, *Hantavirus* pulmonary syndrome is a new viral disease first reported in May 1993. Known for its high mortality, it

Screening for *Hantavirus* pulmonary syndrome

The Centers for Disease Control and Prevention (CDC) has developed a screening procedure to track cases of *Hantavirus* pulmonary syndrome. The screening criteria below identify potential and actual cases.

Potential cases

For a diagnosis of possible *Hantavirus* pulmonary syndrome, a patient must have one of the following:
● a febrile illness in a previously healthy person, characterized by unexplained adult respiratory distress syndrome
● bilateral interstitial pulmonary infiltrates that develop within 1 week of hospitalization, with respiratory compromise that requires supplemental oxygen
● an unexplained respiratory illness resulting in death and autopsy findings showing noncardiogenic pulmonary edema without an identifiable specific cause of death.

Exclusions

Of the patients who meet the above criteria, the CDC excludes those with any of the following:
● a predisposing underlying medical condition; for example, severe underlying pulmonary disease or acquired immunodeficiency syndrome (AIDS), or a medical condition (such as organ transplantation or rheumatoid arthritis) that requires immunosuppressive drug therapy
● an acute illness that provides a likely explanation for the respiratory illness — for example, a recent major trauma, burn, or surgery; recent seizures or a history of aspiration; another respiratory disorder such as respiratory syncytial virus in young children; influenza; or legionella pneumonia.

Confirmed cases

Cases of confirmed *Hantavirus* pulmonary syndrome must include the following:
● at least one serum or tissue specimen available for laboratory testing for evidence of *Hantavirus* infection
● in a patient with a compatible clinical illness, serologic evidence (presence of *Hantavirus*-specific immunoglobulin M [IgM] or rising titers of IgG), polymerase chain reaction for hantavirus ribonucleic acid, or positive immunohistochemistry for the *Hantavirus* antigen.

rapidly progresses from flulike symptoms to respiratory failure and, sometimes, death.

The *Hantavirus* strain that causes disease in Asia and Europe — mainly hemorrhagic fever and renal disease — is distinctly different from the one currently described in North America.

CAUSES

A member of the Bunyaviridae family, the genus *Hantavirus* (first isolated in 1977) is responsible for *Hantavirus* pulmonary syndrome. Disease transmission results from exposure to infected rodents.

Data suggest that the deer mouse is the main source, but pinton mice, brush mice, and western chipmunks living in close proximity to humans in rural areas also are sources. Infected rodents show no apparent illness but shed the virus in feces, urine, and saliva.

Human infection may occur from inhalation, ingestion (of contaminated food or water, for example), contact with rodent excrement, or rodent bites. Transmission from person to person or by mosquitos, fleas, or other arthropods hasn't been reported.

Hantavirus infections have been documented in people whose activities are associated with rodent contact, such as farming, hiking or camping in rodent-infested areas, and occupying rodent-infested dwellings.

SIGNS AND SYMPTOMS

Noncardiogenic pulmonary edema distinguishes the syndrome. Common signs and symptoms include myalgia, fever, headache, nausea and vomiting, and cough. Respiratory distress typically follows onset of a cough. Fever, hypoxia and, in some patients, markedly low blood pressure typify the hospital course.

Other signs and symptoms include a rising respiratory rate (28 breaths per minute or more) and an increased heart rate (120 beats per minute or more).

DIAGNOSTIC TESTS

Doctors are trying to identify the clinical features and laboratory results that distinguish *Hantavirus* pulmonary syndrome from other infections with similar features. For now, diagnosis hinges on patient history and physical examination, along with a protocol developed by the Centers for Disease Control and Prevention (CDC) with the Council of State and Territorial Epidemiologists. (See *Screening for* Hantavirus *pulmonary syndrome*.) The CDC and state health departments can perform definitive testing for *Hantavirus* exposure and antibody formation.

Laboratory tests usually show an elevated white blood cell count with certain white cells predominating, an elevated hematocrit, a decreased platelet count, an elevated partial thromboplastin time, and a normal fibrinogen level. Chest X-rays eventually show characteristic lung changes.

TREATMENT

Treatment consists of maintaining adequate oxygenation, monitoring vital signs, and intervening as needed to stabilize the patient's heart rate and blood pressure.

Drug therapy may involve vasopressors, such as dopamine or epinephrine, to correct hypotension. Fluid volume replacement also may be ordered (although the patient must not be overhydrated).

Clinical trials with ribavirin are currently underway.

SPECIAL CONSIDERATIONS

● A patent airway must be maintained by suctioning, if necessary.
● Adequate humidification is important and ventilator settings should be checked frequently.
● Cases of *Hantavirus* pulmonary syndrome should be reported to the state health department.

Headache

The most common patient complaint, headache usually arises as a symptom of an underlying disorder. About 90% of headaches are vascular, muscle contraction, or a combination; the remaining 10% reflect underlying intracranial, systemic, or psychological disorders.

Migraine headaches — probably the most intensively studied — are throbbing, vascular headaches that usually begin in childhood or adolescence and recur throughout adulthood. Affecting up to 10% of Americans, they have a strong familial incidence.

CAUSES

Most chronic headaches result from tension (muscle contraction) brought on by such conditions as emotional stress, fatigue, menstruation, or environmental stimuli (noise, crowds, bright lights).

Other causes include:
● glaucoma
● inflammation of the eyes or mucosa of the nasal or paranasal sinuses
● diseases of the scalp, teeth, extracranial arteries, or external or middle ear
● muscle spasms of the face, neck, or shoulders
● use of vasodilators (nitrates, alcohol, histamine)
● systemic disease

Drug therapy for migraines

For migraine headache, ergotamine alone or with caffeine may be effective. These drugs and others, such as metoclopramide or naproxen, work best when taken early in the course of an attack. If nausea and vomiting make oral administration impossible, these medications may be given as rectal suppositories.

Many clinicians prefer sumatriptan for acute migraine attacks or cluster headaches.

Migraine prevention

Drugs that can help *prevent* migraine headache include propranolol, atenolol, clonidine, and amitriptyline.

• hypoxia
• hypertension
• head trauma or tumor
• intracranial bleeding, abscess, or aneurysm.

Migraine headaches

The cause of migraines is unknown, but these headaches are associated with constriction and dilation of intracranial and extracranial arteries. Certain biochemical abnormalities are thought to occur during a migraine attack: local leakage of a vasodilator polypeptide called neurokinin through the dilated arteries, and a decrease in the blood serotonin level.

SIGNS AND SYMPTOMS

Migraine headaches and muscle contraction headaches produce different signs and symptoms.

Migraine headaches

Initially, migraine headache usually produces unilateral, pulsating pain, which later becomes more generalized. Commonly, the headache is preceded by visual defects, unilateral paresthesia, or speech disorders. The patient may experience irritability, anorexia, nausea, vomiting, and photophobia.

Muscle contraction headaches

Muscle contraction headaches produce a dull, persistent ache, tender spots on the head and neck, and a feeling of tightness around the head with a "hatband" distribution. Often, the pain is severe and unrelenting.

If caused by intracranial bleeding, these headaches may lead to neurologic deficits, such as paresthesia and muscle weakness; narcotics fail to relieve pain in these cases. If caused by a tumor, pain is most severe when the patient awakens.

DIAGNOSTIC TESTS

Diagnosis requires an investigation of the patient's history of recurrent headaches and examination of the head, neck, and nervous system. If the doctor suspects an underlying systemic disease (such as high blood pressure) or a psychosocial problem, the patient will be evaluated further.

Diagnostic tests may include skull X-rays, electroencephalography, computed tomography scan of the brain, and lumbar puncture.

TREATMENT

Depending on the type of headache, analgesics (ranging from aspirin to codeine or meperidine) may relieve symptoms. A tranquilizer, such as diazepam, may help during acute attacks.

Other measures include identifying and eliminating the underlying cause and, possibly, psychotherapy for headaches caused by emotional stress. Chronic tension headaches may warrant muscle relaxants.

Migraines may be treated with ergotamine or other drugs. (See *Drug therapy for migraines*.)

SPECIAL CONSIDERATIONS

• Measures to relieve headache pain include resting in a dark, quiet room during an attack and placing ice packs on the forehead or a cold cloth over the eyes.

TEACHING TIP: Instruct the patient to take prescribed medication at the onset of migraine symptoms. To prevent dehydration, advise him to drink plenty of fluids after nausea and vomiting subside.

Hearing loss

Loss of hearing results from a mechanical or nervous impediment to the transmission of sound waves. Hearing loss may be partial or complete and occurs in three major forms.

• *Conductive loss* is the interrupted passage of sound from the external ear to the junction of the stapes and oval window.

• *Sensorineural loss* refers to impaired cochlear or acoustic nerve dysfunction, causing failure of transmission of sound impulses within the inner ear or brain.

• *Mixed hearing loss* is a combination of conductive and sensorineural loss.

CAUSES

Hearing loss may be congenital, or it may result from drugs or illness, exposure to loud noise, or aging.

Congenital hearing loss

Congenital hearing loss may be transmitted as a dominant, autosomal dominant, autosomal recessive, or sex-linked recessive trait. In neonates, it also may result from trauma, toxicity, or infection during pregnancy or delivery.

Predisposing factors include a family history of hearing loss or known hereditary disorders, maternal exposure to rubella or syphilis during pregnancy, use of ototoxic drugs during pregnancy, prolonged fetal anoxia during delivery, and congenital abnormalities of the ears, nose, or throat. Trauma during delivery may damage the cochlea or acoustic nerve.

Sudden deafness

Sudden hearing loss may occur in a patient with no prior hearing impairment. This condition is considered a medical emergency because prompt treatment may restore full hearing. Acute infection is a leading cause of sudden deafness. (See *Sudden deafness: Causes and predisposing factors.*)

Noise-induced hearing loss

Hearing loss caused by loud noise may be transient or permanent, or it may follow prolonged exposure to loud noise (85 to 90 dB) or brief exposure to extremely loud noise (more than 90 dB). Such hearing loss is common in workers subjected to constant industrial noise and in military personnel, hunters, and rock musicians.

Presbycusis

An effect of aging, presbycusis results from a loss of hair cells in the organ of Corti. This disorder causes senso-

---

Sudden deafness: Causes and predisposing factors

Sudden hearing loss may result from acute infections, especially mumps, and other bacterial and viral infections—rubella, rubeola, influenza, herpes zoster, infectious mononucleosis, and mycoplasmal infections.

Other causes and predisposing factors include:
• metabolic disorders, including diabetes mellitus, hypothyroidism, and hyperlipoproteinemia
• vascular disorders, such as hypertension and arteriosclerosis
• head trauma or brain tumors
• ototoxic drugs, including tobramycin, streptomycin, quinine, gentamicin, furosemide, and ethacrynic acid
• neurologic disorders, such as multiple sclerosis and neurosyphilis
• blood dyscrasias, such as leukemia and hypercoagulation.

rineural hearing loss, usually of high-frequency tones.

SIGNS AND SYMPTOMS
The four types of hearing loss cause different signs and symptoms:
• With congenital hearing loss, a poor response to auditory stimuli generally becomes apparent within 2 to 3 days of birth. As the child grows older, hearing loss impairs speech development.
• With sudden deafness, clinical features depend on the underlying condition.
• Noise-induced hearing loss causes sensorineural damage. Initially, the patient loses perception of certain frequencies (around 4,000 Hz) but, with continued exposure, eventually loses perception of all frequencies.
• Presbycusis usually produces tinnitus and inability to understand the spoken word.

DIAGNOSTIC TESTS
Usually, the patient's medical, family, and occupational histories and a complete hearing examination provide ample evidence of hearing loss. These histories also may suggest possible causes or predisposing factors.

To determine if the patient has conductive, sensorineural, or mixed hearing loss, a doctor or an audiologist may perform various tests (Weber's test, Rinne test, and specialized hearing tests).

TREATMENT
Therapy depends on the type of hearing loss.

Congenital hearing loss
The underlying condition must be identified. If the condition doesn't improve with surgery, treatment focuses on teaching the patient to communicate through sign language, speech reading, or other effective means.

Sudden deafness
Sudden deafness calls for prompt identification and correction of the underlying cause. Prevention requires educating patients and health care professionals about the many causes of sudden deafness and ways to recognize and treat them.

Noise-induced hearing loss
Overnight rest usually restores normal hearing in those who have been exposed to noise levels greater than 90 dB for several hours, but not in those who have been exposed to such noise repeatedly. As hearing deteriorates, treatment must include speech and hearing rehabilitation.

Prevention of noise-induced hearing loss requires public recognition of the dangers of noise exposure and insistence on the use of protective devices during occupational exposure to noise.

Presbycusis
Patients with presbycusis usually require a hearing aid.

SPECIAL CONSIDERATIONS
• When speaking to a patient with hearing loss who can read lips, stand directly in front of him with the light on your face, and speak slowly and distinctly. Approach him within his visual range, and call attention to yourself by raising your arm. (Touching him may startle him.)

 PREVENTION TIP: To help prevent hearing loss, teach patients about the danger of excessive exposure to noise and potentially ototoxic drugs and chemicals and encourage the use of protective devices in a noisy environment. Caution pregnant women about the danger of exposure to infection (especially German measles).

Heart failure
A syndrome characterized by myocardial dysfunction, heart failure leads to impaired pump performance (reduced cardiac output) or to frank heart failure and abnormal circulatory congestion. Congestion of the systemic venous circulation may result in peripheral edema or an enlarged liver; congestion of pulmonary circulation

may bring on pulmonary edema — an acute, life-threatening emergency.

Pump failure usually occurs in a damaged left ventricle (left-sided heart failure), but may occur in the right ventricle (right-sided heart failure) either as a primary disorder or secondary to left-sided failure. Sometimes, left- and right-sided heart failure develop simultaneously.

Although heart failure may be acute (as a direct result of myocardial infarction), it's generally a chronic disorder associated with renal retention of sodium and water. Diagnostic and therapeutic advances have greatly improved the outlook for patients with heart failure, but the prognosis still depends on the underlying cause and its response to treatment.

CAUSES

Heart failure may result from a primary abnormality of the heart muscle (such as an infarction), inadequate myocardial perfusion due to coronary artery disease, or cardiomyopathy. Other causes include:

• mechanical disturbances in ventricular filling during diastole when there's too little blood for the ventricle to pump, as in mitral stenosis secondary to rheumatic heart disease or constrictive pericarditis and atrial fibrillation

• systolic hemodynamic disturbances, such as excessive cardiac workload due to volume overloading or pressure overload, that limit the heart's pumping ability.

Reduced cardiac output triggers three compensatory mechanisms — ventricular dilation, hypertrophy, and increased sympathetic activity — which improve cardiac output at the expense of increased ventricular work. (See *Compensatory mechanisms in heart failure,* page 134.)

Chronic heart failure may worsen as a result of respiratory tract infections, pulmonary embolism, stress, increased sodium or water intake, or failure to comply with therapy.

SIGNS AND SYMPTOMS

Left-sided heart failure primarily produces pulmonary signs and symptoms; right-sided heart failure causes primarily systemic signs and symptoms. However, heart failure commonly affects both sides of the heart.

Left-sided heart failure

Clinical signs include dyspnea, orthopnea, crackles, possible wheezing, hypoxia, respiratory acidosis, cough, cyanosis or pallor, palpitations, arrhythmias, elevated blood pressure, and pulsus alternans.

Right-sided heart failure

Clinical signs include dependent peripheral edema, hepatomegaly, splenomegaly, jugular vein distention, ascites, slow weight gain, arrhythmias, hepatojugular reflex, abdominal distention, nausea, vomiting, anorexia, weakness, fatigue, dizziness, and syncope.

Complications

Heart failure can lead to pulmonary edema, venostasis with a predisposition to thromboembolism, cerebral insufficiency, and renal insufficiency with severe electrolyte imbalance.

DIAGNOSTIC TESTS

Diagnosis of heart failure requires an electrocardiogram (ECG) and a chest X-ray. ECG usually reveals heart strain, an enlarged heart, or poor blood supply to the heart. It also may indicate an enlarged atrium, a fast heart rate, and premature heartbeats. Chest X-ray may show an enlarged heart and other characteristic findings. Pulmonary artery monitoring usually is done to monitor hemodynamic pressures.

TREATMENT

The aim of therapy is to improve pump function by reversing the compensatory mechanisms producing the symptoms. Heart failure can be controlled quickly by treatment that includes:

• diuresis (to reduce total blood volume and circulatory congestion)

• prolonged bed rest (to decrease demands on the heart)

PATHOPHYSIOLOGY

Compensatory mechanisms in heart failure

As the heart's pumping ability becomes increasingly impaired, cardiac output diminishes. This, in turn, triggers three compensatory mechanisms — ventricular dilation, hypertrophy, and increased sympathetic activity. Although these mechanisms boost cardiac output, they also force the ventricle to work harder.

Cardiac dilation
An increase in end-diastolic ventricular volume (preload) causes increased stroke work and stroke volume during contraction. As a result, cardiac muscle fibers are stretched beyond optimum limits, leading to pulmonary congestion and pulmonary hypertension, which in turn cause right-sided heart failure.

Ventricular hypertrophy
An increase in the muscle mass or diameter of the left ventricle allows the heart to pump against increased resistance (impedance) to the outflow of blood.

Greater ventricular diastolic pressure now is necessary to fill the enlarged ventricle. This may compromise diastolic coronary blood flow, limiting the oxygen supply to the ventricle and causing ischemia and impaired myocardial contractility.

Increased sympathetic activity
As a response to decreased cardiac output and blood pressure, sympathetic activity increases by enhancing peripheral vascular resistance, contractility, heart rate, and venous return.

Signs of increased sympathetic activity, such as cool extremities and clamminess, may indicate impending heart failure. Increased sympathetic activity also restricts blood flow to the kidneys, which respond by reducing the glomerular filtration rate and increasing tubular reabsorption of sodium and water, in turn expanding the circulating blood volume. This renal mechanism, if unchecked, can aggravate congestion and produce overt edema.

• digoxin (to strengthen myocardial contractility)
• vasodilators (to increase cardiac output by reducing impedance to ventricular outflow)
• antiembolism stockings (to prevent venostasis and thromboembolus formation).

SPECIAL CONSIDERATIONS
• During the acute phase, the patient is placed in Fowler's position and receives supplemental oxygen to ease breathing.
• Deep vein thrombosis caused by vascular congestion is a risk for this patient. Range-of-motion exercises, enforced bed rest, and antiembolism stockings can help prevent this condition.

 TEACHING TIP: Before the patient is discharged, reinforce teaching about the need to avoid foods high in sodium, to take a potassium supplement as prescribed, to eat high-potassium foods (such as bananas, apricots, and orange juice), and to take digoxin exactly as prescribed and immediately report signs of toxicity (anorexia, vomiting, and yellow vision). Also instruct him to report unusual pulse irregularities or a pulse less than 60 beats/minute, dizziness, blurred vision, shortness of breath, persistent dry cough, palpitations, increased fatigue, paroxysmal nocturnal dyspnea, swollen ankles, decreased urine output, or rapid weight gain.

Hemophilia

A hereditary bleeding disorder, hemophilia results from deficiency of specific clotting factors. After a platelet plug forms at a bleeding site, the clotting factor deficiency impairs formation of a stable fibrin clot.

Hemophilia A (classic hemophilia), accounting for over 80% of hemophiliac cases, results from deficiency of factor VIII. *Hemophilia B* (Christmas disease), seen in 15% of hemophiliacs, results from deficiency of factor IX. However, recent evidence suggests that nonfunctioning of factors VIII and IX, rather than their deficiency, may explain hemophilia.

The severity and prognosis of hemophilia vary with the degree of clotting factor deficiency and the bleeding site. Treatment advances have greatly improved the prognosis, and many hemophiliacs have normal life spans.

CAUSES

Hemophilia A and B are inherited as X-linked recessive traits. This means that female carriers have a 50% chance of transmitting the gene to each daughter, who would then be a carrier, and a 50% chance of transmitting the gene to each son, who would be born with hemophilia.

SIGNS AND SYMPTOMS

Hemophilia produces abnormal bleeding, which may be mild, moderate, or severe, depending on the degree of factor deficiency.

The mild form of hemophilia commonly goes undiagnosed until adulthood, because the patient doesn't bleed spontaneously or after minor trauma but has prolonged bleeding if challenged by major trauma or surgery.

Severe hemophilia causes spontaneous bleeding. Spontaneous bleeding or severe bleeding after minor trauma may produce large subcutaneous and deep intramuscular hematomas.

Bleeding into joints and muscles causes pain, swelling, extreme tenderness, and possibly permanent deformity. Bleeding near peripheral nerves may result in peripheral neuropathies, pain, paresthesia, and muscle atrophy.

If bleeding impairs blood flow through a major vessel, it may cause ischemia and gangrene. Pharyngeal, lingual, intracardial, intracerebral, and intracranial bleeding may lead to shock and death.

Moderate hemophilia causes symptoms similar to severe hemophilia but produces only occasional spontaneous bleeding episodes.

DIAGNOSTIC TESTS

Typically, hemophilia is diagnosed in a patient who experiences prolonged bleeding after injury or surgery (including tooth extraction) or who has episodes of spontaneous bleeding into the muscles or joints. Tests of specific clotting factors determine the type and severity of hemophilia.

TREATMENT

Hemophilia isn't curable, but treatment can prevent crippling deformities and prolong life expectancy. Correct treatment quickly stops bleeding by increasing plasma levels of deficient clotting factors. Treatment varies with the type of hemophilia:
• In hemophilia A, cryoprecipitated antihemophilic factor (AHF), lyophilized AHF, or both, given in doses large enough to raise clotting factor levels above 25% of normal, can permit normal hemostasis. Before surgery, AHF is administered to raise clotting factors. Levels are then kept within a normal range until the wound has completely healed.
• In hemophilia B, administering factor IX concentrate during bleeding episodes increases factor IX levels. The patient who undergoes surgery needs careful management by a hematologist with expertise in hemophilia care and requires deficient factor replacement before and after

Tips on managing hemophilia

Parents who have a child with hemophilia need thorough teaching to help them cope with the disease and to help the child cope. Provide these instructions.

Reduce the risk of injury and bleeding

● Instruct parents to notify the doctor immediately after even a minor injury — but especially after an injury to the head, neck, or abdomen. Such injuries may call for special blood factor replacement. Also, parents should check with the doctor before allowing dental extractions or any other surgery.
● Stress the importance of regular, careful toothbrushing to prevent the need for dental surgery. The child should use a soft toothbrush.
● Advise parents to stay alert for signs and symptoms of severe internal bleeding: severe pain or swelling in a joint or muscle, stiffness, decreased joint movement, severe abdominal pain, blood in the urine, severe headache, and black, tarry stools.

Minimize other risks

● Inform the parents that because the child receives blood components, he's at risk for hepatitis. Early signs and symptoms — headache, fever, decreased appetite, nausea, vomiting, abdominal tenderness, and pain over the liver — may appear 3 weeks to 6 months after treatment with blood components.
● Discuss the increased risk for human immunodeficiency virus (HIV) infection if the child received a blood product before routine screening for HIV began. Tell the parents to ask the doctor about periodic testing for HIV.

Review precautions and treatment

● Urge parents to make sure their child wears a medical identification bracelet at all times.

● *Warn parents never to give their child aspirin.* It can increase the tendency to bleed. Advise them to give acetaminophen instead.
● Instruct parents to protect their child from injury, but to avoid unnecessary restrictions that impair his development. For example, they can sew padded patches into the knees and elbows of a toddler's clothing to protect these joints during falls. They must forbid an older child to play contact sports such as football but can encourage swimming or golf.
● Teach parents to apply cold compresses or ice bags to an injured area and to elevate it or to apply light pressure to a bleeding site. To prevent recurrence of bleeding, advise parents to restrict their child's activity for 48 hours after his bleeding is under control.
● If parents have been trained to give blood factor components at home to avoid hospitalization, make sure they know venipuncture and infusion techniques and don't delay treatment during bleeding episodes.
● Instruct parents to keep blood factor concentrate and infusion equipment on hand, even on vacation.
● Emphasize the importance of having the child keep routine appointments at the local hemophilia center.

Recommend genetic screening

● Daughters should have genetic screening and testing to determine if they're hemophilia carriers. Affected males should have counseling as well. If they mate with a noncarrier, all of their daughters will be carriers; if they mate with a carrier, each male or female child has a 25% chance of being affected.
● For more information, refer parents to the National Hemophilia Foundation.

surgery — even for minor surgery such as a dental extraction.

In addition, epsilon-aminocaproic acid is commonly used for oral bleeding to inhibit the active fibrinolytic system present in the oral mucosa.

SPECIAL CONSIDERATIONS
• Applying cold compresses or ice bags and raising the injured part helps to stop bleeding.
• If the patient has bled into a joint, the joint should be elevated immediately. Range-of-motion exercises, begun at least 48 hours after the bleeding is controlled, can help restore joint mobility.
• Pain can be controlled with an analgesic. I.M. injections are avoided because of possible hematoma formation at the injection site. Aspirin and aspirin-containing medications are contraindicated because they decrease platelet adherence and may increase the bleeding.
• To prevent recurrence of bleeding, the patient's activity should be restricted for 48 hours after bleeding is under control.
• Genetic counseling helps hemophilia carriers understand how this disease is transmitted. (See *Tips on managing hemophilia*.)

Hemorrhoids

Hemorrhoids (varicosities in the venous plexus) are painful, enlarged bleeding veins in the anal region. Hemorrhoids may be internal or external; external hemorrhoids may protrude from the rectum.

CAUSES
Hemorrhoids probably result from increased intravenous pressure in the hemorrhoidal plexus. Predisposing factors include occupations that require prolonged standing or sitting; straining due to constipation, diarrhea, coughing, sneezing, or vomiting; and heart failure.

Other predisposing factors include:
• hepatic disease
• alcoholism
• anorectal infections

• loss of muscle tone due to old age, rectal surgery, or episiotomy
• anal intercourse
• pregnancy.

SIGNS AND SYMPTOMS
Hemorrhoids are classified as first-degree, second-degree, or third-degree, depending on their severity. Signs and symptoms vary accordingly:
• Although *first-degree* hemorrhoids may produce no symptoms, they commonly cause painless, intermittent bleeding during defecation. Bright-red blood appears in stools or on toilet paper. The hemorrhoids may itch from poor anal hygiene.
• When *second-degree* hemorrhoids prolapse, they're usually painless and return to the anal canal spontaneously after defecation.
• *Third-degree* hemorrhoids cause constant discomfort and prolapse in response to an increase in intra-abdominal pressure. They must be manually reduced. Thrombosis of external hemorrhoids produces sudden rectal pain and a subcutaneous, large, firm lump that the patient can feel.
If hemorrhoids cause severe or recurrent bleeding, they may lead to secondary anemia with pallor, fatigue, and weakness.

DIAGNOSTIC TESTS
Physical examination confirms external hemorrhoids. Proctoscopy confirms internal hemorrhoids and rules out rectal polyps.

TREATMENT
Effective treatment depends on the type and severity of the hemorrhoid and on the patient's overall condition.

Nonsurgical treatment
The doctor may recommend measures to ease pain, combat swelling and congestion, and regulate bowel habits. Patients can relieve constipation by increasing the amount of raw vegetables, fruit, and whole grain cereal in the diet or by using stool softeners.

Venous congestion can be prevented by avoiding prolonged sitting on the toilet; local swelling and pain can be decreased with local anesthetic agents (lotions, creams, or suppositories), astringents, or cold compresses, followed by warm sitz baths or thermal packs.

Other nonsurgical treatments include injection of a sclerosing solution to produce scar tissue that decreases prolapse, manual reduction, and hemorrhoid ligation or laser ablation.

Hemorrhoidectomy

Hemorrhoidectomy (surgical removal of the hemorrhoid) is indicated for patients with severe bleeding, intolerable pain and pruritus, and large prolapse.

SPECIAL CONSIDERATIONS

After hemorrhoid surgery:
• The patient is observed for signs of prolonged rectal bleeding. Treatment includes analgesics and sitz baths.
• Caution the patient to avoid stool softeners soon after hemorrhoidectomy because firm stools act as a natural dilator to prevent anal stricture from the scar tissue.

 TEACHING TIP: Inform the patient that taking a bulk medication such as psyllium about 1 hour after the evening meal helps to ensure a daily bowel movement.

Hepatic encephalopathy

Also called hepatic coma, hepatic encephalopathy is a neurologic syndrome that develops as a complication of chronic liver disease. Most common in patients with cirrhosis, hepatic encephalopathy usually reflects ammonia intoxication of the brain. It may be acute and self-limiting, or chronic and progressive. In advanced stages, the prognosis is extremely poor.

CAUSES

Hepatic encephalopathy results from rising blood ammonia levels, as from improper shunting of blood, excessive protein intake, sepsis, excessive

accumulation of nitrogenous body wastes (caused by constipation or GI bleeding), and bacterial action on protein and urea to form ammonia.

Improper shunting of blood may result from portal hypertension or from surgically created portal-systemic shunts. Cirrhosis further compounds this problem. When portal blood shunts past the liver, it causes ammonia to directly enter the systemic circulation; from there, it is carried to the brain.

SIGNS AND SYMPTOMS

Clinical features of hepatic encephalopathy vary with the severity of neurologic involvement. These features develop in four stages.

Prodromal stage

The prodromal stage is commonly overlooked because early signs and symptoms, such as slight personality changes (disorientation, forgetfulness, slurred speech) and a slight tremor, are subtle.

Impending stage

In the impending stage, tremor progresses to asterixis, the hallmark of hepatic encephalopathy. Asterixis is characterized by quick, irregular extensions and flexions of the wrists and fingers when the wrists are held out straight and the hands flexed upward. Lethargy, aberrant behavior, and apraxia also occur.

Stuporous stage

During the stuporous stage, the patient experiences hyperventilation with stupor; typically, he is noisy and abusive when aroused.

Comatose stage

The comatose stage is marked by hyperactive reflexes, a positive Babinski's sign, coma, and a musty, sweet breath odor.

DIAGNOSTIC TESTS

Along with a history of liver disease, elevated serum ammonia levels in venous and arterial samples confirm hepatic encephalopathy. Slowed brain

activity indicated by electroencephalography supports the diagnosis.

TREATMENT

Treatment involves correcting the
underlying cause and reducing blood
ammonia levels to stop the progression of encephalopathy. Such treatment eliminates ammonia-producing
substances from the GI tract by:
• administration of neomycin to suppress bacterial flora (preventing them
from converting amino acids into
ammonia)
• sorbitol-induced catharsis to produce osmotic diarrhea
• continuous aspiration of blood
from the stomach
• reduction of dietary protein intake
• lactulose administration to reduce
blood ammonia levels.

Other treatments

Treatment also may include potassium supplements to correct alkalosis
(caused by increased ammonia levels). Some patients need hemodialysis
to temporarily clear toxic blood. Exchange transfusions may provide dramatic but temporary improvement;
however, they require a large amount
of blood.

Salt-poor albumin may be used to
maintain fluid and electrolyte balance, replace depleted albumin levels, and restore plasma.

SPECIAL CONSIDERATIONS

• The patient's handwriting should
be checked daily, if possible, to monitor the progression of neurologic involvement.
• The patient must consume a low-
protein diet, with carbohydrates supplying most of the calories.
• Restraints may be used, if necessary,
but sedatives should be avoided.
• Using artificial tears or eye patches
protects the comatose patient's eyes
from corneal injury.

Hepatitis, nonviral

Classified as toxic or drug-induced
(idiosyncratic) hepatitis, nonviral hepatitis is an inflammation of the liv-

er. Most patients recover from this illness, although a few develop fulminating hepatitis or cirrhosis.

CAUSES

Nonviral hepatitis usually results
from exposure to certain chemicals or
drugs.

Toxic hepatitis

Various hepatotoxins (carbon tetrachloride, acetaminophen, trichloro-
ethylene, poisonous mushrooms,
vinyl chloride) can cause toxic hepatitis. After exposure to these
agents, liver damage usually occurs
within 24 to 48 hours, depending on
the dose. Alcohol, anoxia, and preexisting liver disease exacerbate the toxic effects of some of these agents.

Drug-induced hepatitis

Idiosyncratic hepatitis may stem
from a hypersensitivity reaction
unique to the affected person (unlike
toxic hepatitis, which appears to affect all people indiscriminately).
Among the drugs that may cause this
type of hepatitis are niacin, halo-
thane, sulfonamides, isoniazid,
methyldopa, and phenothiazines.

In hypersensitive people, symptoms of hepatic dysfunction may appear at any time during or after exposure to these drugs, but usually
emerge after 2 to 5 weeks of therapy.

SIGNS AND SYMPTOMS

Clinical features of toxic and drug-induced hepatitis vary with the severity
of liver damage and the causative
agent. In most patients, signs and
symptoms resemble those of viral hepatitis: anorexia, nausea, vomiting,
jaundice, dark urine, hepatomegaly,
possible abdominal pain, and clay-
colored stools or pruritus with the
cholestatic form of hepatitis.

Carbon tetrachloride poisoning
also produces headache, dizziness,
drowsiness, and vasomotor collapse.
Halothane-related hepatitis produces
fever, moderate leukocytosis, and
eosinophilia. Chlorpromazine results
in a rash, abrupt fever, arthralgias,

lymphadenopathy, and epigastric or right upper quadrant pain.

DIAGNOSTIC TESTS
Diagnosis requires a thorough patient history and blood tests to detect liver inflammation. A liver biopsy may be done to identify the underlying cause.

TREATMENT
Effective treatment must remove the causative agent by lavage, catharsis, or hyperventilation, depending on the exposure route. Acetylcysteine may serve as an antidote for toxic hepatitis caused by acetaminophen poisoning, but doesn't prevent hepatitis caused by other substances.

Corticosteroids may be given to a patient with drug-induced hepatitis. Thioctic acid, an investigational agent, may be effective in mushroom poisoning.

SPECIAL CONSIDERATIONS
 PREVENTION TIP: Proper use of drugs and proper handling of cleaning agents and solvents are key components in preventing nonviral hepatitis.

Hepatitis, viral
A fairly common systemic disease, viral hepatitis is marked by hepatic cell destruction, necrosis, and autolysis, leading to anorexia, jaundice, and hepatomegaly. In most patients, hepatic cells eventually regenerate with little or no residual damage. However, old age and serious underlying disorders make complications more likely. The prognosis is poor if edema and hepatic encephalopathy develop.

There are five major types of viral hepatitis: hepatitis A, B, C, D, and E. (See *Five types of hepatitis*.)

CAUSES
The five major types of viral hepatitis result from infection with the causative viruses.

Highly contagious, *hepatitis A* usually is transmitted by the fecal-oral route but sometimes can be transmitted parenterally. It usually results from ingesting contaminated food, milk, or water.

Hepatitis B is transmitted by direct exchange of contaminated blood or by contact with human secretions and feces. For this reason, nurses, doctors, laboratory technicians, and dentists are frequently exposed to hepatitis B, commonly as a result of wearing defective gloves. Transmission also occurs during intimate sexual contact and through perinatal transmission.

Hepatitis C is usually transmitted through transfused blood from asymptomatic donors.

Hepatitis D is found only in patients with an acute or chronic episode of hepatitis B and requires the presence of the hepatitis B surface antigen.

Hepatitis E is transmitted enterically, much like type A.

SIGNS AND SYMPTOMS
All types of hepatitis cause similar findings. Typically, signs and symptoms progress in three stages — prodromal (preicteric), clinical (icteric), and recovery (posticteric).

Prodromal stage
In the prodromal stage, the patient typically complains of easy fatigue and anorexia, generalized malaise, depression, headache, weakness, arthralgia, myalgia, photophobia, and nausea with vomiting. He also may run a fever and experience changes in his ability to taste and smell. Dark-colored urine and clay-colored stools may appear.

Clinical stage
The patient who progresses to the clinical stage may have pruritus, abdominal pain or tenderness, and indigestion. Early in this stage, he may complain of anorexia; later, his appetite may return. The sclerae, mucous membranes, and skin may reveal jaundice, which can last for 1 to 2 weeks. The liver and spleen may enlarge.

Recovery stage

During the recovery stage, most signs and symptoms decrease or subside. This stage commonly lasts 2 to 12 weeks.

DIAGNOSTIC TESTS

A hepatitis profile identifies antibodies specific to the causative virus, establishing the type of hepatitis. Additional findings from liver function studies support the diagnosis. Liver biopsy may be performed if chronic hepatitis is suspected.

TREATMENT

No specific drug therapy exists for hepatitis, except for hepatitis C, which has been treated somewhat successfully with interferon alfa. Instead, the patient is advised to rest in the early stages of the illness and to combat anorexia by eating small, high-calorie, high-protein meals. Protein intake should be reduced if signs of precoma (lethargy, confusion, and mental changes) develop.

In acute viral hepatitis, hospitalization usually is required only for patients with severe symptoms or complications. Parenteral nutrition may be needed if the patient experiences persistent vomiting and can't maintain oral intake.

Antiemetics may be given 30 minutes before meals to relieve nausea and prevent vomiting. For severe pruritus, the resin cholestyramine may be given.

SPECIAL CONSIDERATIONS

- Enteric precautions must be used when caring for patients with hepatitis A or E. Visitors should be informed about isolation precautions.
- Adequate patient rest is an important part of care. Rest periods should be provided throughout the day.
- Adequate nutrition and hydration are important. Overloading the patient's meal tray or overmedicating him may diminish his appetite. Chipped ice and effervescent soft drinks help maintain hydration without inducing vomiting.

PATHOPHYSIOLOGY

Five types of hepatitis

Viral hepatitis occurs in five forms:

- *Type A* (infectious or short-incubation hepatitis) is rising among homosexuals and in people with immunosuppression related to human immunodeficiency virus (HIV) infection.
- *Type B* (serum or long-incubation hepatitis) also is increasing among HIV-positive individuals. Routine screening of donor blood for the hepatitis B surface antigen has decreased the incidence of posttransfusion cases, but transmission by needles shared by drug abusers remains a major problem.
- *Type C* accounts for about 20% of all viral hepatitis cases and for most posttransfusion cases.
- *Type D* (delta hepatitis) is responsible for about 50% of cases of fulminant hepatitis. Fulminant hepatitis causes unremitting liver failure with encephalopathy. It progresses to coma and commonly leads to death within 2 weeks. In the United States, hepatitis D is confined to people who are frequently exposed to blood and blood products, such as I.V. drug users and hemophiliacs.
- *Type E* (formerly grouped with type C under the name *non-A, non-B hepatitis*) occurs primarily in people who have recently returned from an endemic area, such as India, Africa, Asia, or Central America.

Herniated disk

A herniated disk (also called ruptured disk, slipped disk, and herniated nucleus pulposus) occurs when all or part of the nucleus pulposus — the soft, gelatinous, central portion of an intervertebral disk — is forced through the disk's weakened or torn outer ring (anulus fibrosus). When this happens, the extruded disk may impinge on spinal nerve roots as they exit from the spinal canal or on the spinal cord itself, resulting in back pain and other signs of nerve root irritation. Herniated disk is most common in adults under age 45.

CAUSES

A herniated disk may result from severe trauma or strain or may be related to intervertebral joint degeneration. In older patients whose disks have begun to degenerate, minor trauma may cause herniation. Most herniated disks occur in the lumbar and lumbosacral regions.

SIGNS AND SYMPTOMS

The overriding symptom of lumbar herniated disk is severe, low back pain, which radiates to the buttocks, legs, and feet (usually unilaterally). When herniation follows trauma, the pain may begin suddenly, subside in a few days, then recur at shorter intervals and with progressive intensity.

Sciatic pain follows, starting as a dull pain in the buttocks. Valsalva's maneuver, coughing, sneezing, and bending intensify the pain, which is often accompanied by muscle spasms. A herniated disk may also cause sensory and motor loss in the area innervated by the compressed spinal nerve root and, in later stages, weakness and atrophy of leg muscles.

DIAGNOSTIC TESTS

A careful patient history, including the mechanisms that intensify disk pain, is vital. The straight-leg-raising test may be done to support the diagnosis.

Spinal X-rays rule out other disorders but may not diagnose a herniated disk. Aside from physical findings and X-rays, myelography, a computed tomography scan, and magnetic resonance imaging provide the most specific diagnostic information.

These tests show spinal canal compression by herniated disk material.

TREATMENT

Initial measures are conservative and consist of several weeks of bed rest (possibly with pelvic traction), heat application, an exercise program, and medication. If neurologic impairment progresses rapidly, surgery may be necessary.

Aspirin reduces inflammation and edema at the injury site. Rarely, corticosteroids such as dexamethasone may be prescribed for the same purpose. Muscle relaxants, especially diazepam or methocarbamol, may also be beneficial.

A patient who fails to respond to conservative treatment may need surgery. The most common procedure, laminectomy, involves excision of a portion of the lamina and removal of the protruding disk.

If laminectomy doesn't alleviate pain and disability, spinal fusion may be necessary to overcome segmental instability. Laminectomy and spinal fusion are sometimes performed concurrently to stabilize the spine.

Other treatments

Chemonucleolysis — injection of the enzyme chymopapain into the herniated disk to dissolve nucleus pulposus — is a possible alternative to laminectomy. Microdiskectomy can be used to remove fragments of the herniated disk.

SPECIAL CONSIDERATIONS

• If the patient requires myelography, reassure him that a sedative can be given before the test, if needed, to reduce anxiety and increase comfort. Before myelography, the patient should be questioned carefully about allergies to iodides, iodine-containing substances, or seafood (such allergies may indicate sensitivity to the test's radiopaque dye).
• After myelography, the patient should remain in bed with his head elevated and drink plenty of fluids. He is monitored for seizures and an allergic reaction.

• Analgesics may be administered 30 minutes before initial attempts at sitting or walking to reduce discomfort.

 TEACHING TIP: Teach the patient who has undergone spinal fusion how to wear a brace and perform straight-leg-raising and toe-pointing exercises as necessary. Explain the importance of proper body mechanics — bending at the knees and hips (never at the waist), standing straight, and carrying objects close to the body.

Herpes simplex

Herpes simplex is a recurrent viral infection caused by *Herpesvirus hominis* (HVH), a widespread infectious agent. Herpes Type 1 affects the skin and mucous membranes and commonly produces cold sores and fever blisters. Herpes Type 2 primarily affects the genital area.

Primary HVH infection is the leading cause of childhood gingivostomatitis in children ages 1 to 3. It can pass to the fetus transplacentally and, in early pregnancy, may cause spontaneous abortion or premature birth.

Herpes occurs worldwide and is most prevalent among children in lower socioeconomic groups who live in crowded environments. Saliva, feces, urine, skin lesions, and purulent eye exudate are potential infection sources.

CAUSES

Herpes Type 1 is transmitted by oral and respiratory secretions. Herpes Type 2 is transmitted by sexual contact. However, cross-infection may result from orogenital sex.

SIGNS AND SYMPTOMS

About 85% of HVH infections cause subtle symptoms that go unnoticed. The others produce localized lesions and systemic reactions.

After the first infection, a patient is a carrier susceptible to recurrent infections, which may be provoked by fever, menses, stress, heat, and cold. In recurrent infections, the patient rarely has constitutional signs and symptoms.

In neonates, signs and symptoms of HVH infection usually appear a week or two after birth. They range from localized skin lesions to a disseminated infection of the liver, lungs, or brain. Common complications include seizures, mental retardation, blindness, chorioretinitis, deafness, microcephaly, diabetes insipidus, and spasticity. Up to 90% of infants with disseminated disease die.

Primary infection may be generalized or localized.

Generalized infection

After an incubation period of 2 to 12 days, the patient experiences fever, pharyngitis, erythema, and edema. A brief prodrome of tingling and itching is followed by eruption of primary lesions, which appear as vesicles on an erythematous base. Eventually, the lesions rupture and leave a painful ulcer, followed by a yellowish crust. Healing begins 7 to 10 days after onset and is complete in 3 weeks.

Vesicles may form on any part of the oral mucosa and may be accompanied by submaxillary lymphadenopathy, increased salivation, halitosis, anorexia, and fever of up to 105° F (40.6° C). Herpetic stomatitis may lead to severe dehydration in children.

A generalized infection usually runs its course in 4 to 10 days. In this form, virus reactivation causes cold sores — single or grouped vesicles in and around the mouth.

Localized infection

Genital herpes usually affects adolescents and young adults. Typically painful, the initial attack produces fluid-filled vesicles that ulcerate and heal in 1 to 3 weeks. Fever, regional lymphadenopathy, and dysuria also may occur.

Herpetic keratoconjunctivitis usually is unilateral and causes only local symptoms: conjunctivitis, regional adenopathy, blepharitis, and vesicles on the lid. The patient may also experience excessive lacrimation, ede-

Herpetic whitlow: Occupational hazard?

Herpetic whitlow, a herpes simplex infection of the finger, commonly affects health care workers.

Identifying clinical features
First, the finger tingles and then becomes red, swollen, and painful. Vesicles with a red halo erupt and may ulcerate or coalesce. Other effects may include satellite vesicles, fever, chills, malaise, and a red streak up the arm.

Preventing transmission
To prevent spread of the herpes virus, abstain from direct patient care if you have an outbreak of herpetic whitlow. Don't share towels or utensils with uninfected people. Also, teach colleagues and other susceptible people about the risk of contracting the disease.

ma, chemosis, photophobia, and purulent exudate.

Herpetic whitlow may occur on the finger. (See *Herpetic whitlow: Occupational hazard?*)

DIAGNOSTIC TESTS
Typical lesions may suggest HVH infection. Confirmation requires isolation of the virus from local lesions and a histologic biopsy. A rise in antibodies and moderate leukocytosis may support the diagnosis.

TREATMENT
Symptomatic and supportive therapy is essential. Generalized primary infection usually requires an analgesic-antipyretic to reduce fever and relieve pain. Anesthetic mouthwashes such as viscous lidocaine may reduce pain from mouth ulcers, enabling the pa-

tient to eat and preventing dehydration. Drying agents such as calamine lotion make labial lesions less painful.

A 5% acyclovir ointment may bring relief to patients with genital herpes or to immunosuppressed patients with HVH skin infections. Acyclovir I.V. helps treat more severe infections.

Patients with eye infections require an ophthalmologist's care. Topical corticosteroids are contraindicated in active infection, but idoxuridine, trifluridine, and vidarabine are effective.

SPECIAL CONSIDERATIONS
 TEACHING TIP: Teach the patient about self-care during an HVH outbreak and ways to avoid infecting others. If the patient has an active outbreak, advise him to use warm compresses or take sitz baths several times a day and to increase his fluid intake. Caution him to avoid all sexual contact during the active stage. Also, tell patients with cold sores not to kiss infants or people with eczema. (Those with genital herpes pose no risk to infants if their hygiene is meticulous.)
• Pregnant women with herpes infections should have weekly viral cultures of the cervix and external genitalia starting at 32 weeks' gestation.

Herpes zoster
Also called shingles, herpes zoster is an acute unilateral and segmental inflammation of the dorsal root ganglia caused by infection with the herpesvirus varicella-zoster — the virus that causes chickenpox. The disorder produces localized vesicular skin lesions confined to a dermatome, and severe neuralgic pain in peripheral areas innervated by the nerves arising in the inflamed root ganglia.

The prognosis is good unless the infection spreads to the brain. Eventually, most patients recover completely, except for possible scarring and, in corneal damage, visual impairment. Occasionally, neuralgia may persist for months or years.

Herpes zoster occurs primarily in adults, especially those past age 50. It seldom recurs.

CAUSES

Herpes zoster results from reactivation of varicella virus that has lain dormant in the cerebral ganglia or the ganglia of posterior nerve roots since a previous episode of chickenpox. Exactly how or why this reactivation occurs isn't clear.

SIGNS AND SYMPTOMS

Herpes zoster usually runs a typical course with classic signs and symptoms. However, serious complications sometimes occur.

Onset of disease

Herpes zoster begins with fever and malaise. Within 2 to 4 days, severe deep pain, pruritus, and paresthesia or hyperesthesia develop, usually on the trunk and occasionally on the arms and legs in a dermatomal distribution. Pain may be continuous or intermittent and usually lasts 1 to 4 weeks.

Skin lesions

Up to 2 weeks after the first symptoms, small red nodular skin lesions erupt on painful areas. Sometimes nodules don't appear, but when they do, they quickly become vesicles filled with clear fluid or pus.

About 10 days after appearing, vesicles dry and form scabs. When they rupture, the lesions often become infected and, in severe cases, may lead to enlargement of regional lymph nodes. Intense pain may precede the rash and follow scab formation.

Nerve involvement

Occasionally, herpes zoster involves the cranial nerves. Vesicles may form in the external auditory canal, and the patient may experience ipsilateral facial palsy, hearing loss, dizziness, and loss of taste.

Complications

In rare cases, herpes zoster leads to generalized central nervous system infection, muscle atrophy, motor paralysis, acute transverse myelitis, and ascending myelitis. More commonly, generalized infection causes acute retention of urine and unilateral paralysis of the diaphragm. In postherpetic neuralgia, intractable neuralgic pain may persist for years.

DIAGNOSTIC TESTS

A positive diagnosis usually isn't possible until characteristic skin lesions develop. Examination of vesicular fluid and infected tissue shows eosinophilic intranuclear inclusions and varicella virus. Lumbar puncture shows increased pressure; examination of cerebrospinal fluid reveals increased protein levels and, possibly, pleocytosis.

Staining antibodies from vesicular fluid and identification under fluorescent light differentiates herpes zoster from localized herpes simplex.

TREATMENT

No specific treatment exists. Supportive treatment aims to relieve itching and neuralgic pain with calamine lotion or another antipruritic. Aspirin may be given, possibly with codeine or another analgesic. If bacteria have infected ruptured vesicles, treatment usually includes an appropriate systemic antibiotic.

Trigeminal zoster with corneal involvement calls for instillation of idoxuridine ointment or another antiviral agent.

Acyclovir seems to stop progression of the rash and prevent visceral complications. In immunocompromised patients, acyclovir therapy may be given I.V.

SPECIAL CONSIDERATIONS

• Care focuses on keeping the patient comfortable, maintaining meticulous hygiene, and preventing infection.
• During the acute phase, the patient needs adequate rest and supportive care to promote healing of lesions.
• Calamine lotion can be applied liberally to lesions. If lesions are severe and widespread, a wet dressing may be used. The patient must avoid

scratching the lesions. If vesicles rupture, a cold compress should be applied.

 TEACHING TIP: To decrease the pain of oral lesions, advise the patient to use a soft toothbrush, eat a soft diet, and use saline mouthwash. Reassure him that herpetic pain eventually will subside.

Hiatal hernia

Hiatal hernia, or hiatus, is a defect in the diaphragm that allow a portion of the stomach to pass through the diaphragmatic opening into the chest. A hiatal hernia can be sliding or paraesophageal ("rolling"). A mixed type, which includes features of both, also occurs. (See *Two types of hiatal hernia.*)

In a *sliding hernia,* both the stomach and the gastroesophageal junction slip up into the chest. In *paraesophageal hernia,* a part of the greater curvature of the stomach rolls through the diaphragmatic defect. Treatment can prevent such complications as strangulation of the herniated intrathoracic portion of the stomach.

CAUSES
Usually, hiatal hernia results from muscle weakening that's common with and may occur secondary to esophageal cancer, kyphoscoliosis, trauma, or certain surgical procedures. Hernia also may result from certain diaphragmatic malformations that cause congenital weakness.

Conditions that increase intra-abdominal pressure (such as pregnancy, obesity, constrictive clothing, straining, coughing, Valsalva's maneuver, or extreme physical exertion) also may cause hiatal hernia.

SIGNS AND SYMPTOMS
With paraesophageal hernia, symptoms include a feeling of fullness in the chest or pain resembling angina pectoris. Even if it produces no symptoms, this type of hernia requires surgical treatment because of the high risk of strangulation.

A sliding hernia without an incompetent sphincter produces no reflux or symptoms and, consequently, doesn't require treatment. When a sliding hernia does cause symptoms, they are typical of gastric reflux:
• pyrosis (heartburn) 1 to 4 hours after eating, which is aggravated by reclining, belching, and increased intra-abdominal pressure
• retrosternal or substernal chest pain (most common after meals or at bedtime), which is aggravated by reclining, belching, and increased intra-abdominal pressure

Other common signs and symptoms reflect possible complications:
• Dysphagia (difficulty swallowing) occurs when the hernia causes esophagitis, esophageal ulceration, or stricture.
• Bleeding may be mild or massive, frank or occult; the source may be esophagitis or erosions of the gastric pouch.
• Severe pain and shock result from incarceration, in which a large portion of the stomach is caught above the diaphragm. Incarceration may lead to perforation of a gastric ulcer and strangulation and gangrene of the herniated stomach portion.

DIAGNOSTIC TESTS
Diagnosis rests on typical clinical features and results of laboratory tests and other studies. For example, chest X-ray may reveal a large hernia and a barium study may show the hernia as a pouch at the lower end of the esophagus. Other studies can confirm stomach acid reflux, bleeding, anemia, or blood in stools.

TREATMENT
The primary goals of treatment are to relieve symptoms by minimizing or correcting the incompetent cardia and to manage and prevent complications.

Medical therapy
Usually, the doctor tries medical therapy first because symptoms usually respond to it and because hiatal hernia tends to recur after surgery. Spe-

PATHOPHYSIOLOGY

Two types of hiatal hernia

A hiatal hernia may be sliding, paraesophageal (rolling), or a combination of the two. Compare these abnormalities with normal anatomy.

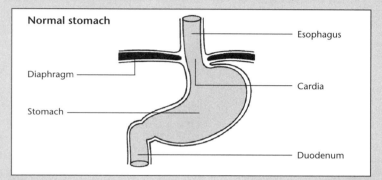

Normal stomach

- Esophagus
- Diaphragm
- Cardia
- Stomach
- Duodenum

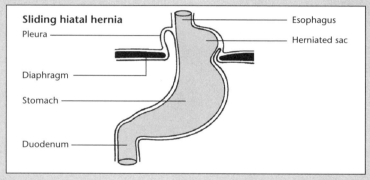

Sliding hiatal hernia

- Pleura
- Esophagus
- Herniated sac
- Diaphragm
- Stomach
- Duodenum

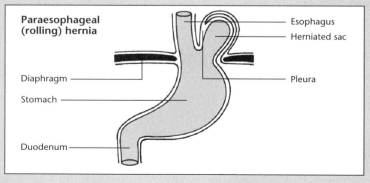

Paraesophageal (rolling) hernia

- Diaphragm
- Esophagus
- Herniated sac
- Pleura
- Stomach
- Duodenum

cific treatment measures may include any of the following:
● restricting any activity that increases intra-abdominal pressure (coughing, straining, bending)
● using antiemetics and cough suppressants
● avoiding constrictive clothing
● modifying the diet
● using stool softeners or laxatives to prevent straining during defecation
● stopping smoking (because it stimulates gastric acid production).

Intensive antacid therapy may call for hourly administration. Antacids modify the fluid refluxed into the esophagus and are probably the best treatment for intermittent reflux. Cimetidine also modifies the refluxed fluid.

To reduce the amount of reflux, the overweight patient should lose weight to decrease intra-abdominal pressure. Elevating the head of the bed about 6" (15 cm) reduces gastric reflux by gravity.

Drug therapy to strengthen cardiac sphincter tone may include a cholinergic agent such as bethanecol. Metoclopramide also has been used to stimulate smooth-muscle contraction, increase cardiac sphincter tone, and decrease reflux after eating.

Surgery

Surgical repair is necessary if medical measures fail to control symptoms or if the patient has complications, such as stricture, bleeding, pulmonary aspiration, strangulation, or incarceration.

Surgery creates an artificial closing mechanism at the gastroesophageal junction to strengthen the lower esophageal sphincter's barrier function. An abdominal or a thoracic approach may be used, or the hernia may be repaired by laparascopic surgery.

SPECIAL CONSIDERATIONS

 Teaching tip: If the doctor prescribes dietary therapy, instruct the patient to eat small, frequent, bland meals at least 2 hours before lying down (no bedtime snacks); to eat slowly; and to avoid spicy foods, fruit juices, alcoholic beverages, and coffee.

Histoplasmosis

Histoplasmosis is a fungal infection caused by *Histoplasma capsulatum.* In the United States, it occurs in three forms: *primary acute histoplasmosis, progressive disseminated histoplasmosis* (acute disseminated or chronic disseminated disease), and *chronic pulmonary (cavitary) histoplasmosis,* which causes cavitations in the lung similar to those in pulmonary tuberculosis.

Histoplasmosis occurs worldwide, especially in the temperate areas of Asia, Africa, Europe, and North and South America. In the United States, it's most prevalent in the central and eastern states.

The prognosis varies with each form. The primary acute disease is benign; the progressive disseminated disease is fatal in approximately 90% of patients. Without proper chemotherapy, chronic pulmonary histoplasmosis is fatal in 50% of patients within 5 years.

CAUSES

H. capsulatum is found in the feces of birds and bats or in soil contaminated by their feces, such as that near roosts, chicken coops, barns, caves, or underneath bridges. Transmission occurs through inhalation of *H. capsulatum* spores or through invasion of spores after minor skin trauma.

The incubation period is 5 to 18 days, although chronic pulmonary histoplasmosis may progress slowly for many years.

SIGNS AND SYMPTOMS

Clinical findings vary with each form of this disease, as follows:
● Primary acute histoplasmosis may be asymptomatic or may cause symptoms of a mild respiratory illness similar to a severe cold or influenza. Typical symptoms include fever, malaise, headache, myalgia, anorexia, cough, and chest pain.
● Progressive disseminated histoplas-

mosis causes hepatosplenomegaly, lymphadenopathy, anorexia, weight loss, fever, and possibly ulcerations of the tongue, palate, epiglottis, and larynx (with resulting pain, hoarseness, and dysphagia). It may also cause endocarditis, meningitis, pericarditis, and adrenal insufficiency.

• Chronic pulmonary histoplasmosis causes a productive cough, dyspnea, and occasional hemoptysis. Eventually, it produces weight loss, extreme weakness, breathlessness, and cyanosis.

DIAGNOSTIC TESTS

A history of exposure to contaminated soil in an area that's native to the organism, miliary calcification in the lung or spleen, and a positive histoplasmin skin test indicate exposure to histoplasmosis. Other important tests include blood studies, biopsy, and culture of *H. capsulatum* from sputum or other specimens.

TREATMENT

Therapy consists of antifungal therapy, surgery, and supportive care. Antifungal therapy is most important. Except for asymptomatic primary acute histoplasmosis (which resolves spontaneously) and the African form, histoplasmosis requires high-dose or long-term (10-week) therapy with amphotericin B or fluconazole. For a patient who also has acquired immunodeficiency syndrome, lifelong therapy with fluconazole is indicated.

Supportive care usually includes oxygen for respiratory distress, glucocorticoids for adrenal insufficiency, and parenteral fluids for dysphagia due to oral or laryngeal ulcerations.

SPECIAL CONSIDERATIONS

• A patient with histoplasmosis does not require isolation.

• Patients with chronic pulmonary or disseminated histoplasmosis need psychological support because of long-term hospitalization.

 PREVENTION TIP: To help prevent histoplasmosis, people living in endemic areas should be taught to watch for early signs and symptoms of this infection and to seek treatment promptly.

Hodgkin's disease

A neoplastic disease, Hodgkin's disease is characterized by painless, progressive enlargement of the lymph nodes, spleen, and other lymphoid tissue due to proliferation of lymphocytes, histiocytes, eosinophils, and Reed-Sternberg giant cells. The latter cells are its special histologic feature.

Untreated, Hodgkin's disease follows a variable but relentlessly progressive and ultimately fatal course. However, recent therapeutic advances make the disease potentially curable, even in advanced stages.

CAUSES

The cause of Hodgkin's disease is unknown. This disease is most common in young adults.

SIGNS AND SYMPTOMS

Clinical features vary with the stage of the disease.

Early signs

The first sign of Hodgkin's disease is usually a painless swelling of one of the cervical lymph nodes (but sometimes the axillary, mediastinal, or inguinal lymph nodes). In older patients, the first indications may be nonspecific persistent fever, night sweats, fatigue, weight loss, and malaise.

Another early feature is pruritus. Mild at first, itching grows acute as the disease progresses. Other symptoms depend on the degree and location of systemic involvement.

Lymph nodes may enlarge rapidly, producing pain and obstruction, or they may enlarge slowly and painlessly for months or years. It's not unusual to see the lymph nodes wax and wane, but they usually don't return to normal.

Late signs

Sooner or later, most patients develop systemic manifestations, including enlargement of retroperitoneal

Precautions for patients with Hodgkin's disease

If your patient is receiving outpatient radiation or chemotherapy to treat Hodgkin's disease, provide the following advice.

● Instruct the patient to promptly report adverse effects of treatment, especially anorexia, nausea, vomiting, diarrhea, fever, and bleeding.

● To minimize adverse effects, urge the patient to maintain good nutrition. If his appetite is poor, he should eat small, frequent meals of favorite foods.

● Encourage him to drink plenty of fluids.

● Advise him to pace activities to counteract therapy-induced fatigue.

● Instruct him to keep skin in radiated areas dry.

● If the patient has mouth pain or sores, he should use a soft toothbrush, cotton swab, or anesthetic mouthwash (such as viscous lidocaine) and should avoid astringent mouthwashes. Applying petroleum jelly to the lips will ease cracking.

nodes and nodular infiltrations of the spleen, liver, and bones. At this late stage, other findings include edema of the face and neck, progressive anemia, possible jaundice, nerve pain, and increased susceptibility to infection.

DIAGNOSTIC TESTS

Confirming Hodgkin's disease requires a thorough history and a complete physical examination, followed by a lymph node biopsy to check for Reed-Sternberg cells and abnormal lymph node changes. To aid diagnosis, the doctor typically orders biopsies of the bone marrow, liver, chest, lymph nodes, and spleen,

along with a routine chest X-ray, an abdominal computed tomography scan, lung and bone scans, and lymphangiography.

The same diagnostic tests are used for staging. A staging laparotomy is necessary for some patients. Diagnosis must rule out other disorders that cause enlarged lymph nodes.

TREATMENT

Appropriate therapy (chemotherapy, radiation, or both, depending on the disease stage) is based on a careful physical examination with accurate histologic interpretation and proper clinical staging. Correct and timely treatment allows longer survival and even induces an apparent cure in many patients.

Chemotherapy and radiation therapy

Radiation therapy is used alone for stage I and stage II disease, and in combination with chemotherapy for stage III. Chemotherapy is used for stage IV, sometimes inducing a complete remission. The well-known MOPP protocol (mechlorethamine, Oncovin [vincristine], procarbazine, and prednisone) was the first to provide significant cures in patients with generalized Hodgkin's.

Another useful combination is ABVD (Adriamycin [doxorubicin], bleomycin, vinblastine, and dacarbazine). Treatment with these drugs may require concomitant antiemetics, sedatives, or antidiarrheals to combat GI adverse effects.

Other treatments

New treatments include high-dose chemotherapeutic agents with autologous bone marrow transplantation or autologous peripheral blood stem cell transfusions. Biotherapy alone hasn't proven effective.

SPECIAL CONSIDERATIONS

● A female patient of childbearing age should delay pregnancy until prolonged remission because radiation and chemotherapy can cause genetic mutations and spontaneous abortions.

• Because the patient with Hodgkin's disease has usually been healthy up until this point, he is likely to be especially distressed. Be sure to provide emotional support.

• Patients receiving outpatient radiation or chemotherapy should take special measures to minimize adverse effects. (See *Precautions for patients with Hodgkin's disease.*)

Hookworm disease

Hookworm disease is an infection of the upper intestine caused by *Ancylostoma duodenale* (found in the eastern hemisphere) or *Necator americanus* (in the western hemisphere). Sandy soil, high humidity, a warm climate, and failure to wear shoes favor its transmission.

Although this disease can cause cardiopulmonary complications, it's rarely fatal, except in debilitated persons and infants under age 1.

CAUSES

Both forms of hookworm disease are transmitted to humans through direct skin penetration (usually in the foot) by hookworm larvae in soil contaminated with feces containing hookworm ova. These ova develop into infectious larvae in 1 to 3 days.

Larvae travel through the lymphatics to the pulmonary capillaries, where they penetrate alveoli and move up the bronchial tree to the trachea and epiglottis. From there, they are swallowed and enter the GI tract. When they reach the small intestine, they mature, attach to the mucosa, and suck blood, oxygen, and glucose from the intestinal wall.

These mature worms then deposit ova, which are excreted in stools, starting the cycle anew. Hookworm larvae mature in approximately 5 to 6 weeks.

SIGNS AND SYMPTOMS

Hookworm disease typically produces few symptoms and may be overlooked until worms are passed in stools. The earliest features include irritation, pruritus, and edema at the entry site.

When larvae reach the lungs, they may cause pneumonitis and hemorrhage with fever, sore throat, crackles, and cough. Finally, intestinal infection may lead to fatigue, nausea, weight loss, dizziness, melena, and uncontrolled diarrhea.

In severe and chronic infection, anemia from blood loss may result in cardiomegaly, heart failure, and generalized massive edema.

DIAGNOSTIC TESTS

Diagnosis includes a complete history, with special attention to travel or residency in endemic areas. The patient's family and other close contacts should be interviewed to see if they too have any symptoms.

Identification of hookworm ova in stools confirms the diagnosis. Anemia suggests severe chronic infection. In infected patients, blood studies show:

• hemoglobin level of 5 to 9 g (in severe cases)

• leukocyte count as high as 47,000/µl

• eosinophil count of 500 to 700/µl.

TREATMENT

The usual treatment includes administering mebendazole or pyrantel and providing an iron-rich diet or iron supplements to prevent or correct anemia.

SPECIAL CONSIDERATIONS

• A patient with confirmed hookworm infestation must be segregated if incontinent.

• For a patient with severe anemia, oxygen may be given at a low to moderate flow rate. The oxygen must be humidified because the patient may already have upper airway irritation from the parasites.

• To combat malnutrition, the patient's diet should include foods high in iron and protein. If he is receiving iron supplements, inform him that the supplements will darken stools.

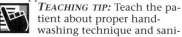 *TEACHING TIP:* Teach the patient about proper handwashing technique and sanitary disposal of feces.

Hydronephrosis

An abnormal dilation of the renal pelvis and the calyces of one or both kidneys, hydronephrosis is caused by an obstruction of urine flow in the genitourinary tract. Although partial obstruction and hydronephrosis may not produce symptoms initially, pressure buildup behind the area of obstruction eventually leads to indications of renal dysfunction.

Obstruction sites

If obstruction is in the urethra or bladder, hydronephrosis is usually bilateral; ureteral obstruction is usually unilateral. Obstructions distal to the bladder cause the bladder to dilate and act as a buffer zone, delaying hydronephrosis.

CAUSES

Almost any type of obstructive urinary tract disease can result in hydronephrosis. The most common causes are benign prostatic hypertrophy, urethral strictures, and calculi. Less common causes are strictures or stenosis of the ureter or bladder outlet, congenital abnormalities, abdominal tumors, blood clots, and neurogenic bladder.

SIGNS AND SYMPTOMS

Clinical features vary with the cause of the obstruction. In some patients, hydronephrosis produces no symptoms or only mild pain and slightly decreased urinary flow. In others, it may cause severe, colicky renal pain or dull flank pain that may radiate to the groin, along with gross urinary abnormalities (hematuria, pyuria, dysuria, alternating oliguria and polyuria, or complete anuria).

Other features include nausea, vomiting, abdominal fullness, pain on urination, dribbling, or hesitancy. Unilateral obstruction may cause pain on only one side, usually in the flank area.

Complications

The most common complication of an obstructed kidney is infection (pyelonephritis), caused by stasis that worsens renal damage and may create a life-threatening crisis. In many cases, paralytic ileus accompanies acute obstructive uropathy.

DIAGNOSTIC TESTS

While clinical findings may suggest hydronephrosis, excretory urography, retrograde pyelography, renal ultrasound, and renal function studies are necessary to confirm it.

TREATMENT

The goals of treatment are to preserve renal function and prevent infection through surgical removal of the obstruction, such as dilation for stricture of the urethra or prostatectomy for benign prostatic hypertrophy.

If renal function is already affected, therapy may include a diet low in protein, sodium, and potassium. This diet is designed to stop the progression of renal failure before surgery.

Inoperable obstructions may call for kidney decompression and drainage using a nephrostomy tube placed in the renal pelvis. Concurrent infection requires appropriate antibiotic therapy.

SPECIAL CONSIDERATIONS

 PREVENTION TIP: To prevent hydronephrosis from progressing to irreversible renal disease, urge older men to have routine medical checkups.

Hyperlipoproteinemia

About one in five people with elevated plasma lipid and lipoprotein levels has hyperlipoproteinemia, an inherited disorder in which plasma concentrations of one or more lipoproteins increase. Hyperlipoproteinemia also may result from other conditions, such as diabetes, pancreatitis, hypothyroidism, and renal disease.

This disorder affects lipid transport in serum and produces varied clinical changes, from relatively mild symptoms that can be corrected by diet to potentially fatal pancreatitis.

PATHOPHYSIOLOGY

Comparing the types of hyperlipoproteinemia

This chart presents the causes, incidence, and diagnostic results for the five main types of hyperlipoproteinemia.

TYPE	CAUSES AND INCIDENCE	DIAGNOSTIC FINDINGS
I (Frederickson's hyperlipoproteinemia, fat-induced hyperlipemia, idiopathic familial)	• Deficient or abnormal lipoprotein lipase, resulting in decreased or absent postheparin lipolytic activity • Relatively rare • Present at birth	• Chylomicrons (very-low-density lipoprotein [VLDL], low-density lipoprotein [LDL], and high-density lipoprotein) in plasma 14 hours or more after last meal • Highly elevated serum chylomicron and triglyceride levels; slightly elevated serum cholesterol level • Lower serum lipoprotein lipase level • Leukocytosis
II (Familial hyperbetalipoproteinemia, essential familial hypercholesterolemia)	• Deficient cell surface receptor that regulates LDL degradation and cholesterol synthesis, causing increased plasma LDL over joints and pressure points • Onset between ages 10 and 30	• Increased plasma concentrations of LDL • Increased serum LDL and cholesterol levels • Amniocentesis shows increased LDL levels.
III (Familial broad-beta disease, xanthoma tuberosum)	• Unknown underlying defect results in deficient conversion of triglyceride-rich VLDL to LDL. • Uncommon; usually occurs after age 20 but can occur earlier in men	• Abnormal serum beta-lipoprotein • Elevated cholesterol and triglyceride levels • Slightly elevated glucose tolerance • Hyperuricemia
IV (Endogenous hypertriglyceridemia, hyperbetalipoproteinemia)	• Usually occurs secondary to obesity, alcoholism, diabetes, or emotional disorders • Relatively common, especially in middle-aged men	• Elevated VLDL levels • Abnormal levels of triglycerides in plasma; variable increase in serum • Normal or slightly elevated serum cholesterol level • Mildly abnormal glucose tolerance • Family history • Early coronary artery disease

PATHOPHYSIOLOGY

Comparing the types of hyperlipoproteinemia *(continued)*

TYPE	CAUSES AND INCIDENCE	DIAGNOSTIC FINDINGS
V (Mixed hypertriglyceridemia, mixed hyperlipidemia)	• Defective triglyceride clearance causes pancreatitis; usually secondary to another disorder, such as obesity or nephrosis • Uncommon; onset usually occurs in late adolescence or early adulthood	• Chylomicrons in plasma • Elevated plasma VLDL levels • Elevated serum cholesterol and triglyceride levels

Hyperlipoproteinemia occurs as five distinct metabolic disorders. Types I and III are transmitted as autosomal recessive traits; types II, IV, and V are transmitted as autosomal dominant traits.

CAUSES
Each type of hyperlipoproteinemia has distinct causes. (See *Comparing the types of hyperlipoproteinemia,* pages 153 and 154.)

SIGNS AND SYMPTOMS
Each type of hyperlipoproteinemia has distinctive symptoms:
• Type I causes attacks of severe abdominal pain, usually occurring when the patient eats fatty foods. It also may cause general discomfort, appetite loss, fever, and eruptions of pinkish yellow fatty deposits (xanthomas) on the skin.
• Type II causes firm masses on the Achilles tendons and the tendons of the hands and feet, tuberous xanthomas, xanthelasma, along with an opaque ring surrounding the cornea.
• Type III may produce soft, inflamed sores over the elbows and knees as well as palmar xanthomas on the hands.
• Type IV predisposes the patient to atherosclerosis and early coronary artery disease.
• Type V causes abdominal pain, pancreatitis, peripheral neuropathy,

eruptive xanthomas on the arms and legs, and reddish white blood vessels in the retinas.

DIAGNOSTIC TESTS
See *Comparing the types of hyperlipoproteinemia,* pages 153 and 154.

TREATMENT
The first goal is to identify and treat any underlying problem such as diabetes. If no underlying problem exists, the primary treatment for types II, III, and IV is dietary management — especially cholesterol restriction. Drug therapy (cholestyramine, clofibrate, or niacin) may be used to lower the blood triglyceride or cholesterol level when diet alone fails.

In type I, treatment requires long-term weight reduction, with fat intake restricted to less than 20 g/day. The patient should avoid alcoholic beverages to decrease plasma triglycerides.

In type V, the most effective treatment is weight reduction and long-term maintenance of a low-fat diet. Alcoholic beverages must be avoided. Niacin, clofibrate, gemfibrozil, and a 20- to 40-g/day medium-chain triglyceride diet may prove helpful.

SPECIAL CONSIDERATIONS
• Patient care emphasizes careful monitoring for adverse reactions to drugs and teaching about the importance of long-term dietary management.

• Cholestyramine is administered before meals or before bedtime; it must not be given with other medications.
• Patients with active peptic ulcers or hepatic disease should not take niacin; patients with diabetes should use niacin with caution.
• For 2 weeks preceding serum cholesterol and serum triglyceride tests, the patient should maintain a steady weight and adhere strictly to the prescribed diet. A fast is also required for 12 hours preceding the test.
• Women with elevated serum lipid levels should avoid oral contraceptives and drugs that contain estrogen.

Hyperparathyroidism

In hyperparathyroidism, one or more of the four parathyroid glands is overactive, leading to excessive secretion of parathyroid hormone (PTH). Such hypersecretion promotes bone resorption and causes hypercalcemia and hypophosphatemia. (See *Bone resorption in primary hyperparathyroidism,* page 156.) In turn, renal and GI absorption of calcium increases.

CAUSES

Hyperparathyroidism may be primary or secondary. In *primary hyperparathyroidism,* one or more of the parathyroid glands enlarges, increasing PTH secretion and elevating serum calcium levels. The most common cause is a single adenoma. Other causes include a genetic disorder or multiple endocrine neoplasia.

In *secondary hyperparathyroidism,* excessive compensatory production of PTH stems from a hypocalcemia-causing abnormality outside the parathyroid gland, which leads to resistance to the metabolic action of PTH. Conditions that cause hypocalcemia include rickets, vitamin D deficiency, chronic renal failure, and osteomalacia due to phenytoin or laxative abuse.

SIGNS AND SYMPTOMS

Clinical effects of primary hyperparathyroidism result from hypercalcemia and typically involve various body systems. A common renal feature is polyuria. Skeletal symptoms include chronic low back pain and easy fractures. GI features may include constant, severe epigastric pain radiating to the back and peptic ulcers, causing abdominal pain, anorexia, nausea, and vomiting.

Neuromuscular signs and symptoms include marked muscle weakness and atrophy, particularly in the legs. Psychomotor and personality disturbances, depression, overt psychosis, stupor and, possibly, coma are neurologic effects.

DIAGNOSTIC TESTS

Primary disease is confirmed by high serum PTH and calcium levels. X-rays typically show diffuse bone demineralization, bone cysts, outer cortical bone absorption, and subperiosteal erosion of the phalanges and distal clavicles. Microscopic examination of the bone typically shows increased bone turnover.

In secondary disease, serum calcium levels are normal or slightly decreased and serum phosphorus levels are variable. The patient may have a family history of kidney disease, seizure disorders, or drug ingestion. Other diagnostic studies and physical findings identify the cause of secondary hyperparathyroidism.

TREATMENT

Effective treatment varies with the cause of the disease.

Primary disease

Treatment may include surgery to remove the adenoma. Such surgery may relieve bone pain within 3 days. However, renal damage may be irreversible.

Preoperatively — or if surgery isn't feasible or necessary — other treatments can decrease calcium levels. These include forcing fluids, limiting dietary intake of calcium, and promoting sodium and calcium excretion through forced diuresis.

Additional treatments include administration of oral sodium or potassium phosphate, S.C. calcitonin, I.V. mithramycin, or I.V. biphosphonates.

PATHOPHYSIOLOGY
Bone resorption in primary hyperparathyroidism

This illustration identifies subperiosteal erosion of the middle phalanx of the finger and demineralization of the phalangeal tuft resulting from primary hyperparathyroidism.

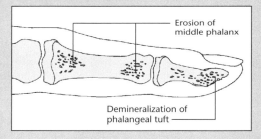

Erosion of middle phalanx

Demineralization of phalangeal tuft

Secondary disease

Treatment must correct the underlying cause of parathyroid hypertrophy. It involves vitamin D therapy or, in a patient with renal disease, an oral calcium preparation for hyperphosphatemia.

A patient with renal failure requires dialysis (possibly lifelong) to lower calcium levels.

SPECIAL CONSIDERATIONS

• Patient care emphasizes prevention of complications from the underlying disease and its treatment.
• The patient should consume at least 3 qt (3 L) of fluid a day, including cranberry or prune juice, to increase urine acidity and prevent kidney stones. Urine is strained to check for stones.
• The patient on digitalis glycosides must be carefully monitored because elevated calcium levels can rapidly produce toxic effects.
• The patient should be encouraged and assisted to ambulate as soon as possible postoperatively, even though it may be uncomfortable, because pressure on bones speeds bone recalcification.

 PREVENTION TIP: Because the patient is prone to pathologic fractures, take safety precautions to minimize the risk for injury. For example, assist the patient with walking, keep the bed at its lowest position, and raise the side rails.

Hypertension

An intermittent or sustained elevation in diastolic or systolic blood pressure, hypertension occurs as two major types: essential (idiopathic) hypertension (more common), and secondary hypertension, which results from renal disease or another identifiable cause. *Malignant hypertension* is a severe, fulminant form of hypertension common to both types. An episode of severely elevated blood pressure (*hypertensive crisis*) may prove fatal.

Hypertension affects 15% to 20% of adults in the United States. It's a major cause of cerebrovascular accident, cardiac disease, and renal failure. Untreated, it carries a high mortality, but the prognosis is good if the disorder is detected early and if treatment begins before complications develop.

CAUSES

Risk factors for essential hypertension include a positive family history, race (most common in blacks), stress, obesity, high intake of saturated fats or sodium, use of tobacco, sedentary lifestyle, and aging.

Secondary hypertension may result from renovascular disease, pheochro-

Controlling hypertension through stepped care

The National Institutes of Health recommend the following stepped-care approach to treating primary hypertension.

Step 1
The patient makes necessary lifestyle modifications: weight reduction, moderation of alcohol intake, regular physical exercise, reduction of sodium intake, and smoking cessation.

Step 2
If the patient fails to achieve the desired blood pressure or make significant progress, lifestyle modifications continue and drug therapy starts. Preferred drugs include diuretics and beta blockers. These drugs have proved effective in reducing cardiovascular morbidity and mortality.

If diuretics or beta blockers are ineffective or unacceptable, the doctor may prescribe angiotensin-converting enzyme inhibitors, calcium antagonists, alpha$_1$-receptor blockers, or alpha-beta blockers. While these agents reduce blood pressure, they have yet to prove effective in reducing morbidity and mortality.

Step 3
If the patient still fails to achieve the desired blood pressure or make significant progress, the doctor increases the drug dosage, substitutes a drug in the same class, or adds a drug from a different class.

Step 4
If the patient still fails to reach the desired blood pressure or to make significant progress, the doctor adds a second or third agent (or adds a diuretic if one isn't already prescribed). Second or third agents may include direct-acting vasodilators, alpha$_1$-antagonists, and peripherally acting adrenergic neuron antagonists.

---

mocytoma, Cushing's syndrome, primary hyperaldosteronism, coarctation of the aorta, pregnancy, neurologic disorders, use of oral contraceptives or other drugs such as cocaine, and thyroid, pituitary, or parathyroid dysfunction.

SIGNS AND SYMPTOMS
Hypertension usually doesn't produce clinical effects until vascular changes in the heart, brain, or kidneys occur. Highly elevated blood pressure damages the inner lining of small vessels, resulting in fibrin build-up, edema and, possibly, intravascular clotting.

Changes produced by this process depend on the location of the damaged vessels:
• brain: cerebrovascular accident
• retina: blindness
• heart: myocardial infarction
• kidneys: proteinuria, edema and, eventually, renal failure.

Hypertension increases the heart's workload, causing left ventricular hypertrophy and, later, left ventricular failure, left- and right-sided heart failure, and pulmonary edema.

DIAGNOSTIC TESTS
Serial blood pressure measurements greater than 140/90 mm Hg in people under age 50 or greater than 150/95 mm Hg in those over age 50 confirm hypertension. Physical examination may reveal bruits over certain arteries; ophthalmoscopy may reveal characteristic changes.

The patient history and additional diagnostic studies may point to certain predisposing factors and help identify an underlying cause or complications. To check for damage to the heart and blood vessels and other complications, the doctor may order the following tests:

• electrocardiogram, which may show an enlarged left ventricle or decreased blood supply to this chamber

• chest X-ray, which may show an enlarged heart

• echocardiography, which may show an enlarged left ventricle.

TREATMENT

Therapy for secondary hypertension focuses on correcting the underlying cause and controlling hypertensive effects.

For primary hypertension, many doctors use the stepped-care approach. (See *Controlling hypertension through stepped care,* page 157.)

Hypertensive emergency

Typically, hypertensive emergency calls for parenteral administration of a vasodilator or an adrenergic inhibitor, or oral administration of a selected drug, such as nifedipine or captopril, to rapidly reduce blood pressure.

SPECIAL CONSIDERATIONS

 TEACHING TIP: Inform the patient that uncontrolled hypertension may cause stroke or heart attack and that compliance with therapy is essential. Urge him to establish a daily routine for taking medication. Caution him to avoid high-sodium antacids and over-the-counter cold and sinus medications, which contain vasoconstrictors.

• Many patients must avoid high-sodium foods (pickles, potato chips, canned soups, cold cuts) and table salt. Lifestyle modifications, such as increased exercise and reduced stress, also play a major role.

Hyperthyroidism

Hyperthyroidism is a metabolic imbalance resulting from thyroid hormone overproduction. The most common form is Graves' disease, which increases thyroxine production, enlarges the thyroid gland (goi-

ter), and causes changes in many body systems.

Incidence of Graves' disease is highest between ages 30 and 40, especially in people with family histories of thyroid abnormalities. With treatment, most patients can lead normal lives. Thyroid storm — an acute exacerbation of hyperthyroidism — is a medical emergency that may lead to life-threatening cardiac, hepatic, or renal failure.

CAUSES

Hyperthyroidism may result from both genetic and immunologic factors. In latent hyperthyroidism, excessive dietary intake of iodine and, possibly, stress can trigger clinical hyperthyroidism. In a person with inadequately treated hyperthyroidism, stress can trigger thyroid storm.

SIGNS AND SYMPTOMS

The classic features of Graves' disease are an enlarged thyroid, nervousness, heat intolerance, weight loss despite increased appetite, sweating, diarrhea, tremor, and palpitations. Exophthalmos (bulging of the eyes) is characteristic, although not always present. Many other signs and symptoms are also common. (See *Far-ranging effects of hyperthyroidism.*)

When hyperthyroidism escalates to thyroid storm, the patient may also experience extreme irritability, hypertension, tachycardia, vomiting, temperature up to 106° F (41.1° C), delirium, and coma.

DIAGNOSTIC TESTS

Diagnosis usually is straightforward and depends on patient history, physical findings, a high index of suspicion, and routine hormone studies. Radioimmunoassay, thyroid scan, thyroid-stimulating hormone levels, and the thyroid-releasing hormone stimulation test may confirm hyperthyroidism.

TREATMENT

The primary forms of therapy are antithyroid drugs, ^{131}I, and surgery. Appropriate treatment depends on the

Far-ranging effects of hyperthyroidism

Hyperthyroidism profoundly affects virtually every body system, causing the following signs and symptoms.

Central nervous system
Difficulty concentrating; excitability or nervousness; fine tremor, shaky handwriting, and clumsiness; emotional instability and mood swings

Skin, hair, and nails
Smooth, warm, flushed skin; fine, soft hair; premature graying and increased hair loss; friable nails and separation of the distal nail from the nail bed; thickened skin; raised red patches of skin that are itchy and sometimes painful

Cardiovascular system
Tachycardia; full, bounding pulse; wide pulse pressure; enlarged heart; increased cardiac output and blood volume; arrhythmias

Respiratory system
Dyspnea on exertion and at rest

GI system
Possible anorexia; nausea and vomiting; increased defecation; soft stools or, with severe disease, diarrhea; liver enlargement

Musculoskeletal system
Weakness, fatigue, muscle atrophy

Reproductive system
In females, oligomenorrhea or amenorrhea, decreased fertility; in males, gynecomastia due to increased estrogen levels; in both sexes, diminished libido

Eyes
Exophthalmos; occasional inflammation of the conjunctivae, corneas, or eye muscles; diplopia; increased tearing

---

size of the goiter, underlying causes, the patient's age and parity, and how long surgery will be delayed (if the patient is an appropriate candidate).

Antithyroid therapy
Antithyroid drugs are used for children, young adults, pregnant women, and patients who refuse surgery or ^{131}I treatment. Options include thyroid hormone antagonists (propylthiouracil and methimazole) and propranolol (which may be given concomitantly to manage tachycardia and other peripheral effects).

[131]I
A single oral dose of ^{131}I is the treatment of choice for patients not planning to have children. The thyroid picks up this radioactive element as it would regular iodine. The radioactivity destroys some of the cells that normally concentrate iodine and produce T_4, thus decreasing thyroid hormone production.

In most patients, hypermetabolic symptoms diminish from 6 to 8 weeks after such treatment.

Surgery
Subtotal (partial) thyroidectomy, which decreases the thyroid's capacity for hormone production, is indicated for patients with a large goiter whose hyperthyroidism has repeatedly relapsed after drug therapy, or patients who refuse or aren't candidates for ^{131}I treatment. Preoperatively, the patient may receive iodides, antithyroid drugs, or propranolol to help prevent thyroid storm.

After ablative treatment with ^{131}I or surgery, patients require regular medical supervision for the rest of their lives because they usually develop hypothyroidism.

Treatment for thyroid storm
Thyroid storm calls for administration of an antithyroid drug, I.V. pro-

pranolol, a corticosteroid, and an io-dide to block release of thyroid hormone. Supportive measures include administration of nutrients, vitamins, fluids, and sedatives.

SPECIAL CONSIDERATIONS

• Encourage the patient to rest in a cool, quiet, and dark room.

• Reassure the patient and family that any bizarre behavior probably will subside with treatment. Sedatives may be necessary.

• If the doctor prescribes iodide, it can be mixed with milk, juice, or water to prevent GI distress and administered through a straw to prevent tooth discoloration.

• Advise the patient and family to stay alert for signs and symptoms of thyroid storm: tachycardia, poor concentration, fever, vomiting, and hypertension.

• If the patient has exophthalmos, sunglasses or eye patches can protect his eyes from light.

For the patient on drug therapy or [131]I:

• Taking propylthiouracil or methimazole with meals minimizes GI distress. Also, the patient should avoid over-the-counter cough preparations containing iodine.

 TEACHING TIP: After ^{131}I therapy, instruct the patient not to expectorate or cough freely because his saliva is radioactive for 24 hours. Also, tell him to report any symptoms of hypothyroidism.

Hypoglycemia

An abnormally low blood glucose level, hypoglycemia occurs when glucose burns up too rapidly, when the glucose release rate falls behind tissue demands, or when excessive insulin enters the bloodstream.

Hypoglycemia is classified as reactive or fasting. *Reactive hypoglycemia* results from the reaction to the disposition of meals or administration of excessive insulin. *Fasting hypoglycemia* causes discomfort during long periods of abstinence from food — for example, before breakfast.

Although hypoglycemia is a specific endocrine imbalance, symptoms commonly are vague and depend on how quickly the glucose levels drop. If not corrected, severe hypoglycemia may result in coma, irreversible brain damage, and death.

CAUSES

The two forms of hypoglycemia have different causes and occur in different types of patients.

Reactive hypoglycemia

Several forms of reactive hypoglycemia occur. In a diabetic patient, the disorder may result from administration of too much insulin or too much oral hypoglycemia medication. In a mildly diabetic patient, reactive hypoglycemia may result from delayed and excessive insulin production after carbohydrate ingestion.

Similarly, a nondiabetic patient may suffer reactive hypoglycemia from a sharp increase in insulin output after a meal. Sometimes called *postprandial hypoglycemia,* this condition usually disappears on ingestion of something sweet.

In some patients, reactive hypoglycemia may have no known cause (idiopathic reactive) or may result from hyperalimentation due to gastric dumping syndrome or from impaired glucose tolerance.

Fasting hypoglycemia

Fasting hypoglycemia most commonly stems from an excess of insulin or insulin-like substance or from a decrease in counterregulatory hormones. It can be *exogenous,* resulting from such external factors as alcohol or drug ingestion, or *endogenous,* resulting from organic problems.

SIGNS AND SYMPTOMS

Reactive hypoglycemia causes fatigue, malaise, nervousness, irritability, trembling, tension, headache, hunger, cold sweats, and a rapid heart rate. These same signs and symptoms usually occur in fasting hypoglycemia.

Managing a hypoglycemic episode

A sudden hypoglycemic episode (also called insulin shock) may make it hard for a patient to recognize his own symptoms and take care of himself. If you're caring for a patient who is at risk for such an episode, it will be up to you to manage the crisis for him and raise his blood glucose level immediately to prevent permanent brain damage and possibly even death.

If the patient is conscious

If a glucose product, such as Glutose, Glutol, or Instant Glucose, is available, squeeze it into the patient's mouth — taking care not to block his airway. If you can't obtain one of these products, place some honey on his tongue or squeeze prepared cake icing between his gum and cheek.

Other foods and fluids you may give include:
- a glass of fruit juice (such as apple juice or orange juice)
- nondiet soft drink (such as cola or ginger ale)
- 1 tbsp of corn syrup, honey, or grape jelly
- water with 3 tbsp of table sugar added to it
- six jelly beans, 5 to 6 pieces of hard candy, or 10 gumdrops.

After giving the sugary food, call for medical help at once.

If the patient is unconscious or has trouble swallowing

Give an S.C. injection of glucagon if you've been trained to administer it. This will raise the blood glucose level rapidly. Then get immediate medical attention for the patient.

Fasting hypoglycemia also may cause central nervous system disturbances — for example, blurry or double vision, confusion, motor weakness, hemiplegia, seizures, or coma.

In infants and children, signs and symptoms of hypoglycemia are vague. A newborn's refusal to feed may be the primary clue.

DIAGNOSTIC TESTS

Reagent or glucose reagent strips provide quick screening methods for determining the blood glucose level. A color change that corresponds to less than 45 mg/dl indicates the need for a venous blood sample.

Laboratory testing showing decreased blood glucose values confirms the diagnosis. The following values indicate hypoglycemia:
- *full-term infants:* less than 30 mg/dl before a feeding; less than 40 mg/dl after a feeding
- *preterm infants:* less than 20 mg/dl before a feeding; less than 30 mg/dl after a feeding
- *children and adults:* less than 40 mg/

dl before a meal; less than 50 mg/dl after a meal.

A 5-hour glucose tolerance test may be administered to provoke reactive hypoglycemia. After a 12-hour fast, laboratory testing to detect plasma insulin and plasma glucose levels may identify fasting hypoglycemia.

TREATMENT

Reactive hypoglycemia and fasting hypoglycemia require different treatments.

Reactive hypoglycemia

Treatment involves dietary modification to delay glucose absorption and gastric emptying. Usually, this involves small, frequent meals; ingestion of complex carbohydrates, fiber, and fat; and avoidance of simple sugars, alcohol, and fruit drinks. The patient also may receive anticholinergic drugs to slow gastric emptying and intestinal motility and to inhibit vagal stimulation of insulin release.

In a sudden hypoglycemic episode, the patient must ingest glucose immediately. (See *Managing a hypoglycemic episode,* page 161.)

Fasting hypoglycemia

In fasting hypoglycemia, surgery and drug therapy usually are required. In patients with insulinoma, tumor removal is the treatment of choice. Drug therapy may include nondiuretic thiazides such as diazoxide to inhibit insulin secretion, streptozocin, and hormones, such as glucocorticoids and long-acting glycogen.

SPECIAL CONSIDERATIONS

 TEACHING TIP: Advise the patient to eat a diet high in complex carbohydrates, fiber, and fat and to avoid simple sugars and alcohol.

Hypogonadism

A condition resulting from decreased androgen production in males, hypogonadism may impair spermatogenesis (causing infertility) and inhibit the development of normal secondary sex characteristics.

Depending on the patient's age at onset, hypogonadism may cause eunuchism (complete gonadal failure) or eunuchoidism (partial failure).

CAUSES

Hypogonadism may be primary or secondary; each type has different causes.

Primary hypogonadism

Primary hypogonadism results directly from interstitial cellular or seminiferous tubular damage caused by faulty development or mechanical damage. Termed *hypergonadotropic hypogonadism,* this condition leads to increased secretion of gonadotropins by the pituitary in an attempt to increase the testicular functional state.

Primary hypogonadism may take the form of Klinefelter's syndrome, Reifenstein's syndrome, male Turner's syndrome, Sertoli-cell–only syndrome, anorchism, orchitis, or sequelae of irradiation.

Secondary hypogonadism

Secondary hypogonadism results from faulty interaction within the hypothalamic-pituitary axis, leading to failure to secrete normal levels of gonadotropins. Therefore, it's termed hypogonadotropic hypogonadism.

Secondary hypogonadism includes the following: hypopituitarism, isolated follicle-stimulating hormone deficiency, isolated luteinizing hormone deficiency, Kallmann's syndrome, and Prader-Willi syndrome.

SIGNS AND SYMPTOMS

Although clinical effects vary with the specific cause of hypogonadism, typical findings may include delayed closure of epiphyses and immature bone age; delayed puberty; infantile penis and small, soft testes; below-average muscle development and strength; fine, sparse facial hair; scant or absent axillary, pubic, and body hair; and a high-pitched, effeminate voice.

In an adult, hypogonadism diminishes sex drive and potency and causes regression of secondary sex characteristics.

DIAGNOSTIC TESTS

Accurate diagnosis requires a detailed history, physical examination, and hormonal studies. Chromosomal analysis may show the specific cause. Testicular biopsy and semen analysis evaluate sperm production, identify impaired sperm formation, and assess low testosterone levels.

TREATMENT

Depending on the underlying cause, treatment may involve hormonal replacement, especially with testosterone, methyltestosterone, or human chorionic gonadotropin (HCG) for primary hypogonadism, and with HCG for secondary hypogonadism.

Fertility can't be restored after permanent testicular damage. However, eunuchism that results from hypothalamic-pituitary lesions can be corrected when administration of gonadotropins stimulates normal testicular function.

SPECIAL CONSIDERATIONS

• Promote self-confidence in an adolescent boy with hypogonadism.

 TEACHING TIP: Urge the patient and family to express their concerns, and reassure them that effective treatment is available. Make sure they understand hormonal replacement therapy fully, including expected adverse reactions, such as acne and water retention.

Hypoparathyroidism

A deficiency of parathyroid hormone (PTH), hypoparathyroidism is caused by disease, injury, or congenital malfunction of the parathyroid glands. Because these glands primarily regulate calcium balance, hypoparathyroidism causes hypocalcemia, producing neuromuscular changes ranging from paresthesia to tetany.

Clinical effects of hypoparathyroidism usually are correctable with replacement therapy. However, some complications of long-term hypocalcemia such as cataracts are irreversible.

CAUSES

Hypoparathyroidism may be acute or chronic. It is classified as idiopathic or acquired, as follows:

• *Idiopathic hypoparathyroidism* may result from an autoimmune genetic disorder or congenital absence of the parathyroid glands.

• *Acquired hypoparathyroidism* commonly results from accidental removal of or injury to one or more parathyroid glands during thyroidectomy or other neck surgery or, rarely, from massive thyroid irradiation. It also may result from ischemic infarction of the parathyroid glands during surgery, or from hemochromatosis, sarcoidosis, amyloidosis, tuberculosis, neoplasms, or trauma.

• *Acquired, reversible hypoparathyroidism* may result from hypomagnesemia-induced impairment of hormone synthesis, suppression of normal gland function due to hypercalcemia, or delayed maturation of parathyroid function.

SIGNS AND SYMPTOMS

Although mild hypoparathyroidism may be asymptomatic, it usually produces hypocalcemia and high serum phosphate levels that affect the central nervous system and other body systems.

Chronic hypoparathyroidism

The chronic form typically causes neuromuscular irritability, increased deep tendon reflexes, Chvostek's sign (hyperirritability of the facial nerve, producing a characteristic spasm when tapped), dysphagia, organic brain syndrome, psychosis, mental deficiency in children, and tetany.

Chronic tetany is usually unilateral. It may cause difficulty in walking and a tendency to fall and may lead to laryngospasm, stridor and, eventually, cyanosis and seizures.

Acute hypoparathyroidism

More severe than chronic tetany, acute (overt) tetany begins with a tingling in the fingertips, around the mouth and, occasionally, in the feet. This tingling spreads and becomes more severe, producing muscle tension and spasms and adduction of the thumbs, wrists, and elbows. Pain varies with the degree of muscle tension, but rarely affects the face, legs, and feet. Like chronic tetany, acute tetany may cause laryngospasm, stridor, cyanosis, and seizures.

Other clinical effects include abdominal pain; dry, lusterless hair; spontaneous hair loss; brittle fingernails that develop ridges or fall out; dry, scaly skin; cataracts; and weakened tooth enamel, which causes the teeth to stain, crack, and decay easily.

Also, hypocalcemia may induce arrhythmias and eventually lead to congestive heart failure.

DIAGNOSTIC TESTS

Test results that confirm the diagnosis include:

• decreased PTH concentration shown by radioimmunoassay for PTH
• decreased serum calcium level
• increased serum phosphorus level

What your patient should know about hypoparathyroidism

To help the patient cope with hypoparathyroidism, advise him to consume a high-calcium, low-phosphorus diet (he should ask the doctor which foods are permitted.)

If the doctor has prescribed drug therapy, emphasize the importance of having serum calcium levels measured at least three times a year. Instruct the patient to watch for signs of overcorrection (hypercalcemia). These include confusion, appetite loss, abdominal pain, muscle pain, and weakness. Caution him to keep medications away from light and heat.

If the patient has scaly skin, instruct him to apply creams. To prevent his nails from splitting, recommend that he keep them trimmed.

• prolonged QT and ST intervals on electrocardiogram (due to hypocalcemia).

To provoke clinical evidence of hypoparathyroidism, the doctor may inflate a blood pressure cuff on the patient's upper arm to between diastolic and systolic blood pressure and maintain this inflation for 3 minutes. Trousseau's sign (carpal spasm) is a positive finding.

TREATMENT

Because calcium absorption from the small intestine requires the presence of vitamin D, treatment includes vitamin D and calcium supplements. Such therapy usually is lifelong, except in the reversible form of the disease. If the patient can't tolerate the pure form of vitamin D, alternatives include dihydrotachysterol and calcitriol.

Acute, life-threatening tetany requires immediate I.V. administration of 10% calcium gluconate to raise serum calcium levels. The patient who's awake and able to cooperate can help raise serum calcium levels by breathing into a paper bag and then inhaling his own carbon dioxide; this produces hypoventilation and mild respiratory acidosis.

Sedatives and anticonvulsants may control spasms until calcium levels rise. Chronic tetany calls for maintenance therapy with oral calcium and vitamin D supplements.

SPECIAL CONSIDERATIONS

• A patient with a history of tetany awaiting a diagnosis of hypoparathyroidism is vulnerable to seizures and requires seizure precautions.

• In a patient with chronic disease, minor muscle twitching and signs of laryngospasm (respiratory stridor or dysphagia) may signal onset of tetany. This patient also must be watched for heart block and signs of decreasing cardiac output. (See *What your patient should know about hypoparathyroidism*.)

• The patient receiving both digitalis glycosides and calcium must be carefully monitored for signs and symptoms of digitalis toxicity (arrhythmias, nausea, fatigue, and visual changes).

Idiopathic thrombocytopenic purpura

Idiopathic thrombocytopenic purpura (ITP) refers to thrombocytopenia (low platelet level) resulting from immunologic platelet destruction. ITP may be acute (postviral thrombocytopenia) or chronic (Werlhof's disease, purpura hemorrhagica, essential thrombocytopenia, autoimmune thrombocytopenia). Acute ITP usually affects children between ages 2 and 6; chronic ITP mainly affects adults under age 50.

The prognosis for acute ITP is excellent; nearly four of five patients recover without treatment. The prognosis for chronic ITP is good; remissions lasting weeks or years are common.

CAUSES
ITP may be an autoimmune disorder; antibodies that reduce the life span of platelets have been found in nearly all patients.

Acute ITP typically follows a viral infection, such as rubella or chickenpox, and may follow immunization with a live virus vaccine. Chronic ITP rarely follows infection; it's often associated with immunologic disorders such as systemic lupus erythematosus. It's also been linked to drug reactions.

SIGNS AND SYMPTOMS
Clinical features common to all disease forms include petechiae, ecchymoses, and mucosal bleeding from the mouth, nose, or GI tract. Hemorrhage is rare. Purpuric lesions may occur in vital organs, such as the lungs, kidneys, or brain, and may prove fatal.

In acute ITP, onset usually is sudden, and the patient experiences easy bruising, epistaxis, and bleeding gums. Chronic ITP has a gradual onset.

DIAGNOSTIC TESTS
A platelet count below 20,000/µl and prolonged bleeding time suggest ITP. Platelet size and morphologic appearance may be abnormal; anemia may be present if bleeding has occurred.

Bone marrow studies show an abundance of megakaryocytes and a shortened circulating platelet survival time (hours or days).

TREATMENT
Acute ITP may be allowed to run its course without intervention, or may be treated with glucocorticoids or immune globulin.

For chronic ITP, corticosteroids may be the initial treatment of choice. Patients who fail to respond within 1 to 4 months or who need high steroid dosages are candidates for splenectomy (about 85% successful). Alternative treatments include immunosuppression, high-dose I.V. gamma globulin, and immunoabsorption apheresis using staphylococcal protein-A columns.

Before splenectomy, the patient may require blood, blood components, and vitamin K to correct anemia and coagulation defects. After splenectomy, he may need blood and component replacement and platelet concentrate. Normally, the platelet count increases spontaneously after splenectomy.

SPECIAL CONSIDERATIONS
 Teaching tip: Advise the patient to watch for petechiae, ecchymoses, and other signs of recurrence and to avoid aspirin and ibuprofen.

Viewing impetigo crusts

In impetigo, when the vesicles break, crust forms from the exudate. This infection is especially contagious among children.

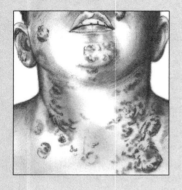

Impetigo

A contagious, superficial skin infection, impetigo can take a nonbullous or bullous form. This vesiculopustular eruptive disorder spreads most easily among infants, young children, and elderly people.

Predisposing factors — poor hygiene, anemia, malnutrition, and a warm climate — favor outbreaks of this infection, most of which occur during the late summer and early fall. Impetigo may complicate chickenpox, eczema, or other skin conditions marked by open lesions.

CAUSES

Coagulase-positive *Staphylococcus aureus* and, less commonly, group A beta-hemolytic streptococci, usually cause nonbullous impetigo. *S. aureus* generally causes bullous impetigo.

SIGNS AND SYMPTOMS

Common nonbullous impetigo typically begins with a small red macule that turns into a vesicle, becoming pustular with a honey-colored crust

within hours. When the vesicle breaks, a thick yellow crust forms from the exudate. (See *Viewing impetigo crusts*.)

Autoinoculation may lead to satellite lesions. Other features include pruritus, burning, and regional lymphadenopathy.

A rare but serious complication of streptococcal impetigo is glomerulonephritis. Infants and young children may develop aural impetigo or otitis externa; lesions usually clear without treatment in 2 to 3 weeks, unless an underlying disorder such as eczema is present.

In *bullous impetigo,* a thin-walled vesicle opens and a thin, clear crust forms from the exudate. The lesion, which commonly appears on the face or other exposed areas, consists of a central clearing, circumscribed by an outer rim.

Both nonbullous and bullous forms usually produce painless itching. They may appear simultaneously and be clinically indistinguishable.

DIAGNOSTIC TESTS

Characteristic lesions suggest impetigo. Microscopic visualization of the causative organism in a Gram stain of vesicle fluid usually confirms *S. aureus* infection and justifies antibiotic therapy.

Culture and sensitivity testing of fluid or denuded skin may indicate the most appropriate antibiotic, but therapy shouldn't be delayed for laboratory results, which can take 3 days. If an infection is present, the white blood cell count may be elevated.

TREATMENT

Usually, treatment involves a 10-day course of systemic antibiotics (usually a penicillinase-resistant penicillin, cephalosporin, or erythromycin). A topical antibiotic such as mupirocin ointment may be used for minor infections.

Therapy also includes removal of the exudate by washing the lesions two or three times daily with soap and water or, for stubborn crusts, application of warm soaks or compresses of normal saline or a diluted soap solution.

SPECIAL CONSIDERATIONS

 TEACHING TIP: Stress the need to continue taking prescribed medications for the entire prescribed course, even after the lesions have healed.

• As difficult as it may be, the patient should avoid scratching because impetigo spreads through scratching. Cutting a child's fingernails can help reduce injury from scratching.

• All family members should be checked for impetigo if one family member has been diagnosed. If this infection is present in a schoolchild, the school should be notified.

 PREVENTION TIP: To limit the spread of this highly contagious infection, encourage the patient to use proper hand-washing technique, to bathe frequently with a bactericidal soap, and to avoid sharing towels, washcloths, or bed linens with family members.

Inactive colon

Also called lazy colon, inactive colon is a state of chronic constipation. If untreated, it may lead to fecal impaction.

Inactive colon is common in elderly persons and invalids because of their inactivity. Often, it can be relieved through diet and exercise.

CAUSES

Inactive colon usually results from some deficiency in the three elements necessary for normal bowel activity: dietary bulk, fluid intake, and exercise. Other possible causes include habitual disregard of the urge to defecate, emotional conflicts, chronic laxative use, and prolonged dependence on enemas (which dull rectal sensitivity to the presence of feces).

SIGNS AND SYMPTOMS

The primary sign of inactive colon is chronic constipation. The patient typically strains to produce dry, hard stools, which are accompanied by mild abdominal discomfort. Straining may aggravate other rectal conditions such as hemorrhoids.

DIAGNOSTIC TESTS

A patient history of dry, hard stools and infrequent bowel movements suggests inactive colon. A digital rectal examination reveals stools in the lower portion of the rectum and a palpable colon. Proctoscopy may show an unusually small colon lumen, prominent veins, and an abnormal amount of mucus.

Diagnostic tests to rule out other causes include an upper GI series, barium enema, and examination of stools for occult blood resulting from neoplasms.

TREATMENT

Effective treatment varies with the patient's age and condition. Increasing dietary bulk and fluid intake and getting sufficient exercise commonly relieve constipation. (See *Breaking the constipation habit,* page 168.)

Treatment for severe constipation may include bulk-forming laxatives such as psyllium or well-lubricated glycerin suppositories. For fecal impaction, manual removal of feces is necessary. An oil-retention enema usually precedes feces removal; an enema is also necessary afterward.

For lasting relief of constipation, the patient with inactive colon must modify his bowel habits.

SPECIAL CONSIDERATIONS

• The patient should respond promptly to the urge to defecate and may use methods such as autosuggestion, relaxation exercises, or reading enjoyable material to enhance comfort during defecation. Using a small footstool to promote thigh flexion while sitting on the toilet may also be helpful.

• If the patient has a history of arteriosclerosis, congestive heart failure, or hypertension, constipation and straining at stool may induce a

Breaking the constipation habit

Patient education may help to break the constipation habit. Provide patients with the following guidelines.

Increase fluid intake
● Drink at least eight to ten glasses (at least 2 qt [2 L]) of liquid every day because fluids help keep the intestinal contents in a semisolid state for easier passage. This becomes particularly important with age.
● Stimulate the bowel with a drink of hot coffee, warm lemonade, iced liquids (plain or with lemon), or prune juice before breakfast or in the evening.

Eat more fiber
● Add fiber to your diet with foods such as whole grain cereals (rolled oats, bran, shredded wheat, brown rice, whole wheat bread, oatmeal). Fiber contributes bulk and stimulates bowel activity. However, too much bran can create an irritable bowel, so check labels on foods for fiber content (low fiber — 0.3 to 1 g; moderate fiber — 1.1 to 2 g; high fiber — 2.1 to 4.2 g).
● Increase the bulk content of your diet slowly to prevent flatulence — a possible temporary effect of a high-bulk diet. For additional bulk, consume fresh fruits with skins as well as raw and coarse vegetables (broccoli, brussels sprouts, cabbage, cauliflower, cucumbers, lettuce, and turnips).

Avoid fats and highly refined foods
● Limit your consumption of fat-containing foods, such as bacon, butter, cream, and oil. Although they will help to soften intestinal contents, they sometimes cause diarrhea.
● Avoid highly refined foods, such as white rice, cream of wheat, farina, white bread, pie or cake, macaroni, spaghetti, noodles, candy, cookies, and ice cream.

Other advice
● Rest at least 6 hours every night.
● Get moderate exercise such as walking every day.
● Avoid overuse of laxatives.
● Maintain a regular time for bowel movements (usually after breakfast).

"bathroom coronary" or cerebrovascular accident.

 TEACHING TIP: if the patient is using bulk-forming laxatives such as psyllium, advise him to take them with at least 8 oz (237 ml) of liquid. Juices, soft drinks, or other pleasant-tasting liquids help mask this drug's grittiness.
● Occasional digital rectal stimulation or abdominal massage near the sigmoid area may help stimulate a bowel movement.
● If the patient requires enemas, sodium biphosphate enema should not be used too often. Its hypertonic solution can absorb as much as 10% of the colon's sodium content or draw intestinal fluids into the colon, causing dehydration.

Influenza

Also called the grippe or flu, influenza is an acute, highly contagious infection of the respiratory tract that results from three different types of *Myxovirus influenzae.* It occurs sporadically or in epidemics (usually during the colder months). Epidemics tend to peak within 2 to 3 weeks after initial cases and subside within a month.

Although influenza affects all age-groups, its incidence is highest in schoolchildren. However, its severity is greatest in the very young, in the elderly, and in those with chronic diseases. In these groups, influenza may even lead to death.

CAUSES

Influenza transmission occurs through inhalation of a respiratory droplet from an infected person or by indirect contact such as use of a contaminated drinking glass. The influenza virus then invades the epithelium of the respiratory tract, causing inflammation and desquamation.

The influenza virus is able to change in subtle or major ways, resulting in infection by strains to which the population at risk has little or no resistance. Minor changes may occur yearly or every few years; major changes can lead to major outbreaks (pandemics). (See *How an influenza virus multiplies,* page 170.)

Influenza viruses are classified into three groups:
• type A, the most prevalent, which strikes every year, with new serotypes causing epidemics every 3 years
• type B, which also strikes annually but causes epidemics only every 4 to 6 years
• type C, which is endemic and causes only sporadic cases.

SIGNS AND SYMPTOMS

After an incubation period of 24 to 48 hours, flu signs and symptoms begin to appear: sudden onset of chills, temperature of 101° to 104° F (38.3° to 40° C), headache, malaise, myalgia, nonproductive cough and, occasionally, laryngitis, hoarseness, conjunctivitis, rhinitis, and rhinorrhea.

These signs and symptoms usually subside in 3 to 5 days, but cough and weakness may persist. In some patients, lack of energy and easy fatigability may persist for several weeks.

Complications

Fever that lasts longer than 3 to 5 days signals onset of complications. The most common complication is pneumonia.

DIAGNOSTIC TESTS

At the start of a flu epidemic, early cases commonly are mistaken for other respiratory disorders. Because signs and symptoms of the flu are not highly distinctive, isolation of

M. influenzae in the nasal secretions of infected people is essential at the first sign of an epidemic. Nose and throat cultures and increased serum antibody titers help confirm the diagnosis.

After these measures confirm a flu epidemic, diagnosis requires only observation of signs and symptoms.

TREATMENT

Uncomplicated influenza is treated with bed rest, adequate fluid intake, aspirin or acetaminophen (in children) to relieve fever and muscle pain, and guaifenesin or another expectorant to relieve nonproductive coughing.

Amantadine, an antiviral agent, has been effective in shortening the duration of signs and symptoms in influenza A infection. Patients with influenza complicated by pneumonia require supportive care (fluid and electrolyte supplements, oxygen, assisted ventilation) and appropriate antibiotics to treat bacterial superinfection.

SPECIAL CONSIDERATIONS

• Patient comfort measures include mouthwashes, increased fluid intake, warm baths or heating pads to relieve myalgia, and nonnarcotic analgesics and antipyretics as needed.

 PREVENTION TIP: Visitors should be screened to protect the patient from bacterial infection and the visitors from influenza. Also, the patient should be taught about proper disposal of tissues and proper hand-washing technique to prevent the virus from spreading.
• High-risk patients should receive annual inoculations at the start of the flu season.
• Influenza vaccines are made from chicken embryos and must not be given to people who are hypersensitive to eggs, feathers, or chickens. Although the vaccine has not been proven harmful to the fetus, it's not recommended for pregnant women, except those who are highly susceptible to influenza.

PATHOPHYSIOLOGY

How an influenza virus multiplies

An influenza virus contains only a portion of ribonucleic or deoxyribonucleic acid, on which are strung the genes that carry instructions for viral replication. Fragmentation of the genetic material accounts for its ability to undergo genetic mutation.

Having only a partial genetic component, the virus can't reproduce or carry out chemical reactions on its own; it needs a host cell. Once inhaled, this airborne virus seeks the necessary host.

Inside the respiratory tract

Here, the virus attaches to a healthy host cell. In an attempt to destroy the invader, the healthy cell engulfs the virus and sends chemicals to dissolve the wall of the virus cell. This attempt at destruction releases the genetic material of the virus into the healthy cell.

Inside the host cell

In the host cell, viral genes find fertile conditions in which to replicate, arranging themselves into identical bundles. These new viruses (up to 1,000 reproduced within 6 hours) burst forth to invade other healthy cells.

The viral invasion destroys the host cells, impairing respiratory defenses and predisposing the patient to secondary bacterial infection.

1. Virus attaches to host

Virus

Healthy host root

2. Host engulfs virus

3. Virus cell wall is destroyed; genes spill into host

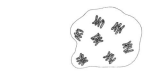

4. Virus genes multiply and bundle

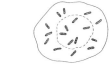

5. New viruses break out

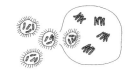

Inguinal hernia

A hernia occurs when part of an internal organ protrudes through an abnormal opening in the containing wall of its cavity. Most hernias occur in the abdominal cavity. Although many kinds of abdominal hernias are possible, inguinal hernias are the most common. (See *Common hernia sites*.)

In an inguinal hernia, the large or small intestine, omentum, or bladder protrudes into the inguinal canal. Hernias can be reducible (if the hernia can be manipulated back into place with relative ease), incarcerated (if the hernia can't be reduced because adhesions have formed in the hernial sac), or strangulated (part of the herniated intestine becomes twisted or edematous, interfering with normal blood flow and peristalsis, and possibly leading to intestinal obstruction and necrosis).

CAUSES
In males, during the seventh month of gestation, the testicle normally descends into the scrotum, preceded by the peritoneal sac. If the sac closes improperly, it leaves an opening through which the intestine can slip.

In either sex, a hernia can result from weak abdominal muscles (caused by congenital malformation, trauma, or aging) or increased intra-abdominal pressure (due to heavy lifting, pregnancy, obesity, or straining).

SIGNS AND SYMPTOMS
Inguinal hernia usually causes a lump to appear over the herniated area when the patient stands or strains; the lump disappears when he is supine. Tension on the herniated contents may cause a sharp, steady pain in the groin, which fades when the hernia is reduced.

Strangulation produces severe pain, and may lead to partial or complete bowel obstruction and even intestinal necrosis. Partial bowel obstruction may cause anorexia, vomiting, pain and tenderness in the groin, an irreducible mass, and diminished

Common hernia sites

Hernias commonly occur in the sites shown below.

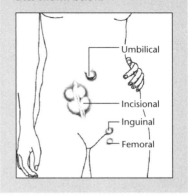

bowel sounds. Complete obstruction may lead to shock, high fever, absent bowel sounds, and bloody stools.

DIAGNOSTIC TESTS
If the hernia is large, an obvious swelling or lump is visible in the groin. With a small hernia, the area may just seem full and the hernia may be palpable when the patient moves. Palpation of the inguinal area during Valsalva's maneuver confirms the diagnosis.

To detect a hernia in a male, the doctor inserts a finger into the scrotum, asks him to cough, and determines the hernia's location by pressure on the finger.

A suspected bowel obstruction calls for X-rays and a white blood cell count.

TREATMENT
If the hernia is reducible, pushing the hernia back into place may relieve pain temporarily. A truss may keep abdominal contents from protruding into the hernial sac.

For infants, adults, and otherwise healthy elderly patients, herniorrhaphy is the treatment of choice.

Herniorrhaphy replaces the contents of the hernial sac into the abdominal cavity and closes the opening.

Another effective surgical procedure for hernia repair is hernioplasty, which reinforces the weakened area with steel mesh, fascia, or wire.

A strangulated or necrotic hernia necessitates bowel resection.

SPECIAL CONSIDERATIONS

● A truss should be applied only after a hernia has been reduced. For best results, it should be applied in the morning, before the patient gets out of bed. It should not be applied over clothing.

● Skin irritation can be prevented by daily bathing and application of cornstarch or baby powder.

 TEACHING TIP: After surgery, caution the patient not to lift or strain. Instruct him to report signs and symptoms of infection (oozing, tenderness, warmth, redness) at the incision site. Advise him to keep the incision clean and covered until the sutures are removed.

Intestinal obstruction

An intestinal obstruction is a partial or complete blockage of the lumen of the small or large bowel. A small-bowel obstruction is far more common and usually more serious. Intestinal obstructions are most likely to occur after abdominal surgery and in people with congenital bowel deformities.

A complete obstruction in any part of the bowel, if untreated, can cause death within hours from shock and vascular collapse.

The three forms of intestinal obstruction are:

● *simple:* blockage prevents intestinal contents from passing, with no other complications

● *strangulated:* blood supply to part or all of the obstructed section is cut off, in addition to blockage of the lumen

● *close-looped:* both ends of a bowel section are occluded, isolating it from the rest of the intestine.

CAUSES

Adhesions and strangulated hernias usually cause small-bowel obstructions; carcinomas usually cause large-bowel obstructions. A mechanical intestinal obstruction results from foreign bodies (fruit pits, gallstones, worms) or compression of the bowel wall caused by stenosis, intussusception, volvulus of the sigmoid or cecum, tumors, or atresia.

A nonmechanical obstruction results from physiologic disturbances, such as paralytic ileus, electrolyte imbalances, toxicity, and neurogenic abnormalities.

SIGNS AND SYMPTOMS

Clinical features depend on the location and extent of the obstruction.

Partial small-bowel obstruction

Colicky pain, nausea, vomiting, constipation, and abdominal distention characterize small-bowel obstruction. The patient also may experience drowsiness, intense thirst, malaise, aching, and dryness of the tongue and oral mucous membranes.

Complete small-bowel obstruction

Vigorous peristaltic waves propel bowel contents toward the mouth instead of the rectum. Spasms may occur every 3 to 5 minutes and last about 1 minute each, with persistent epigastric or periumbilical pain. Passage of small amounts of mucus and blood may occur. Vomitus initially contains gastric juice, then bile, and finally fecal contents of the ileum.

Partial large-bowel obstruction

Signs and symptoms of large-bowel obstruction develop more slowly. Constipation may be the only sign for days. Colicky abdominal pain then may appear suddenly, producing spasms that recur every few minutes. Continuous hypogastric pain and nausea may develop.

Large-bowel obstruction may cause visible loops of large bowel on the abdomen.

Complete large-bowel obstruction

Eventually, a complete large-bowel obstruction may cause fecal vomiting, continuous pain, or localized peritonitis.

Patients with a partial obstruction may display any of the above symptoms in a milder form, along with leakage of liquid stools around the obstruction.

DIAGNOSTIC TESTS

Progressive, colicky, abdominal pain and distention, with or without nausea and vomiting, suggest bowel obstruction; characteristic X-ray findings confirm it.

TREATMENT

Preoperative therapy includes correction of fluid and electrolyte imbalances, bowel decompression to relieve vomiting and distention, and treatment of shock and peritonitis. A strangulated obstruction usually necessitates blood replacement and I.V. fluids. Passage of a nasogastric (NG) tube, followed by use of a Miller-Abbott or Cantor tube, usually accomplishes decompression.

If the patient fails to improve or if his condition deteriorates, surgery is necessary. In large-bowel obstruction, surgical resection with anastomosis, colostomy, or ileostomy commonly follows decompression with an NG tube.

SPECIAL CONSIDERATIONS

 ACTION STAT: Get immediate help if the patient has signs of shock: pallor, rapid pulse, or hypotension.

• Fastidious mouth and nose care is important if the patient has vomited or undergone decompression by intubation.

• The patient should remain in Fowler's position as much as possible to promote pulmonary ventilation and ease respiratory distress.

• An enterostomal therapist should be scheduled to visit the patient who has had an ostomy.

Intussusception

In intussusception, a portion of the bowel (the intussusceptum) telescopes, or invaginates, into an adjacent distal portion. Peristalsis propels the segment along the bowel, pulling more bowel along with it. This invagination produces edema, hemorrhage (from venous engorgement), incarceration, and obstruction.

If treatment is delayed longer than 24 hours, strangulation of the intestine usually occurs, with gangrene, shock, perforation, and possibly death.

Intussusception is most common in infants; 87% of children with intussusception are under age 2.

CAUSES

Studies suggest that intussusception may be linked to viral infections. In infants, the cause usually remains unknown. In older children, polyps, alterations in intestinal motility, hemangioma, lymphosarcoma, lymphoid hyperplasia, or Meckel's diverticulum may trigger the process.

In adults, intussusception usually results from benign or malignant tumors. Other causes include polyps, Meckel's diverticulum, gastroenterostomy with herniation, or an appendiceal stump.

SIGNS AND SYMPTOMS

In adults, intussusception produces nonspecific, chronic, and intermittent signs and symptoms, including colicky abdominal pain and tenderness, vomiting, diarrhea (occasionally constipation), bloody stools, and weight loss. Abdominal pain usually localizes in the right lower quadrant, radiates to the back, and increases with eating. Adults with severe intussusception may develop strangulation with excruciating pain, abdominal distention, and tachycardia.

Identifying intussusception in a child

In an infant or a child, intussusception produces four cardinal signs and symptoms:

● intermittent attacks of colicky pain, which cause the child to scream, draw his legs up to his abdomen, turn pale and diaphoretic and, possibly, display grunting respirations

● initially, vomiting of stomach contents; later, vomiting of bile-stained or fecal material

● "currant jelly" stools, which contain a mixture of blood and mucus

● tender, distended abdomen, with a palpable, sausage-shaped abdominal mass.

In children, intussusception has four distinct hallmarks. (See *Identifying intussusception in a child*.)

DIAGNOSTIC TESTS

Barium enema confirms colonic intussusception when it shows the characteristic coiled spring sign; it also delineates the extent of intussusception.

Upright abdominal X-rays may show a soft-tissue mass and signs of complete or partial obstruction, with dilated loops of bowel.

A white blood cell count up to 15,000/µl indicates obstruction; more than 15,000/µl, strangulation; more than 20,000/µl, possible bowel infarction.

TREATMENT

In children, therapy may include hydrostatic reduction or surgery. Surgery is indicated for children with recurrent intussusception, for those who show signs of shock or peritonitis, and for those whose symptoms have been present longer than 24 hours. In adults, surgery is always the treatment of choice.

Hydrostatic reduction

In hydrostatic reduction, the radiologist drips a barium solution into the rectum; fluoroscopy traces barium progress. In a successful procedure, the barium backwashes into the ileum and the mass disappears. If this does not happen, the procedure is stopped and the patient is prepared for surgery.

Surgery

Manual reduction is attempted first. If manual reduction fails, or if the bowel is gangrenous or strangulated, the doctor resects the affected bowel segment. He may also perform a prophylactic appendectomy.

SPECIAL CONSIDERATIONS

● In a child, intussusception is considered an emergency. Provide encouragement and reassurance to the child and parents.

Iron deficiency anemia

In iron deficiency anemia, the body's iron supply is inadequate for optimal formation of red blood cells (RBCs). RBC mass is depleted, causing a decreased hemoglobin concentration and diminished oxygen-carrying capacity of the blood.

A common disease worldwide, iron deficiency anemia affects 10% to 30% of the adult population of the United States. The disorder is most common in premenopausal women, infants, children, and adolescents.

CAUSES

Iron deficiency anemia may result from:

● inadequate dietary intake of iron

● iron malabsorption, as in chronic diarrhea, gastrectomy, and malabsorption syndromes such as celiac disease

● blood loss secondary to drug-induced GI bleeding (from anticoagulants, aspirin, steroids) or due to heavy menses, hemorrhage from trauma, GI ulcers, cancer, or varices

• pregnancy, which diverts maternal iron to the fetus for erythropoiesis
• intravascular hemolysis-induced hemoglobinuria or paroxysmal nocturnal hemoglobinuria
• mechanical erythrocyte trauma caused by a prosthetic heart valve or vena cava filters
• use of pancreatic enzymes or vitamin E, which may interfere with iron metabolism and absorption.

SIGNS AND SYMPTOMS

Because iron deficiency anemia progresses gradually, many patients initially lack symptoms, except for those of any underlying condition. They tend not to seek medical treatment until anemia is severe.

At advanced stages, the patient experiences dyspnea on exertion, fatigue, listlessness, pallor, inability to concentrate, irritability, headache, and susceptibility to infection. Decreased oxygen perfusion causes the heart to compensate with increased cardiac output and tachycardia.

In chronic iron deficiency anemia, nails become spoon-shaped and brittle, the corners of the mouth crack, the tongue turns smooth, and the patient complains of dysphagia or may develop pica. Neuromuscular effects may include vasomotor disturbances, numbness and tingling of the extremities, and neuralgic pain.

DIAGNOSTIC TESTS

Blood studies (hemoglobin, hematocrit, serum iron, serum ferritin, RBC count) and bone marrow analysis may confirm iron deficiency anemia. However, test results may be misleading because of complicating factors, such as infection, pneumonia, blood transfusion, or iron supplements. Therefore, other forms of anemia must be ruled out.

TREATMENT

The first priority is to determine the underlying cause of anemia. Then iron replacement therapy begins. The treatment of choice is an oral iron preparation or a combination of iron

---

Preventing iron deficiency anemia

The following suggestions can help patients avert iron deficiency anemia.

Eating a balanced diet

• Advise the patient to consume a nutritionally balanced diet — one that includes red meats, green vegetables, eggs, whole wheat iron-fortified bread, and milk. However, keep in mind that no food in itself contains enough iron to *treat* iron deficiency anemia: An average-sized person with anemia would have to eat at least 10 lb (4.5 kg) of steak daily to receive therapeutic amounts of iron.
• If the patient's iron intake is deficient, he should eat meat, fish, or poultry; whole or enriched grain; and foods high in ascorbic acid.

Taking supplemental iron

• A person who is at high risk for iron deficiency should take prophylactic oral iron if prescribed by the doctor. High-risk groups include premature infants, children under age 2, and pregnant women.
• Children under age 2 should also receive supplemental cereals and formulas high in iron.

---

and ascorbic acid (which enhances iron absorption).

In some cases, iron must be given parenterally — for instance, if the patient is noncompliant, if he needs more iron than he can take orally, or if malabsorption prevents adequate iron absorption.

SPECIAL CONSIDERATIONS

 TEACHING TIP: Inform the patient that iron supplement therapy takes some time, and that he shouldn't stop prescribed therapy even if he feels better. Tell him that vitamin C enhances iron absorption and that milk and antacids interfere with its absorption. To prevent tooth staining, advise him to drink liquid supplemental iron through a straw.

• Adverse reactions to iron, such as nausea, vomiting, diarrhea, constipation, fever, or severe stomach pain, may indicate the need for a dosage adjustment.

 PREVENTION TIP: Because an iron deficiency may recur, advise the patient to get regular checkups. Health professionals can play a vital role in preventing iron deficiency anemia. (See *Preventing iron deficiency anemia,* page 175.)

• A dietician may assess a family's dietary habits for iron intake, noting the influence of childhood eating patterns, cultural food preferences, and family income on adequate nutrition.

Irritable bowel syndrome

Also known as spastic colon or spastic colitis, irritable bowel syndrome is a common condition marked by chronic or periodic diarrhea, alternating with constipation and accompanied by straining and abdominal cramps.

The prognosis is good. Supportive treatment or avoidance of known food irritants commonly relieves symptoms.

CAUSES

This functional disorder is generally associated with psychological stress. However, it may result from physical factors, such as diverticular disease, ingestion of irritants (coffee, raw fruits or vegetables), lactose intolerance, laxative abuse, food poisoning, or colon cancer.

SIGNS AND SYMPTOMS

Irritable bowel syndrome typically produces lower abdominal pain (usually relieved by defecation or passage of gas) and day-time diarrhea. These symptoms alternate with constipation or normal bowel function. Stools often are small and contain visible mucus.

DIAGNOSTIC TESTS

A careful patient history is required to determine contributing psychological factors such as a recent stressful life change. Diagnosis must rule out other disorders, such as amebiasis, diverticulitis, colon cancer, and lactose intolerance. Diagnostic procedures include sigmoidoscopy, colonoscopy, barium enema, a rectal biopsy, and stool examination for blood, parasites, and bacteria.

TREATMENT

Therapy aims to relieve symptoms and includes counseling to help the patient understand the relationship between stress and his illness. Strict dietary restrictions aren't beneficial, but food irritants should be investigated and the patient instructed to avoid them.

Rest and heat applied to the abdomen are helpful, as is judicious use of sedatives (such as phenobarbital) and antispasmodics (such as propantheline). However, with chronic use, the patient may become dependent on these drugs. If the cause of irritable bowel syndrome is chronic laxative abuse, bowel training may help correct the condition.

SPECIAL CONSIDERATIONS

 TEACHING TIP: Instruct the patient to avoid irritating foods and to develop regular bowel habits. Advise him to develop methods for dealing with stress, without developing a dependence on sedatives or antispasmodics. Urge him to get regular checkups because irritable bowel syndrome is associated with an increased incidence of diverticulitis and colon cancer.

• Patients over age 40 should have annual sigmoidoscopy and rectal examinations.

Kaposi's sarcoma

Initially, this cancer of the lymphatic cell wall was described as a rare blood vessel sarcoma, occurring mostly in elderly Italian and Jewish men. In recent years, the incidence of Kaposi's sarcoma has risen dramatically along with that of acquired immunodeficiency syndrome (AIDS). Currently, it's the most common AIDS-related cancer.

Kaposi's sarcoma causes both structural and functional damage. When associated with AIDS, it progresses aggressively, involving the lymph nodes, viscera and, possibly, GI structures.

CAUSES
The exact cause of Kaposi's sarcoma is unknown, but the disease may be related to immunosuppression. Genetic or hereditary predisposition also is suspected.

SIGNS AND SYMPTOMS
The initial sign is one or more obvious lesions in various shapes, sizes, and colors ranging from red-brown to dark purple. Lesions most commonly appear on the skin, buccal mucosa, hard and soft palates, lips, gums, tongue, tonsils, conjunctiva, and sclera. In advanced disease, lesions may join to become one large plaque. Untreated lesions may appear as large, ulcerative masses.

The patient also may have pain and additional signs and symptoms. (See *Additional indicators of Kaposi's sarcoma,* page 178.)

The most common extracutaneous sites are the lungs and GI tract (esophagus, oropharynx, and epiglottis).

DIAGNOSTIC TESTS
Diagnosis hinges on a tissue biopsy that identifies the lesion's type and stage. Then, a computed tomography scan may be performed to detect and evaluate possible metastasis.

TREATMENT
Treatment isn't indicated for all patients. Indications include painful, obstructive, or cosmetically offensive lesions of rapidly progressing disease.

Radiation therapy, chemotherapy, and biotherapy with biological response modifiers are treatment options. Besides relieving symptoms, radiation therapy may be used for cosmetic improvement.

Chemotherapy includes combinations of doxorubicin, vinblastine, vincristine, and etoposide (VP-16).

Biotherapy with interferon alfa-2b may be given for AIDS-related Kaposi's sarcoma. This treatment reduces the number of skin lesions but is ineffective in advanced disease.

SPECIAL CONSIDERATIONS
● Besides pain from the lesions, the patient may experience distress over changes in appearance and anxiety related to diagnostic procedures, treatments, and outcomes. Listen to his concerns and answer his questions honestly. Family members also may need help in coping with his disease.
● If lesions are painful, help the patient into a more comfortable position. Pain also may be reduced through the use of distraction, relaxation techniques, and medication, when necessary.
● Eating frequent, small meals high in calories and protein helps ensure sufficient caloric intake. A dietitian can help plan a diet and schedule meals around the patient's treatment.
● Planning daily periods of alternating activity and rest may reduce fatigue.
● If the prognosis is poor, the patient

Additional indicators of Kaposi's sarcoma

Besides the characteristic lesions, some patients with Kaposi's sarcoma experience such signs and symptoms as:
● pain (if the sarcoma advances beyond the early stages or if a lesion breaks down or impinges on nerves or organs)
● edema from lymphatic obstruction
● dyspnea (in cases of pulmonary involvement), wheezing, hypoventilation, and respiratory distress from bronchial blockage. With disease progression and metastasis, the patient may have severe pulmonary involvement and GI involvement leading to digestive problems.

may wish to consider advance directives, durable power of attorney orders, and hospice care options.

Kidney cancer

Kidney cancer usually occurs in older adults. About 85% of these tumors originate in the kidneys; others result from metastasis from other primary sites. Renal pelvic tumors and Wilms' tumor occur primarily in children.

Kidney tumors usually are large, firm, nodular, encapsulated, unilateral, and solitary. Histologically, they are classified as the clear cell, granular, or spindle cell type.

The prognosis probably depends on the cancer stage. The 5-year survival rate is about 50%.

CAUSES

The cause of kidney cancer remains unknown. However, the incidence of this cancer is rising. Even so, kidney cancer accounts for only about 2% of all adult cancers.

SIGNS AND SYMPTOMS

Kidney cancer produces a classic clinical triad — hematuria, pain, and a palpable mass — but any one of these features may be the first sign. All three coexist in only about 10% of patients. Microscopic or gross hematuria suggests that the cancer has spread to the renal pelvis.

Constant abdominal or flank pain may be dull or, if the cancer causes bleeding or blood clots, acute and colicky. The mass typically is smooth, firm, and nontender.

Other clinical features include fever, hypertension, rapidly progressing hypercalcemia, and urine retention. Weight loss, edema in the legs, nausea, and vomiting signal advanced kidney cancer.

DIAGNOSTIC TESTS

Studies to identify kidney cancer usually include a computed tomography scan, excretory urography and retrograde pyelography, ultrasonography, cystoscopy (to rule out associated bladder cancer), and nephrotomography or renal angiography to distinguish a cyst from a tumor.

TREATMENT

Radical nephrectomy, with or without regional lymph node dissection, offers the only chance of cure. The disease resists radiation, so radiation is used only if the cancer has spread to the perinephric region or the lymph nodes or if the primary tumor or metastatic sites can't be fully excised.

Chemotherapy has been only erratically effective against kidney cancer. Biotherapy (lymphokine-activated killer cells with recombinant interleukin-2) shows promise but causes adverse reactions. Interferon is somewhat effective in advanced disease.

SPECIAL CONSIDERATIONS

● Before surgery, emphasize that the patient's body will adapt to the loss of a kidney.
● After surgery, the patient should be placed on the operative side. If possible, he should walk within 24 hours.

Labyrinthitis

An inflammation of the labyrinth of the inner ear, labyrinthitis is a rare disorder. Commonly, it incapacitates the patient by causing severe vertigo for 3 to 5 days. Signs and symptoms gradually subside over 3 to 6 weeks.

CAUSES
Labyrinthitis usually results from viral infection. It may be a primary infection (such as upper respiratory tract infection), the result of trauma, or a complication of influenza, otitis media, or meningitis. Toxic drug ingestion is another possible cause of labyrinthitis.

In chronic otitis media, a cystlike mass (cholesteatoma) forms. The mass erodes the bone of the labyrinth and allows bacteria to enter from the middle ear.

SIGNS AND SYMPTOMS
Because the inner ear controls hearing and balance, labyrinthitis typically produces severe vertigo and sensorineural hearing loss. Vertigo begins gradually but peaks within 48 hours, causing loss of balance and falling in the direction of the affected ear.

Other features of labyrinthitis include spontaneous nystagmus, with jerking movements of the eyes toward the unaffected ear; nausea and vomiting; giddiness; signs of middle ear disease, in cholesteatoma; and purulent drainage, in severe bacterial infection.

DIAGNOSTIC TESTS
Typical clinical features and a history of upper respiratory tract infection suggest labyrinthitis. Diagnostic studies usually include culture and sensitivity testing to identify the infecting organism (if purulent drainage is present) and audiometric testing.

When an infectious agent can't be found, additional testing is done to rule out a brain lesion or Ménière's disease.

TREATMENT
Symptomatic treatment includes bed rest, with the patient's head immobilized between pillows; oral meclizine to control vertigo; and massive antibiotic doses to combat diffuse purulent labyrinthitis. Oral fluids can prevent dehydration from vomiting. For severe nausea and vomiting, I.V. fluids may be necessary.

When conservative management fails, the cholesteatoma is surgically excised and infected areas of the middle and inner ear are drained.

SPECIAL CONSIDERATIONS
• The side rails of the patient's bed should be kept up to prevent falls.
• Antiemetics may be used to control vomiting. The patient may require I.V. fluids to combat dehydration.

 TEACHING TIP: During recovery, which may take up to 6 weeks, instruct the patient to limit activities that vertigo may make hazardous.

• If recovery doesn't occur within 4 to 6 weeks, a computed tomography scan may be performed to rule out an intracranial lesion.

 PREVENTION TIP: Early and vigorous treatment of predisposing conditions, such as otitis media and local or systemic infection, can help prevent labyrinthitis.

Laryngeal cancer

The most common form of cancer of the larynx is squamous cell carcinoma (95%). Rare forms include adenocarcinoma and sarcoma.

Laryngeal cancer may be intrinsic or extrinsic. An *intrinsic* tumor is on

Helping the patient after larynx removal

After total laryngectomy, the following measures may increase the patient's comfort.

• The patient should lie on one side with his head elevated 30 to 45 degrees. His neck must be supported when he is moved.

• Adequate room humidification can help prevent crusting and secretions around the stoma. Secretions should be removed with petrolatum, antimicrobial ointment, and moist gauze.

• Speech rehabilitation may help the patient speak again. The International Association of Laryngectomees is a source of support.

the true vocal cord and tends not to spread. An *extrinsic* tumor is on some other part of the larynx and tends to spread early.

Laryngeal cancer also is classified by location:

• supraglottis (false vocal cords)
• glottis (true vocal cords)
• subglottis (downward extension from the vocal cords [rare]).

CAUSES

Major predisposing factors include smoking and alcoholism. Minor factors are chronic inhalation of noxious fumes and familial tendency.

SIGNS AND SYMPTOMS

In intrinsic laryngeal cancer, the dominant and earliest symptom is hoarseness lasting more than 3 weeks. In extrinsic cancer, it's a lump in the throat or pain or burning in the throat when drinking citrus juice or hot liquid. With metastasis, later clinical features include dysphagia, dyspnea, cough, enlarged cervical lymph nodes, and pain radiating to the ear.

DIAGNOSTIC TESTS

Laryngoscopy is required for patients who experience hoarseness lasting more than 2 weeks. Xeroradiography, biopsy, laryngeal tomography, a computed tomography scan, or laryngography defines the lesion's borders. A chest X-ray may detect metastasis.

TREATMENT

Early lesions are treated with surgery or radiation; advanced lesions with surgery, radiation, and chemotherapy. The treatment goal is to eliminate cancer and preserve speech.

If speech preservation isn't possible, speech rehabilitation may include esophageal speech devices or prosthetic devices. (Surgical techniques to construct a new voice box are still experimental.)

Surgical procedures vary with tumor size and may include cordectomy, partial or total laryngectomy, supraglottic laryngectomy, or total laryngectomy with laryngoplasty.

SPECIAL CONSIDERATIONS

 TEACHING TIP: Before partial or total laryngectomy, the patient should select a temporary nonspeaking method of communication (such as writing). Also, the health care team should prepare him for other functional losses, such as inability to smell, blow the nose, whistle, gargle, sip, or suck on a straw.

After partial laryngectomy

The tracheostomy tube is kept in place until edema subsides. The patient should not use his or her voice until medical permission is granted (usually 2 to 3 days postoperatively). Then, he should whisper until healing is complete.

After total laryngectomy

Carotid artery rupture can occur in patients who have had preoperative radiation, particularly those with a fistula that constantly bathes the carotid artery with oral secretions. If rupture occurs, apply pressure to the site and call for help immediately. The patient must go to the operating room for carotid ligation. (For more information on patient care after a total laryngectomy, see *Helping the patient after larynx removal*.)

Laryngitis

A common disorder, laryngitis is an acute or chronic inflammation of the vocal cords. Acute laryngitis may occur as an isolated infection or as part of a generalized bacterial or viral upper respiratory tract infection. Repeated attacks of acute laryngitis cause inflammatory changes associated with chronic laryngitis.

CAUSES

Acute laryngitis usually results from infection (primarily viral) or excessive use of the voice — an occupational hazard of teachers, public speakers, and singers. It also may result from leisure activities (such as cheering at a sports event), inhaling smoke or fumes, or aspirating caustic chemicals.

Causes of chronic laryngitis include chronic upper respiratory tract disorders (sinusitis, bronchitis, nasal polyps, allergy), mouth breathing, smoking, constant exposure to dust or other irritants, and alcohol abuse.

SIGNS AND SYMPTOMS

Acute laryngitis typically begins with hoarseness, ranging from mild to complete loss of voice. Associated features include pain (especially when swallowing or speaking), dry cough, fever, laryngeal edema, and malaise. In chronic laryngitis, persistent hoarseness usually is the only symptom.

DIAGNOSTIC TESTS

Indirect laryngoscopy confirms the diagnosis by revealing red, inflamed and, occasionally, hemorrhagic vocal cords, with rounded rather than sharp edges and exudate. Bilateral swelling may be present. In severe cases or if toxicity is suspected, a culture of the exudate is obtained for analysis.

TREATMENT

Primary treatment consists of resting the voice. For viral infection, symptomatic care includes analgesics and throat lozenges for pain relief. Bacterial infection calls for antibiotic therapy. In chronic laryngitis, the underlying cause must be eliminated.

Severe, acute laryngitis may necessitate hospitalization. When laryngeal edema results in airway obstruction, tracheotomy may be necessary.

SPECIAL CONSIDERATIONS

• Using medicated throat lozenges and avoiding smoking can promote patient comfort.

 TEACHING TIP: To improve compliance, explain to the patient why he shouldn't talk. Urge him to use another communication method, such as a Magic Slate or a pad and pencil. Placing a sign over his bed will remind others of his speech restriction.

• To minimize the patient's need to talk, anticipate his needs.

• The intercom panel should be marked so that other hospital personnel are aware that the patient can't answer.

 PREVENTION TIP: Using a vaporizer or humidifier during the winter and avoiding air conditioning during the summer (because it dehumidifies) may help prevent laryngitis.

Legionnaires' disease

An acute bronchopneumonia, legionnaires' disease may occur epidemically or sporadically, usually in late summer or early fall. Its severity ranges from a mild illness, with or without pneumonitis, to multilobar pneumonia, with a mortality as high as 15%.

A milder, self-limiting form (Pontiac syndrome) subsides within a few days but leaves the patient fatigued for several weeks. This form causes few or no respiratory symptoms, no pneumonia, and no fatalities.

CAUSES

The causative agent, *Legionella pneumophila,* is an aerobic, gram-negative bacillus that's probably transmitted by an airborne route. In past epi-

Risk factors for legionnaires' disease

Legionnaires' disease is most likely to strike the following:
- middle-aged to elderly people
- immunocompromised patients, especially those receiving corticosteroids (for example, after a transplant)
- patients with lymphoma or other disorders associated with delayed hypersensitivity
- patients with a chronic underlying disease, such as diabetes, chronic renal failure, or chronic obstructive pulmonary disease
- alcoholics
- cigarette smokers (they are three to four times more likely to develop the disease than non-smokers).

demics, it has spread through cooling towers or evaporation condensers in air-conditioning systems. However, *Legionella* bacilli also flourish in soil and excavation sites. The disease does not spread from person to person.

Certain conditions can predispose a person to legionnaires' disease. (See *Risk factors for legionnaires' disease.*)

SIGNS AND SYMPTOMS
Clinical features of legionnaires' disease follow a predictable sequence, although disease onset may be gradual or sudden. After a 2- to 10-day incubation period, the patient may experience diarrhea, anorexia, malaise, diffuse myalgias, generalized weakness, headache, recurrent chills, and an unremitting fever (which arises within 12 to 48 hours and may reach 105° F [40.5° C]). A cough then develops; initially nonproductive, it eventually may produce grayish, nonpurulent sputum.

Other signs and symptoms include nausea, vomiting, disorientation, mental sluggishness, confusion, mild temporary amnesia, pleuritic chest pain, tachypnea, dyspnea, fine crackles, and bradycardia. Complications may include hypotension, delirium, congestive heart failure, arrhythmias, acute respiratory failure, renal failure, and shock.

DIAGNOSTIC TESTS
Patient history focuses on possible sources of infection and predisposing conditions. Physical examination, chest X-rays, and blood studies may reveal evidence of legionnaires' disease. Bronchial washings and blood, pleural fluid, and sputum tests rule out other infections. (Definitive test results, including bacterial culture, aren't available until convalescence.)

TREATMENT
Antibiotic therapy begins as soon as legionnaires' disease is suspected and diagnostic material is collected. If erythromycin, the drug of choice, is not effective alone, rifampin may be added. If erythromycin is contraindicated, rifampin or rifampin with tetracycline may be used.

Supportive therapy includes antipyretics, fluid replacement, circulatory support with pressor drugs if necessary, and oxygen administration by mask, cannula, or mechanical ventilation.

SPECIAL CONSIDERATIONS
- The patient is observed for signs of shock: decreased blood pressure, thready pulse, diaphoresis, and clammy skin.
- Patient comfort measures include avoiding chills and exposure to drafts, providing frequent mouth care, and applying cream to the nostrils.

 TEACHING TIP: Teach the patient how to perform effective coughing and deep-breathing exercises, and instruct him to continue to use these measures until recovery is complete.

Leukemia, acute
Acute leukemia is a malignant proliferation of white blood cell (WBC) precursors (blasts) in bone marrow or

lymph tissue and their accumulation in peripheral blood, bone marrow, and body tissues. Among children, acute leukemia is the most common form of cancer.

Common forms of acute leukemia are:

• acute lymphoblastic (lymphocytic) leukemia (ALL), characterized by abnormal growth of lymphocyte precursors (lymphoblasts)

• acute myeloblastic (myelogenous) leukemia (AML), in which myeloid precursors (myeloblasts) rapidly accumulate

• acute monoblastic (monocytic) leukemia, characterized by a marked increase in monocyte precursors (monoblasts).

Untreated, acute leukemia is invariably fatal, usually from complications caused by leukemic cell infiltration of bone marrow or vital organs. With treatment, the prognosis varies.

In ALL, treatment induces remissions in 90% of children and in 65% of adults. Children between ages 2 and 8 have the best survival rate with intensive therapy.

In AML, average survival time is 1 year after diagnosis, even with aggressive treatment. In acute monoblastic leukemia, treatment induces remissions lasting 2 to 10 months in 50% of children; adults survive only about 1 year after diagnosis, even with treatment.

CAUSES

Research on predisposing factors suggests some combination of viruses, genetic and immunologic factors as well as exposure to radiation and certain chemicals.

Pathogenesis isn't clearly understood, but immature, nonfunctioning WBCs appear to accumulate first in the tissue where they originate and then spill into the bloodstream and infiltrate other tissues, eventually causing organ malfunction due to encroachment or hemorrhage. (See *What happens in leukemia,* page 184.)

SIGNS AND SYMPTOMS

Acute leukemia causes sudden onset of high fever accompanied by thrombocytopenia and abnormal bleeding (nosebleeds, gingival bleeding, purpura, ecchymoses, petechiae, easy bruising after minor trauma, and prolonged menses). Nonspecific symptoms, such as low-grade fever, weakness, and lassitude, may persist for days or months before visible symptoms appear.

Other subtle indicators include pallor, chills, and recurrent infections. In addition, ALL, AML, and acute monoblastic leukemia may cause dyspnea, anemia, fatigue, malaise, tachycardia, palpitations, systolic ejection murmur, and abdominal or bone pain. When leukemic cells cross the blood-brain barrier and escape the effects of systemic chemotherapy, the patient may develop meningeal leukemia (confusion, lethargy, headache).

DIAGNOSTIC TESTS

Diagnosis is based on patient history, physical findings, and bone marrow aspirate showing proliferation of immature WBCs. If the marrow is free of leukemic cells, a bone marrow biopsy is performed. Blood studies typically show a deficiency of platelets and neutrophils. Lumbar puncture can determine if the meninges are involved.

TREATMENT

Systemic chemotherapy aims to eradicate leukemic cells and induce remission. Chemotherapy varies with the type of leukemia.

A bone marrow transplant may be an option for some patients. Treatment also may include antibiotic, antifungal, and antiviral drugs and granulocyte injections to control infection. Transfusions may be given of platelets (to prevent bleeding) and red blood cells (to prevent anemia).

SPECIAL CONSIDERATIONS

 TEACHING TIP: Teach the patient about adverse effects of medications, how to recognize signs and symptoms of infection (fever, chills, cough, sore throat) and

PATHOPHYSIOLOGY

What happens in leukemia

As this illustration shows, blood cells (agranulocytes and granulocytes) proliferate in the bloodstream of a patient with leukemia, overwhelming red blood cells (RBCs) and platelets.

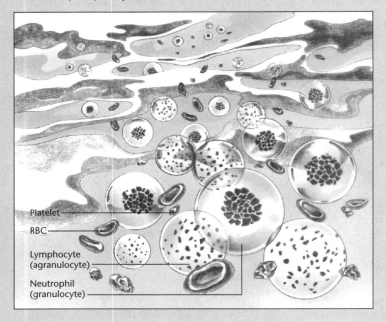

Platelet

RBC

Lymphocyte (agranulocyte)

Neutrophil (granulocyte)

abnormal bleeding (bruising, petechiae), and how to stop such bleeding (by applying pressure and ice to the area).

• A high-calorie, high-protein diet may help to limit the effects of chemotherapy, such as weight loss and anorexia.

• Placing the patient in a private room and imposing reverse isolation, if necessary, can reduce the risk of infection. Patient care should be coordinated so he doesn't come in contact with staff who also care for patients with infections or infectious diseases.

• Bleeding can be controlled by applying ice compresses and pressure and elevating the extremity. I.M. injections, aspirin and aspirin-containing drugs, rectal temperatures, rectal suppositories, and digital examinations should be avoided.

• Mouth ulceration can be controlled by checking often for obvious ulcers and gum swelling and by providing frequent mouth care and saline rinses. The patient should use a soft toothbrush and avoid hot, spicy foods and overuse of commercial mouthwashes.

Leukemia, chronic granulocytic

Chronic granulocytic leukemia (CGL) is characterized by abnormal overgrowth of granulocytic precursors (myeloblasts, promyelocytes, metamyelocytes, and myelocytes) in the bone marrow, peripheral blood, and body tissues. CGL is also known as chronic myelogenous (or myelocytic) leukemia.

The clinical course of CGL proceeds in two distinct phases: the *insidious chronic phase,* with anemia and bleeding abnormalities and, eventually, the *acute phase (blastic crisis),* in which myeloblasts proliferate rapidly.

The disease is invariably fatal. Average survival time is 3 to 4 years after onset of the chronic phase and 3 to 6 months after onset of the acute phase.

CAUSES
Almost 90% of patients with CGL have the Philadelphia (Ph[1]) chromosome, an abnormality of chromosome 22. Radiation and carcinogenic chemicals may induce this abnormality.

Other proposed causes of CGL are myeloproliferative diseases and an unidentified virus.

SIGNS AND SYMPTOMS
Typically, CGL causes:
● anemia (fatigue, weakness, decreased exercise tolerance, pallor, dyspnea, tachycardia, and headache)
● thrombocytopenia, with resulting bleeding and clotting disorders (retinal hemorrhage, ecchymoses, hematuria, melena, bleeding gums, nosebleeds, and easy bruising)
● hepatosplenomegaly, with abdominal discomfort and pain in splenic infarction.

Other signs and symptoms may include sternal and rib tenderness, lowgrade fever, weight loss, anorexia, kidney stones, and gouty arthritis.

DIAGNOSTIC TESTS
Chromosomal analysis of peripheral blood or bone marrow showing Ph[1] and low leukocyte-alkaline-phosphatase levels typically confirms CGL. Other relevant laboratory results include:
● white blood cell abnormalities, such as leukocytosis (an abnormally high leukocyte count), occasional leukopenia (an abnormally low leukocyte count), neutropenia (an abnormally low neutrophil count) despite a high leukocyte count, and increased circulating myeloblasts
● bone marrow aspirate or biopsy, which typically shows bone marrow infiltration by an increased number of myeloid elements.

TREATMENT
Because aggressive chemotherapy has failed to produce remission, the treatment goal in the chronic phase is to control leukocytosis and thrombocytosis. The most commonly used oral agents are busulfan and hydroxyurea. Aspirin may be given to prevent stroke if the platelet count is over 1 million/µl.

Additional treatments may involve radiation, leukapheresis, and drugs. (See *Adjunctive treatments for CGL,* page 186.)

During the acute phase of CGL, lymphoblastic or myeloblastic leukemia may develop. Treatment resembles that for acute lymphoblastic leukemia. In the early phase of illness, bone marrow transplantation may produce long asymptomatic periods. Despite vigorous treatment, CGL usually progresses after onset of the acute phase.

SPECIAL CONSIDERATIONS
● Assist the patient with walking if necessary, if he experiences fatigue related to anemia.
● The patient's skin and mucous membranes must be checked for pallor, petechiae, and bruising. To minimize bleeding, suggest use of a soft-bristled toothbrush and an electric razor.

 TEACHING TIP: Instruct the patient about adverse effects of chemotherapy, especially dangerous ones such as bone marrow suppression. Also tell him how to recognize signs and symptoms of infection (fever over 100° F [37.8° C],

Adjunctive treatments for CGL

Besides chemotherapy, some patients with chronic granulocytic leukemia (CGL) may receive the following treatments:
• local splenic radiation or splenectomy, to increase the platelet count and ease adverse effects of splenomegaly
• leukapheresis (selective leukocyte removal), to reduce the leukocyte count
• allopurinol, to prevent secondary hyperuricemia, or colchicine, to relieve gout caused by elevated serum uric acid levels.

Also, a patient who experiences bone marrow suppression from chemotherapy must be treated promptly for any infections that arise.

chills, redness or swelling, sore throat, and cough). Emphasize the importance of getting adequate rest and eating a high-calorie, high-protein diet to reduce toxic effects of chemotherapy.

Leukemia, chronic lymphocytic

A generalized, progressive disease that's common in elderly people, chronic lymphocytic leukemia (CLL) is marked by the uncontrollable spread of abnormal, small lymphocytes in lymphoid tissue, blood, and bone marrow. The prognosis is poor if the patient has anemia, thrombocytopenia, neutropenia, bulky lymphadenopathy, and severe lymphocytosis.

Nearly all patients with CLL are men over age 50. CLL accounts for almost one-third of new leukemia cases annually.

CAUSES
Although the cause of CLL is unknown, researchers suspect heredi-tary factors, still-undefined chromosome abnormalities, and certain immunologic defects. The disease doesn't seem to be associated with radiation exposure.

SIGNS AND SYMPTOMS
CLL is the most benign and most slowly progressive form of leukemia. Clinical features result from infiltration of leukemic cells in bone marrow, lymphoid tissue, and organ systems.

In early disease stages, patients typically complain of fatigue, malaise, fever, and nodal enlargement. They are particularly susceptible to infection.

In advanced stages, patients may experience severe fatigue and weight loss, with liver or spleen enlargement, bone tenderness, and edema from lymph node obstruction. Pulmonary infiltrates may appear when the lung parenchyma is involved. Skin infiltrations (macular to nodular eruptions) occur in about one-half of CLL cases.

As the disease progresses, bone marrow involvement may lead to anemia, pallor, weakness, dyspnea, tachycardia, palpitations, bleeding, and infection. Opportunistic fungal, viral, and bacterial infections commonly occur in late stages.

DIAGNOSTIC TESTS
Typically, CLL is an incidental finding during a routine blood test that reveals numerous abnormal lymphocytes. In early stages, the white blood cell (WBC) count is mildly but persistently elevated. A reduced granulocyte count is typical, but the WBC count climbs as the disease progresses. Bone marrow biopsy shows lymphocytic invasion.

TREATMENT
Systemic chemotherapy includes alkylating agents (usually chlorambucil or cyclophosphamide) and, sometimes, steroids when autoimmune hemolytic anemia or thrombocytopenia occurs. When CLL causes obstruction or organ impairment or enlargement, local radiation may be used to reduce organ size.

SPECIAL CONSIDERATIONS

• Patient care focuses on relieving symptoms, preventing infection, and identifying complications. Signs and symptoms of infection include a temperature over 100° F (37.8° C), chills, redness, and swelling of any body part. Thrombocytopenia causes easy bruising, nosebleeds, bleeding gums, and black, tarry stools. Anemia leads to pallor, weakness, fatigue, dizziness, and palpitations.

 TEACHING TIP: Instruct the patient to avoid aspirin and products containing aspirin. If he is undergoing chemotherapy, teach him about its purpose and possible adverse effects, and review precautions he should take, such as avoiding contact with obviously ill people, eating high-protein foods and drinking high-calorie beverages, scheduling follow-up care and frequent blood tests, and taking all medications exactly as prescribed.

• Advise the patient to report signs and symptoms of recurrence (swollen lymph nodes in the neck, axilla, and groin and increased abdominal size or discomfort) to the doctor immediately.

Liver abscess

A liver abscess occurs when bacteria or protozoa destroy hepatic tissue. producing a cavity. The cavity fills with infectious organisms, liquefied liver cells, and leukocytes. Necrotic tissue then walls off the cavity from the rest of the liver.

A liver abscess is relatively uncommon and carries a mortality of 30% to 50%. This rate soars to more than 80% with multiple abscesses and to more than 90% with complications, such as rupture into the peritoneum, pleura, or pericardium.

CAUSES

In pyogenic liver abscess, common infecting organisms are *Escherichia coli, Klebsiella, Enterobacter, Salmonella, Staphylococcus,* and *Enterococcus.* Such organisms may invade the liver directly after a liver wound, or they may spread from the lungs, skin, or other organs by the hepatic artery, portal vein, or biliary tract.

An amebic abscess results from infection with the protozoa *Entamoeba histolytica,* the organism that causes amebic dysentery.

SIGNS AND SYMPTOMS

Clinical features depend on the degree of involvement. Some patients are acutely ill; in others, the abscess is recognized only at autopsy, after death from another illness.

With a pyogenic abscess, symptom onset usually is sudden; in an amebic abscess, onset is more gradual. Common signs and symptoms include right abdominal and shoulder pain, weight loss, fever, chills, diaphoresis, nausea, vomiting, and anemia. Evidence of right pleural effusion, such as dyspnea and pleural pain, develops if the abscess extends through the diaphragm. Liver damage may cause jaundice.

DIAGNOSTIC TESTS

A liver scan showing filling defects at the area of the abscess more than ¾" (2 cm) in diameter, together with characteristic clinical features, confirms this diagnosis. A liver ultrasound may indicate defects caused by the abscess but is less definitive than a liver scan. In a chest X-ray, the diaphragm on the affected side appears raised and fixed. A computed tomography scan confirms the diagnosis.

Relevant laboratory values include elevated levels of serum aspartate aminotransferase, alanine aminotransferase, alkaline phosphatase and bilirubin; an increased white blood cell count; and decreased serum albumin levels.

In pyogenic abscess, a blood culture can identify the bacterial agent; in amebic abscess, a stool culture and serologic and hemagglutination tests can isolate *E. histolytica.*

TREATMENT

If the organism causing the liver abscess is unknown, long-term antibiotic therapy begins immediately with

Environmental agents and liver cancer

Although the precise cause of liver cancer remains a mystery, some researchers suspect that in adults, the disease may be linked to environmental exposure to one of the following carcinogens:
● the chemical compound aflatoxin, a mold that grows on rice and peanuts
● thorium dioxide, a contrast medium formerly used in liver radiography
● alkaloids of the *Senecio* genus
● androgens and oral estrogens.

aminoglycosides, cephalosporins, clindamycin, or chloramphenicol.

If cultures demonstrate that the infectious organism is *E. coli,* treatment includes ampicillin; if they show *E. histolytica,* treatment includes emetine, chloroquine, or metronidazole. Drug therapy continues for 2 to 4 months. An abscess that fails to respond is surgically removed.

SPECIAL CONSIDERATIONS
● After surgery, the patient is observed for such complications as hemorrhage and infection.

 TEACHING TIP: Stress the importance of complying with therapy.

Liver cancer

A rare form of cancer, liver cancer (primary and metastatic hepatic carcinoma) has a high mortality. It is rapidly fatal, usually within 6 months, from GI hemorrhage, progressive cachexia, hepatic failure, or metastasis.

Most primary liver tumors (90%) originate in the parenchymal cells and are hepatomas (hepatocellular carcinoma). Some originate in the intrahepatic bile ducts and are known as cholangiomas. Rarer tumors include a mixed-cell type, Kupffer cell sarcoma, and hepatoblastomas.

The liver is one of the most common sites of metastasis from other primary cancers such as colorectal cancer. In the United States, metastatic liver carcinoma is 20 times more common than primary carcinoma.

CAUSES
The immediate cause of liver cancer is unknown, but it may be a congenital disease in children. This cancer may be associated with exposure to certain environmental agents in adults. (See *Environmental agents and liver cancer.*)

Risk factors
Roughly 30% to 70% of patients with hepatomas also have cirrhosis. Whether cirrhosis is a premalignant state or alcohol and malnutrition predispose the liver to develop hepatomas, is unclear. Another risk factor is exposure to the hepatitis B virus.

SIGNS AND SYMPTOMS
Clinical features of liver cancer include:
● a mass in the right upper abdominal quadrant
● tender, nodular liver on palpation
● severe pain in the epigastrium or right upper quadrant
● bruit, hum, or rubbing sound, if the tumor involves a large part of the liver
● weight loss, weakness, anorexia, fever
● dependent edema
● occasional jaundice or ascites.

DIAGNOSTIC TESTS
The confirming test for liver cancer is a needle or open liver biopsy. Liver cancer is hard to diagnose in the presence of cirrhosis, but several tests can help identify it. For instance, liver function studies show abnormal liver function, and the alpha-fetoprotein level increases above 500 µg/ml.

A liver scan may reveal filling defects; arteriography may define large tumors. Electrolyte studies may show abnormalities such as increased sodium retention. A chest X-ray may rule out metastasis.

TREATMENT

Some hepatic tumors are resectable. Typically, a resectable tumor must be a single tumor in one lobe, without cirrhosis, jaundice, or ascites.

Radiation therapy for unresectable tumors usually is palliative. However, because of the liver's low tolerance for radiation, this therapy hasn't increased survival.

Another treatment method is chemotherapy, administered I.V. or by regional infusion (catheter placement directly into the hepatic artery or left brachial artery for continuous infusion for 7 to 21 days, or permanent implantable pumps used on an outpatient basis for long-term infusion).

Treatment for liver metastasis may include resection by lobectomy or chemotherapy. Liver transplantation is an alternative for some patients.

SPECIAL CONSIDERATIONS

• Elevating the patient's legs whenever possible helps to control edema.
• Most patients need a special diet that restricts sodium, fluids (no alcohol allowed), and protein.
• Administering sponge baths and aspirin suppositories (if there are no signs of GI bleeding) reduces fever. Acetaminophen should be avoided because the diseased liver can't metabolize it. A high fever indicates infection and the need for antibiotics.
• Meticulous skin care includes turning the patient frequently and keeping the skin clean to prevent pressure ulcers. Antipruritics can be used to manage severe itching.

Lung abscess

A lung abscess is a lung infection accompanied by pus accumulation and tissue destruction. The abscess may be putrid (due to anaerobic bacteria) or nonputrid (due to anaerobes or aerobes). It often has a well-defined border. The availability of effective antibiotics has made lung abscesses much less common than they were in the past.

CAUSES

A lung abscess is a manifestation of necrotizing pneumonia, commonly the result of aspiration of oropharyngeal contents. Poor oral hygiene with dental or gum disease is strongly associated with a putrid lung abscess. Septic pulmonary emboli commonly produce cavitary lesions. Infected cystic lung lesions and cavitating bronchial carcinoma must be distinguished from lung abscesses.

SIGNS AND SYMPTOMS

The patient may have a cough that produces bloody, purulent, or foul-smelling sputum; pleuritic chest pain; dyspnea; excessive sweating; chills; fever; headache; malaise; diaphoresis; and weight loss.

Complications include rupture into the pleural space, which results in empyema and, rarely, massive hemorrhage. A chronic lung abscess may cause localized bronchiectasis. Failure of an abscess to improve with antibiotic treatment suggests an underlying neoplasm or other cause of obstruction.

DIAGNOSTIC TESTS

A chest X-ray typically shows a localized infiltrate with one or more clear spaces, usually containing air-fluid levels. Percutaneous aspiration of an abscess or bronchoscopy may be used to obtain cultures to identify the causative organism. Blood cultures, Gram stain, and sputum culture also are used to detect the underlying organism.

TREATMENT

Antibiotic therapy commonly lasts for months until X-rays show resolution or definite stability occurs. Symptoms usually disappear in a few weeks. Postural drainage may promote discharge of necrotic material into the upper airways, where expectoration is possible. Oxygen therapy may relieve hypoxemia. A poor response to therapy warrants lesion resection or removal of the diseased lung section. All patients need rigorous follow-up and serial chest X-rays.

SPECIAL CONSIDERATIONS
• Increasing fluid intake helps to loosen secretions.
• The patient benefits from a quiet, restful atmosphere.

Lung cancer
Lung cancer usually develops within the wall or epithelium of the bronchial tree. The most common types are squamous cell carcinoma, small cell (oat cell) carcinoma, adenocarcinoma, and large cell carcinoma.

Prognosis varies with the extent of spread at the time of diagnosis and the growth rate of the specific cell type. Only about 13% of patients survive 5 years after diagnosis. Lung cancer is the most common cause of cancer death in men and is fast becoming the most common cause in women.

CAUSES
Lung cancer is 10 times more common in smokers than in nonsmokers. About 80% of lung cancer patients are smokers. The most susceptible smokers are those over age 40 — especially those who began smoking before age 15, who smoked a whole pack or more per day for 20 years, or who work with or near asbestos.

Familial factors and exposure to air pollutants and industrial carcinogens also may increase the risk of lung cancer. (See *Lung cancer: Danger in the workplace*.)

SIGNS AND SYMPTOMS
Because early-stage lung cancer usually produces no symptoms, the disease is commonly in an advanced state at diagnosis. The following late-stage signs and symptoms often lead to diagnosis:
• with squamous cell and small cell carcinomas: smoker's cough, hoarseness, wheezing, dyspnea, hemoptysis, and chest pain
• with adenocarcinoma and large cell carcinoma: fever, weakness, weight loss, anorexia, and shoulder pain.

Signs and symptoms of metastatic liver cancer vary greatly, depending on how the tumor affects intrathoracic and distant structures.

DIAGNOSTIC TESTS
Chest X-ray usually shows an advanced tumor, but can detect a tumor up to 2 years before symptoms appear; it also indicates tumor size and location. Sputum cytology requires a specimen coughed up from the lungs. Computed tomography (CT) scans of the chest may help determine the tumor's size and whether it affects surrounding structures. Bronchoscopy can locate the tumor site.

Needle biopsy of the lung can detect tumors in the outer lung portion. Tissue biopsy can be done if the site of cancer spread is accessible. Thoracentesis allows analysis of pleural fluid.

Other tests to detect cancer spread include bone scans, bone marrow biopsy, and CT scans of the brain and abdomen.

TREATMENT
Various combinations of surgery, radiation, and chemotherapy may improve the prognosis and prolong survival. However, because treatment usually begins at an advanced stage, it's largely palliative.

Unless the tumor is nonresectable or other conditions rule out surgery, partial or total lung removal is the primary treatment for stage I, stage II, or selected stage III squamous cell carcinoma, adenocarcinoma, and large cell carcinoma.

Preoperative radiation therapy may reduce tumor bulk to allow surgical resection. Preradiation chemotherapy helps improve the response. Radiation ordinarily is recommended for stage I and stage II lesions, if surgery is contraindicated, and for certain stage III lesions.

Otherwise, radiation therapy generally is delayed until 1 month after surgery. High-dose radiation therapy or radiation implants also may be used.

Another treatment is chemotherapy, typically using a combination of drugs. Laser therapy, still largely experimental, involves directing laser

Lung cancer: Danger in the workplace

Although smoking is the leading risk factor for lung cancer, other airborne pollutants are villains, too. In particular, exposure to industrial carcinogens increases susceptibility to lung cancer. The list below identifies known workplace carcinogens:

● Acrylonitrile — found in fiber mills (blankets, carpets, clothing, draperies, synthetic furs, and wigs)

● Arsenic — found in copper smelting and metallurgic industries, mines, insecticide and pesticide plants, and tanning factories

● Asbestos — found in asbestos factories and asbestos removal work sites; insulation, rubber, and textile plants; mines; and shipyards

● Beryllium — found in beryllium plants and electronic-parts and missile-parts factories

● Cadmium — found in cadmium factories; battery, chemical, jewelry, paint, and pigment plants; and electroplating and metallurgic industries

● Coal tar pitch volatiles — found in steel mills and foundries

● Coke oven emissions — found in coke plants and steel mills

● Dimethylsulfate — found in chemical, drug, and dye plants

● Epichlorohydrin — found in chemical plants

● Hematite — found in hematite mines

● Mineral oils, soot, and tars — found in construction sites, roofing plants, chimney sweep businesses, and heavy industry

● Nickel — found in nickel refineries

● Vinylchloride — found in plastics and vinylchloride polymer plants.

energy through a bronchoscope to destroy local tumors.

SPECIAL CONSIDERATIONS

● During radiation therapy, practicing good skin care helps minimize skin breakdown.

 TEACHING TIP: If the patient is undergoing chemotherapy or radiation, teach him ways to minimize adverse effects, such as eating soft, nonirritating foods that are high in protein, consuming high-calorie between-meal snacks, and using antiemetics and antidiarrheals as needed.

 PREVENTION TIP: High-risk individuals can reduce their risk of developing lung cancer by stopping smoking.

Lupus erythematosus

A chronic inflammatory disorder of the connective tissues, lupus erythematosus appears in two forms: *discoid lupus erythematosus,* which affects only the skin, and *systemic lupus erythematosus (SLE),* which affects multiple organ systems (as well as the skin) and can be fatal. SLE is characterized by recurring remissions and exacerbations.

SLE is eight times more common in women than in men. It occurs worldwide but is most prevalent among Asians and blacks. The prognosis improves with early detection and treatment but remains poor for patients who develop cardiovascular, renal, or neurologic complications or severe bacterial infections.

CAUSES

The exact cause of SLE remains a mystery, but evidence points to interrelated immunologic, environmental, hormonal, and genetic factors. Autoimmunity is thought to be the prime causative mechanism. In autoimmunity, the body produces antibodies, such as the antinuclear antibody (ANA), against its own cells.

Certain predisposing factors may increase susceptibility to SLE: physical or mental stress, streptococcal or viral infections, exposure to sunlight or ultraviolet light, immunization, pregnancy, and abnormal estrogen metabolism. SLE also may be triggered or aggravated by various drugs.

SIGNS AND SYMPTOMS
SLE onset may be acute or insidious. Common signs and symptoms include fever, weight loss, malaise, fatigue, rashes, and polyarthralgia. SLE may involve every organ system.

Joint and skin effects
In 90% of patients, joint involvement resembles that of rheumatoid arthritis. The most common skin lesion is an erythematous rash in areas exposed to light. The classic butterfly rash over the nose and cheeks occurs in less than half of patients. Patchy alopecia and mucous membrane ulcers are common.

Cardiopulmonary and renal effects
About 50% of patients develop cardiopulmonary abnormalities, such as pleuritis, pericarditis, and dyspnea. Renal effects and proteinuria, may progress to total kidney failure.

Neurologic effects
Seizures and mental dysfunction may indicate neurologic damage. Central nervous system involvement may produce emotional instability, psychosis, and organic brain syndrome. Headaches, irritability, and depression are common.

Systemic effects
The patient may experience aching, malaise, fatigue, low-grade or spiking fever, chills, anorexia, weight loss, lymph node enlargement, abdominal pain, nausea, vomiting, diarrhea, and constipation.

DIAGNOSTIC TESTS
Typically, a complete blood count with differential shows anemia and a decreased white blood cell count. Other laboratory findings include a decreased platelet count, an elevated erythrocyte sedimentation rate, and hypergammaglobulinemia.

ANA, anti-deoxyribonucleic acid, and lupus erythematosus cell tests are positive in active SLE. Blood studies also reveal decreased serum complement (C3 and C4) levels, which indicate active disease.

Other studies may detect cardiovascular or renal effects; kidney biopsy determines the disease stage and the extent of renal involvement.

TREATMENT
Patients with mild disease require little or no medication. Nonsteroidal anti-inflammatory compounds, including aspirin, may control arthritis symptoms. Skin lesions call for topical treatment.

Corticosteroids are used for systemic symptoms, acute generalized exacerbations, or serious disease related to vital organ systems.

Diffuse proliferative glomerulonephritis, a major complication of SLE, requires high-dose steroid treatment. If renal failure occurs, dialysis or a kidney transplant may be necessary.

SPECIAL CONSIDERATIONS
• The patient may experience fatigue and should try to get plenty of rest.
• Heat packs may be applied to relieve joint pain and stiffness; regular exercise helps to maintain full range of motion and prevent contractures.
• The patient may benefit from physical therapy and occupational counseling.

Lyme disease
A multisystemic disorder, Lyme disease is caused by the spirochete *Borrelia burgdorferi,* which is carried by the minute tick *Ixodes dammini* or another tick in the Ixodidae family. It often begins in the summer with the classic skin lesion called erythema chronicum migrans (ECM). Weeks or months later, cardiac or neurologic abnormalities may develop, possibly followed by arthritis.

Lyme disease has been reported in 43 states and 20 other countries. It's endemic to three parts of the United States:

- the northeast, from Massachusetts to Maryland
- the midwest, in Wisconsin and Minnesota
- the west, in California and Oregon.

CAUSES
Lyme disease occurs when a tick injects spirochete-laden saliva into the bloodstream or deposits fecal matter on the skin. After incubating for 3 to 32 days, spirochetes migrate out to the skin, causing ECM. Then they spread to other skin sites or organs by the bloodstream or lymph system.

SIGNS AND SYMPTOMS
Typically, Lyme disease has three stages.

Stage 1
ECM heralds stage 1 with a red macule or papule, often at the site of a tick bite. This lesion often feels hot and itchy and may grow to more than 20" (50 cm) in diameter. Within a few days, more lesions may erupt along with a malar rash, conjunctivitis, or diffuse urticaria. In 3 to 4 weeks, lesions are replaced by small red blotches, which last several more weeks.

Malaise and fatigue are constant, but other findings are intermittent: headache, fever, chills, achiness, and regional lymphadenopathy. Less common effects are meningeal irritation, mild encephalopathy, migrating musculoskeletal pain, and hepatitis.

Stage 2
Weeks to months later, the second stage begins with neurologic abnormalities that usually resolve after days or months. Facial palsy is especially noticeable. Cardiac abnormalities also may develop.

Stage 3
Stage 3 begins weeks or years later. Musculoskeletal pain leads to arthritis with marked swelling, especially in large joints. Recurrent attacks may precede chronic arthritis with severe cartilage and bone erosion.

DIAGNOSTIC TESTS
Because isolation of *B. burgdorferi* is unusual and because indirect immunofluorescent antibody tests are marginally sensitive, diagnosis commonly rests on the characteristic ECM lesion and related clinical findings. Mild anemia and elevations in the erythrocyte sedimentation rate, leukocyte count, serum immunoglobulin M level, and aspartate aminotransferase level support the diagnosis.

TREATMENT
A 10- to 20-day course of oral tetracycline is the treatment of choice for adults; penicillin and erythromycin are alternates. Oral penicillin usually is prescribed for children. When given in early disease stages, these drugs can minimize later complications. For late stages, high-dose penicillin I.V. may be effective.

SPECIAL CONSIDERATIONS
- Antibiotic therapy is monitored carefully because the patient may experience adverse reactions.
- Neurologic status and level of consciousness are checked frequently and the patient is watched for indications of increased intracranial pressure and cranial nerve involvement.

 TEACHING TIP: Advise patients with arthritis to perform range-of-motion and strengthening exercises, but to avoid overexertion.

Lymphomas, malignant

Also known as non-Hodgkin's lymphomas or lymphosarcomas, malignant lymphomas are a heterogeneous group of malignant diseases originating in the lymph glands and other lymphoid tissue. Nodular lymphomas have a better prognosis than the diffuse form of the disease. However, in both, the prognosis is worse than in Hodgkin's disease.

Up to 35,000 new cases of malignant lymphoma appear annually in the United States. Malignant lymphomas occur in all age-groups.

CAUSES
The cause of malignant lymphomas is unknown, although some theories suggest a virus.

SIGNS AND SYMPTOMS
Usually, the first signs of malignant lymphoma are swelling of the lymph glands, enlarged tonsils and adenoids, and painless, rubbery nodes in the cervical supraclavicular areas. In children, these nodes usually are in the cervical region, and the disease causes dyspnea and coughing.

As lymphoma progresses, the patient experiences fatigue, malaise, weight loss, fever, and night sweats as well as symptoms specific to the area involved.

DIAGNOSTIC TESTS
Biopsies of lymph nodes, tonsils, bone marrow, liver, bowel, or skin aid diagnosis and differentiate malignant lymphoma from Hodgkin's disease. Other tests may include bone and chest X-rays, lymphangiography, liver and spleen scan, computed tomography scan of the abdomen, and excretory urography. Common laboratory tests include a complete blood count and uric acid, blood calcium, blood protein, and liver function studies.

TREATMENT
Radiation therapy is used mainly in the early localized stage of the disease. Total nodal irradiation is often successful. Chemotherapy is most effective with multiple combinations of antineoplastic agents.

SPECIAL CONSIDERATIONS
• The patient who's undergoing radiation or chemotherapy is likely to experience anorexia, nausea, vomiting, or diarrhea. Small, frequent meals scheduled around treatment help minimize these adverse effects.
• Provide emotional support to the patient and family. The local chapter of the American Cancer Society is a good resource for information and counseling.

Macular degeneration

In this condition, the macular disk of the retina undergoes atrophy or degeneration. Macular degeneration accounts for about 12% of all cases of blindness in the United States and for about 17% of new cases. It's one cause of severe irreversible loss of central vision in elderly people.

Age-related macular degeneration has two forms. In the *dry (atrophic) form* (most often associated with a slow, progressive, mild visual loss), atrophic pigment epithelial changes occur. The *wet (exudative) form* causes rapidly progressive and severe vision loss; subretinal neovascularization causes leakage, hemorrhage, and fibrovascular scar formation, leading to significant central vision loss.

CAUSES
Age-related macular degeneration results from hardening and obstruction of retinal arteries. No predisposing conditions have been identified. However, the condition may be hereditary.

SIGNS AND SYMPTOMS
The patient notices a change in central vision — for example, a blank spot in the center of the page when reading. Drusen (bumps), which are common in elderly people, appear as yellow deposits beneath the pigment epithelium and may be prominent in the macula.

DIAGNOSTIC TESTS
Indirect ophthalmoscopy may reveal gross macular changes. I.V. fluorescein angiography may show leaking vessels as fluorescein dye flows into the tissues from the subretinal neovascular net. Amsler's grid reveals visual field loss.

TREATMENT
Laser photocoagulation reduces the incidence of severe visual loss in patients with subretinal neovascularization.

SPECIAL CONSIDERATIONS
• To improve vision to some degree, the patient with bilateral central vision loss can take advantage of visual rehabilitation services. A patient with good peripheral vision can use devices such as low-vision optical aids.

Magnesium imbalance

Magnesium is the second most common cation in intracellular fluid. Besides enhancing neuromuscular integration, it regulates skeletal muscles, activates many enzymes for proper metabolism, promotes cell metabolism and sodium and potassium transport across cell membranes, and influences serum sodium, potassium, calcium, and protein levels.

CAUSES
Magnesium deficiency (*hypomagnesemia*) may result from the following conditions:
• decreased magnesium intake or absorption, as in malabsorption syndrome or chronic diarrhea
• chronic alcoholism
• prolonged diuretic therapy, nasogastric suctioning, or administration of parenteral fluids without magnesium salts
• starvation or malnutrition
• excessive magnesium loss, as in severe dehydration.
Magnesium excess (*hypermagnesemia*) may result from such conditions as:
• chronic renal insufficiency

Clinical features of magnesium imbalance

This chart presents the signs and symptoms of hypomagnesemia and hypermagnesemia grouped by body system.

Body system	Hypomagnesemia	Hypermagnesemia
Neuromuscular	• Hyperirritability, tetany, leg and foot cramps, Chvostek's sign (facial muscle spasms induced by tapping branches of the facial nerve)	• Diminished reflexes, muscle weakness, flaccid paralysis, respiratory muscle paralysis
Central nervous	• Confusion, delusions, hallucinations, seizures	• Drowsiness, flushing, lethargy, confusion, diminished sensorium
Cardiovascular	• Arrhythmias, vasodilation, hypotension; occasionally, hypertension	• Bradycardia, weak pulse, hypotension, heart block, cardiac arrest

• use of magnesium-containing laxatives
• overuse of magnesium-containing antacids
• severe dehydration
• overcorrection of hypomagnesemia.

SIGNS AND SYMPTOMS

Hypomagnesemia may cause neuromuscular irritability and cardiac arrhythmias. Hypermagnesemia may lead to central nervous system and respiratory depression, and neuromuscular and cardiac changes. (See *Clinical features of magnesium imbalance.*)

DIAGNOSTIC TESTS

Decreased serum magnesium levels (less than 1.5 mEq/L) confirm hypomagnesemia; increased levels (greater than 2.5 mEq/L) confirm hypermagnesemia.

TREATMENT

The goal of therapy is to identify and correct the underlying cause of the magnesium imbalance.

Treatment of *mild hypomagnesemia* consists of daily magnesium supplements. Treatment of *severe hypomag-* *nesemia* calls for magnesium sulfate I.V. Magnesium intoxication (a possible adverse effect) warrants calcium gluconate I.V. administration.

Therapy for *hypermagnesemia* includes increased fluid intake and loop diuretics for impaired renal function; calcium gluconate, a magnesium antagonist, for temporary relief of symptoms in an emergency; and dialysis if renal function fails or if excess magnesium can't be eliminated.

SPECIAL CONSIDERATIONS
For patients with hypomagnesemia

• Magnesium replacement is infused slowly; the patient is observed for bradycardia, heart block, and decreased respiratory rate.

 TEACHING TIP: Advise the patient to eat foods rich in magnesium, such as fish and green vegetables.

For patients with hypermagnesemia

• The patient receiving digitalis glycosides and calcium gluconate simultaneously is observed for digitalis toxicity.

PREVENTION TIP: To help prevent hypermagnesemia, caution patients not to abuse laxatives or antacids containing magnesium — particularly elderly patients and those with compromised renal function.

Malignant melanoma

A neoplasm that arises from melanocytes, malignant melanoma occurs in three forms — *superficial spreading melanoma, nodular malignant melanoma,* and *lentigo maligna melanoma.* Incidence of melanoma peaks between ages 50 and 70.

Common melanoma sites are on the head and neck in men, on the legs in women, and on the backs of people exposed to excessive sunlight. Up to 70% of malignant melanoma tumors arise from a preexisting nevus.

Melanoma may spread to the regional lymph nodes, skin, liver, lungs, and central nervous system. Its course is unpredictable, and recurrence and metastasis may occur more than 5 years after resection of the primary lesion.

The prognosis varies with tumor thickness. Generally, superficial lesions are curable, while deeper lesions tend to metastasize.

CAUSES

Several factors may influence melanoma development. (See *Risk factors for melanoma.*)

SIGNS AND SYMPTOMS

Clinical features of melanoma include a skin lesion or nevus that enlarges, changes color, becomes inflamed or sore, itches, ulcerates, bleeds, undergoes textural changes, or shows signs of surrounding pigment regression (halo nevus or vitiligo).

DIAGNOSTIC TESTS

A skin biopsy with histologic examination can distinguish malignant melanoma from other lesions and can determine tumor thickness. Physical findings may point to metastatic involvement.

Risk factors for melanoma

Melanoma is more likely to develop in people with the following risk factors:

● *Excessive exposure to sunlight.* Melanoma is most common in sunny, warm climates and on parts of the body that are exposed to the sun.

● *Skin type.* Most persons who develop melanoma have blond or red hair, fair skin, and blue eyes; are prone to sunburn; and are of Celtic or Scandinavian ancestry.

● *Hormonal factors.* Pregnancy may increase the risk and exacerbate melanoma growth.

● *Family history.* Melanoma occurs slightly more commonly within families.

● *Past history of melanoma.* A person who has had one melanoma is at greater risk of developing a second.

Laboratory studies include a complete blood count with differential, erythrocyte sedimentation rate, platelet count, liver function studies, and urinalysis. Depending on depth of tumor invasion and metastasis, the doctor also may order a chest X-ray, bone scans, and computed tomography scans of the chest and abdomen.

TREATMENT

The lesion is removed surgically. Closure of a wide resection may require a skin graft. Surgical treatment may include regional lymphadenectomy.

Deep primary lesions may warrant adjuvant chemotherapy and biotherapy. Radiation therapy usually is reserved for metastatic disease; it does not prolong survival but may reduce tumor size and relieve pain.

Melanomas require close, long-term follow-up to detect metastasis and recurrences. About 13% of recurrences develop more than 5 years after the primary surgery.

SPECIAL CONSIDERATIONS

• Emphasize the need for close follow-up to detect recurrences early, and teach the patient how to recognize signs and symptoms of recurrence.

 PREVENTION TIP: To help prevent malignant melanoma, warn all patients about the detrimental effects of exposure to the sun. Recommend use of a sunblock or sunscreen.

Mallory-Weiss syndrome

In Mallory-Weiss syndrome, a tear in the mucosa or submucosa of the cardia or lower esophagus causes mild to massive and usually painless bleeding. Such a tear, usually singular and longitudinal, typically results from prolonged or forceful vomiting. Mallory-Weiss syndrome is most common in men over age 40, especially alcoholics.

CAUSES

The direct cause of a tear in Mallory-Weiss syndrome is forceful or prolonged vomiting, probably when the upper esophageal sphincter fails to relax during vomiting. Lack of sphincter coordination seems more common after excessive alcohol intake.

Other factors that may predispose the patient to esophageal tearing include coughing, straining during bowel movements, trauma, seizures, childbirth, hiatal hernia, esophagitis, gastritis, and atrophic gastric mucosa.

SIGNS AND SYMPTOMS

Typically, Mallory-Weiss syndrome begins with vomiting blood or passing large amounts of blood rectally a few hours to several days after normal vomiting. Such bleeding, which may be accompanied by epigastric or back pain, may range from mild to massive. Massive bleeding may quickly lead to fatal shock.

DIAGNOSTIC TESTS

Identifying esophageal tears by fiberoptic endoscopy confirms Mallory-Weiss syndrome. These lesions appear as erythematous longitudinal cracks in the mucosa when recently produced and as raised, white streaks surrounded by erythema in older tears.

Selective celiac arteriography can determine the bleeding site but not the cause; this study is used when endoscopy isn't available. Gastrotomy may be performed at the time of surgery. Hematocrit helps quantify blood loss.

TREATMENT

Appropriate treatment varies with the severity of bleeding. Usually, GI bleeding stops spontaneously, requiring supportive measures and careful observation but no definitive treatment. However, if bleeding continues, treatment may include:

• angiographic infusion of a vasoconstrictor (vasopressin) into the superior mesenteric artery or direct infusion into a vessel that leads to the bleeding artery

• transcatheter embolization or thrombus formation with an autologous blood clot or other hemostatic material (insertion of artificial material, such as a shredded absorbable gelatin sponge or, less commonly, the patient's own clotted blood through a catheter into the bleeding vessel to aid thrombus formation)

• surgery to suture each laceration (for massive recurrent or uncontrollable bleeding).

SPECIAL CONSIDERATIONS

• Oxygen is given as necessary.

• The patient should not consume substances that may cause nausea or vomiting, such as medication, alcohol, or aspirin.

Ménière's disease

A dysfunction of the labyrinth of the inner ear, Ménière's disease causes severe vertigo, sensorineural hearing loss, and tinnitus. It usually affects adults between ages 30 and 60. After

PATHOPHYSIOLOGY

What happens in Ménière's disease

In Ménière's disease, overproduction or decreased absorption of endolymph (the fluid in the labyrinth [cochlea, semicircular canals] of the inner ear) causes pressure within the labyrinth to increase. This results in hearing loss, dizziness, and related signs and symptoms.

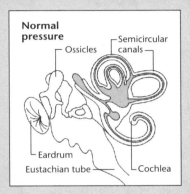

Normal pressure
- Ossicles
- Semicircular canals
- Eardrum
- Eustachian tube
- Cochlea

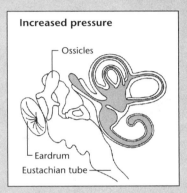

Increased pressure
- Ossicles
- Eardrum
- Eustachian tube

multiple attacks over several years, the disorder leads to residual tinnitus and hearing loss.

CAUSES
Ménière's disease may result from overproduction or decreased absorption of endolymph, which causes endolymphatic hydrops or endolymphatic hypertension. (See *What happens in Ménière's disease*.)

The condition may stem from an autonomic nervous system dysfunction that temporarily narrows the blood vessels supplying the inner ear. In some women, premenstrual edema may trigger attacks of Ménière's disease.

SIGNS AND SYMPTOMS
Ménière's disease produces three characteristic effects: severe vertigo, tinnitus, and sensorineural hearing loss. Fullness or a blocked feeling in the ear is also common.

Violent paroxysmal attacks last from 10 minutes to several hours. During an acute attack, other features include severe nausea, vomiting, sweating, giddiness, and nystagmus. Vertigo may cause loss of balance and falling to the affected side. To ease these symptoms, the patient may lie on the unaffected ear and look in the direction of the affected ear.

Initially, the patient may be asymptomatic between attacks, except for residual tinnitus that worsens during an attack. Such attacks may occur several times a year, or remissions may last as long as several years. Attacks become less frequent as hearing loss progresses; they may cease when hearing loss is total.

DIAGNOSTIC TESTS
The presence of all three characteristic symptoms described above suggests Ménière's disease. Hearing tests and X-rays of the inner ear also may be required.

TREATMENT
Atropine may stop an attack in 20 to 30 minutes. Epinephrine or diphenhydramine may be necessary in a severe attack; dimenhydrinate, meclizine, diphenhydramine, or diazepam may be effective in a milder attack.

Long-term management includes diuretic or vasodilator therapy and restricted sodium intake. Prophylactic antihistamines or mild sedatives also may be helpful. Surgery may be necessary if Ménière's disease persists after 2 years of treatment, produces incapacitating vertigo, or resists medical management. Destruction of the affected labyrinth permanently relieves symptoms but causes irreversible hearing loss. Systemic streptomycin is reserved for patients with bilateral disease when no other treatment can be considered.

SPECIAL CONSIDERATIONS
• If the patient is in the hospital during an attack, the side rails of the bed must be kept up to prevent falls.
• The patient should not attempt to get out of bed without assistance.
 TEACHING TIP: To reduce dizziness, advise the patient to avoid reading and exposure to glaring lights. Also, because an attack can come on rapidly, warn him to avoid sudden position changes and any tasks that vertigo makes hazardous.

Meningitis
In meningitis, the meninges (the membranes that cover the brain and spinal cord) become inflamed, usually as a result of bacterial infection. The prognosis is good and complications are rare, especially if the disease is recognized early and the infecting organism responds to antibiotics. However, mortality in untreated meningitis is 70% to 100%.

CAUSES
Meningitis usually arises a complication of another bacterial infection (bacteremia, sinusitis, otitis media, encephalitis, myelitis, or brain ab-

scess), which is usually caused by *Neisseria meningitidis, Haemophilus influenzae, Streptococcus pneumoniae,* or *Escherichia coli.*

Meningitis also may follow skull fracture, a penetrating head wound, lumbar puncture, or a ventricular shunting procedure. Aseptic meningitis may result from a virus or other organism. Sometimes no causative organism can be found.

SIGNS AND SYMPTOMS
Cardinal features of meningitis are those of infection (fever, chills, malaise) and of increased intracranial pressure (headache, vomiting, seizures, changes in motor function and vital signs, papilledema [rare]).

Signs of meningeal irritation also may occur. These include nuchal rigidity, positive Brudzinski's and Kernig's signs, exaggerated and symmetrical deep tendon reflexes, and opisthotonos (a spasm in which the back and extremities arch backward so that the body rests on the head and heels). As the illness progresses, twitching, seizures, or coma may develop.

DIAGNOSTIC TESTS
A lumbar puncture showing typical findings in cerebrospinal fluid (CSF) and positive Brudzinski's and Kernig's signs usually establish the diagnosis. (See *Two telltale signs of meningitis.*)

CSF may appear cloudy or milky white, with an above-normal protein level and a below-normal glucose level. CSF culture and sensitivity tests usually identify the infecting organism, unless it's a virus.

Determining major infection sites requires a chest X-ray, an electrocardiogram, and cultures of blood, urine, and nose and throat secretions.

TREATMENT
Treatment includes appropriate antibiotic therapy and vigorous supportive care. Usually, I.V. antibiotics are given for at least 2 weeks and are followed by oral antibiotics. Other drugs may include a digitalis glycoside to

Two telltale signs of meningitis

To test for *Brudzinski's sign,* the patient is placed in a dorsal recumbent position. The examiner puts his hands behind the patient's neck and bends it forward. Pain and resistance may indicate meningeal inflammation, neck injury, or arthritis. But if the patient also flexes the hips and knees in response to this manipulation, chances are he has meningitis.

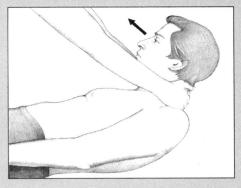

To test for *Kernig's sign,* the patient is placed in a supine position. The examiner flexes the patient's leg at the hip and knee and then straightens the knee. Pain or resistance points to meningitis.

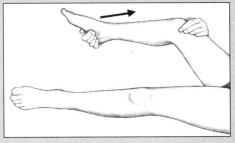

control arrhythmias, mannitol to decrease cerebral edema, an anticonvulsant or a sedative to reduce restlessness, and aspirin or acetaminophen to relieve headache and fever.

Supportive therapy includes bed rest, fever reduction, and measures to prevent dehydration. Isolation is necessary if nasal cultures are positive. Treatment also includes appropriate therapy for coexisting conditions, such as endocarditis or pneumonia.

SPECIAL CONSIDERATIONS
• Patient comfort measures include maintaining a quiet environment, darkening the room to decrease photophobia, and relieving headache with a nonnarcotic analgesic.
• If a severe neurologic deficit appears permanent, the patient may be referred to a rehabilitation program once the acute phase of illness has passed.

Meningococcal infections

Two major meningococcal infections — meningitis and meningococcemia — result from the gramnegative bacteria *Neisseria meningitidis,* which also causes primary pneumonia, purulent conjunctivitis, endocarditis, sinusitis, and genital infection.

Meningococcemia occurs as simple bacteremia, fulminant meningococcemia and, rarely, chronic meningococcemia. It often accompanies meningitis. Meningococcal infections may occur sporadically or in epidemics. Virulent infections may be fatal within hours.

Identifying fulminant and chronic meningococcemia

Fulminant meningococcemia

If meningococcal bacteremia progresses to fulminant meningococcemia, the patient may experience:
- extreme prostration
- enlargement of skin lesions
- disseminated intravascular coagulation
- shock.

Without prompt treatment, fulminant meningococcemia results in death in 6 to 24 hours.

Chronic meningococcemia

If meningococcemia becomes chronic, the patient may experience an intermittent fever, maculopapular rash, joint pain, and an enlarged spleen.

CAUSES

N. meningitidis is commonly present in upper respiratory flora. Transmission takes place by inhaling an infected droplet from a carrier (an estimated 2% to 38% of the population). The bacteria then localize in the nasopharynx.

After an incubation period of several days, bacteria spread through the bloodstream to the joints, skin, adrenal glands, lungs, and central nervous system. The resulting tissue damage produces clinical changes and, in fulminant meningococcemia and meningococcal bacteremia, progresses to hemorrhage, thrombosis, and necrosis.

SIGNS AND SYMPTOMS

Meningococcal bacteremia causes a sudden, spiking fever; headache; sore throat; cough; chills; myalgia in the back and legs; arthralgia; tachycardia; tachypnea; mild hypotension; and a petechial, nodular, or maculopapular rash.

In 10% to 20% of patients, this progresses to fulminant meningococcemia. (See *Identifying fulminant and chronic meningococcemia.*)

DIAGNOSTIC TESTS

Isolation of *N. meningitidis* through a positive blood culture, cerebrospinal fluid culture, or lesion scraping confirms the diagnosis.

TREATMENT

As soon as meningococcal infection is suspected, appropriate antibiotic treatment begins. Therapy also may include mannitol for cerebral edema, heparin I.V. for disseminated intravascular coagulation, dopamine for shock, and digoxin and a diuretic if congestive heart failure develops.

Supportive measures may include administration of fluids and electrolytes, proper ventilation (a patent airway and oxygen, if necessary), and insertion of an arterial or central venous pressure line to monitor cardiovascular status.

SPECIAL CONSIDERATIONS

- Bed rest is enforced during early disease stages. The patient benefits from a dark, quiet, restful environment.
- All meningococcal infections must be reported to the public health department.

 PREVENTION TIP: To help prevent the spread of meningococcal infection, respiratory isolation should be imposed until the patient has received antibiotic therapy for 24 hours. Prophylaxis with rifampin or minocycline is useful for hospital workers who come in close contact with the patient.

Metabolic acidosis

A state of excess acid accumulation and deficient base bicarbonate, metabolic acidosis is produced by an un derlying pathologic disorder. Clinical effects result from the body's attempt to correct the acidosis through compensatory mechanisms in the lungs, kidneys, and cells. Severe or untreated metabolic acidosis can be fatal.

CAUSES

Metabolic acidosis usually results from excessive burning of fats in the absence of usable carbohydrates, as may occur with diabetic ketoacidosis, chronic alcoholism, malnutrition, or a low-carbohydrate, high-fat diet.

Other causes of metabolic acidosis include:
● anaerobic carbohydrate metabolism, as occurs with pump failure after myocardial infarction, or when pulmonary or hepatic disease, shock, or anemia forces a shift from aerobic to anaerobic metabolism
● renal insufficiency and failure
● diarrhea and intestinal malabsorption.

Less commonly, metabolic acidosis stems from salicylate intoxication (overuse of aspirin), exogenous poisoning, or Addison's disease.

SIGNS AND SYMPTOMS

In mild acidosis, features of the underlying disease may mask those of acidosis. Metabolic acidosis typically begins with headache and lethargy progressing to drowsiness, central nervous system depression, Kussmaul's respirations, and stupor, and, if the condition is severe and goes untreated, coma and death.

Associated GI distress usually produces anorexia, nausea, vomiting, and diarrhea and may lead to dehydration. Underlying diabetes mellitus may cause fruity breath odor.

DIAGNOSTIC TESTS

Arterial pH below 7.35 confirms metabolic acidosis. In severe acidosis, pH may fall to 7.10; partial pressure of arterial carbon dioxide may be normal or less than 34 mm Hg as compensatory mechanisms take hold. The bicarbonate level may measure less than 22 mEq/L.

TREATMENT

Treatment consists of sodium bicarbonate I.V. for severe cases, evaluation and correction of electrolyte imbalances and, ultimately, correction of the underlying cause.

SPECIAL CONSIDERATIONS

● Sodium bicarbonate ampules should be kept handy for emergency administration.
● Seizure precautions should be taken.
● Sodium bicarbonate washes may be used to neutralize mouth acids, and lemon and glycerine swabs can be used to lubricate the patient's lips.

 PREVENTION TIP: Patients receiving I.V. therapy, those who have intestinal tubes in place, and those suffering from shock, hyperthyroidism, hepatic disease, circulatory failure, or dehydration are at risk for metabolic acidosis and should be observed carefully.

Metabolic alkalosis

Metabolic alkalosis is a clinical state marked by decreased amounts of acid or increased amounts of base bicarbonate. The metabolic, respiratory, and renal responses to this state produce characteristic signs and symptoms — most notably, hypoventilation.

Metabolic alkalosis always occurs secondary to an underlying cause. With early diagnosis and prompt treatment, the prognosis is good. However, untreated metabolic alkalosis may lead to coma and death.

CAUSES

Metabolic alkalosis results from loss of acid, retention of base, or renal mechanisms associated with decreased serum levels of potassium and chloride. (See *What causes acid loss and base retention,* page 204.)

SIGNS AND SYMPTOMS

Clinical features of metabolic alkalosis result from the body's attempt to correct the acid-base imbalance, primarily through hypoventilation. Other manifestations include irritability, picking at bedclothes, twitch-

What causes acid loss and base retention

Causes of critical *acid loss* include hyperadrenocorticism, vomiting, nasogastric tube drainage or lavage without adequate electrolyte replacement, fistulas, and use of steroids and certain diuretics (furosemide, thiazides, and ethacrynic acid).

Excessive *base retention* may result from excessive intake of bicarbonate of soda or other antacids, excessive intake of absorbable alkali (as in milk-alkali syndrome), administration of excessive amounts of I.V. fluids with high concentrations of bicarbonate or lactate, and respiratory insufficiency.

ing, confusion, nausea, vomiting, and diarrhea.

Cardiovascular abnormalities (such as atrial tachycardia) and respiratory disturbances (such as cyanosis and apnea) also occur.

DIAGNOSTIC TESTS
Arterial blood gas results — blood pH greater than 7.45 and a bicarbonate level above 29 mEq/L — confirm the diagnosis. Partial pressure of carbon dioxide greater than 45 mm Hg indicates attempts at respiratory compensation. Serum electrolyte levels show a potassium level of 3.5 mEq/L and a chloride level of 98 mEq/L.

TREATMENT
The goal of treatment is to correct the underlying cause of metabolic alkalosis. Therapy for severe alkalosis may include cautious administration of ammonium chloride I.V. (to release hydrogen chloride and restore the concentration of extracellular fluid and chloride levels).

Potassium chloride and normal saline solution (except in the presence of congestive heart failure) are usually sufficient to replace losses from gastric drainage. Electrolyte replacement with potassium chloride and discontinuation of diuretics may correct metabolic alkalosis brought on by potent diuretic therapy.

SPECIAL CONSIDERATIONS
• Patient monitoring includes vital signs, fluid intake, and signs of muscle weakness, tetany, or decreased activity.
• Seizure precautions must be taken.

 TEACHING TIP: To help prevent metabolic alkalosis, tell patients with ulcers to watch for signs and symptom of milk-alkali syndrome: a distaste for milk, anorexia, weakness, and lethargy.

Mononucleosis

Infectious mononucleosis is an acute infectious disease caused by the Epstein-Barr virus (EBV), a member of the herpes group. It primarily affects young adults and children, although in children it's usually so mild that it's commonly overlooked.

Infectious mononucleosis is fairly common in the United States, Canada, and Europe. The prognosis is excellent, and major complications are rare.

CAUSES
Infectious mononucleosis probably spreads by the oropharyngeal route. It can also be transmitted by blood transfusion and has been reported after cardiac surgery as the "post–pump perfusion" syndrome. The disease is probably contagious from before symptoms develop until the fever subsides and oropharyngeal lesions disappear.

SIGNS AND SYMPTOMS
Clinical features mimic those of many other infectious diseases. Typically, after an incubation period of about 10 days in children and 30 to 50 days in adults, infectious mononucleosis produces prodromal symptoms, such as headache, malaise, and fatigue.

After 3 to 5 days, patients typically develop a triad of features: sore throat, cervical lymphadenopathy, and temperature fluctuations, with an evening peak of 101° to 102° F (38.3° to 38.9° C). Spleen and liver enlargement, stomatitis, exudative tonsillitis, or pharyngitis also may develop.

Early in the illness, a maculopapular rash resembling rubella may appear. In about 5% of patients, jaundice occurs. Signs and symptoms usually subside about 6 to 10 days after disease onset but may persist for weeks.

DIAGNOSTIC TESTS
Physical examination demonstrating the clinical triad suggests infectious mononucleosis. Abnormal laboratory results confirm it. (See *Confirming infectious mononucleosis.*)

TREATMENT
Infectious mononucleosis resists prevention and antimicrobial treatment. Therefore, therapy is essentially supportive and focuses on relief of symptoms, bed rest during the acute febrile period, and aspirin or another salicylate for headache and sore throat.

If severe throat inflammation causes airway obstruction, steroids can be used to relieve swelling and avoid tracheotomy. Splenic rupture, marked by sudden abdominal pain, requires splenectomy. About 20% of patients with infectious mononucleosis also have streptococcal pharyngotonsillitis; these patients should receive antibiotic therapy for at least 10 days.

SPECIAL CONSIDERATIONS
• During the acute illness, the patient must get sufficient bed rest.
• To minimize throat discomfort, the patient can drink milk shakes, fruit juices, and broths and eat cool, bland foods. Saline gargles and aspirin may be used as needed.

Multiple myeloma
Multiple myeloma is a disseminated neoplasm of marrow plasma cells that infiltrates bone to produce osteolytic lesions throughout the skeleton. In late stages, the neoplasm infiltrates the liver, spleen, lymph

---

Confirming infectious mononucleosis

The following laboratory results confirm infectious mononucleosis:
• The white blood cell (WBC) count increases 10,000 to 20,000/µl during the second and third weeks of illness. Lymphocytes and monocytes account for 50% to 70% of the total WBC count; 10% of the lymphocytes are atypical.
• Heterophil antibodies in serum drawn during the acute illness and at 3- to 4-week intervals rise to four times normal.
• Indirect immunofluorescence shows antibodies to Epstein-Barr virus and cellular antigens.
• Liver function studies are abnormal.

---

nodes, lungs, adrenal glands, kidneys, skin, and GI tract.

Prognosis is usually poor because the disease is commonly diagnosed after skeletal destruction is widespread. About 52% of patients die within 3 months of diagnosis and 90% die within 2 years.

Early diagnosis and treatment prolong the lives of many patients by 3 to 5 years. Death usually follows complications, such as infection, renal failure, or hematologic disorders.

SIGNS AND SYMPTOMS
The earliest indication is severe, constant back pain that increases with exercise. Joint aching, swelling, and tenderness also may occur. Other effects include fever, malaise, signs of peripheral neuropathy (such as paresthesia), and pathologic fractures.

With disease progression, symptoms of vertebral compression may become acute, accompanied by anemia, weight loss, thoracic deformities, and decreased height. Renal complications and severe, recurrent infection may occur.

DIAGNOSTIC TESTS
Complete blood count shows moderate or severe anemia. The differential may show 40% to 50% lymphocytes but seldom more than 3% plasma cells. Rouleaux formation results from an elevated erythrocyte sedimentation rate.

Urine studies may show Bence Jones protein and hypercalciuria. Presence of Bence Jones protein almost invariably confirms the disease.

Other tests may include bone marrow aspiration, serum electrophoresis, X-rays (which may reveal multiple, sharply circumscribed punched-out lesions, particularly on the skull, pelvis, and spine), and excretory urography (to assess renal involvement).

TREATMENT
Long-term treatment consists mainly of chemotherapy. Adjuvant local radiation reduces acute lesions and relieves localized pain.

Other treatment may involve a melphalan-prednisone combination, with analgesics for pain. For spinal cord compression, the patient may require a laminectomy; for renal complications, dialysis.

SPECIAL CONSIDERATIONS
● Prednisone commonly masks infection, so patients taking this drug must be observed closely for signs of infection.
● Complications can be prevented by watching for fever, malaise, severe anemia, and fractures.

 TEACHING TIP: Encourage the patient to walk to slow bone demineralization and decrease the risk of pneumonia. However, caution him not to walk unaccompanied. Advise him to use a walker or other supportive aid to prevent falls.

Multiple sclerosis
A progressive disease, multiple sclerosis (MS) results from demyelination of the white matter of the brain and spinal cord. Sporadic patches of demyelination throughout the central nervous system lead to varied neurologic dysfunction. (See *How MS affects the body.*)

MS is a major cause of chronic disability in young adults. It usually begins between ages 20 and 40.

The disease course is characterized by exacerbations and remissions. The prognosis varies. MS may progress rapidly, causing disability by early adulthood or causing death within months of onset. However, 70% of patients lead active, productive lives with prolonged remissions.

CAUSES
The cause of MS is unknown. Current theories suggest a slow-acting or latent viral infection and an autoimmune response. Other theories suggest that environmental and genetic factors may play a role.

A family history of MS and living in a cold, damp climate seem to increase the risk of MS. Emotional stress, overwork, fatigue, pregnancy, or acute respiratory infection may precede onset of the illness.

SIGNS AND SYMPTOMS
Clinical manifestations may be transient, or they may last hours or weeks. They may wax and wane with no predictable pattern, vary from day to day, and be bizarre and hard for the patient to describe.

In most patients, visual problems and sensory impairment (such as paresthesia) are the first signs that something may be wrong. Other typical changes include:
● visual disturbances (such as double vision or blurred vision)
● muscle dysfunction (such as weakness, paralysis, spasticity, or hyperreflexia)
● urinary disturbances (such as incontinence, frequency, and urgency)
● emotional lability (such as mood swings, irritability, or depression).

DIAGNOSTIC TESTS
Because early symptoms may be mild, years may elapse between onset

of initial symptoms and diagnosis. Diagnosing MS requires evidence of multiple neurologic attacks and characteristic remissions and exacerbations.

Periodic testing and close patient observation are necessary, perhaps for years. Diagnostic studies may include magnetic resonance imaging to detect MS lesions, electroencephalography, lumbar puncture, and electrophoresis.

Differential diagnosis must rule out spinal cord compression, foramen magnum tumor, multiple small strokes, infection, and psychological disturbances.

TREATMENT

The goal of therapy is to shorten exacerbations and ease neurologic deficits so the patient can resume a normal lifestyle. Corticotropin, prednisone, or dexamethasone is used to reduce edema of the myelin sheath during exacerbations.

Other drugs may include chlordiazepoxide to ease mood swings, baclofen or dantrolene to relieve spasticity, and bethanechol or oxybutynin to relieve urine retention and minimize frequency and urgency.

Interferon beta-1b has been used to reduce frequency of exacerbations in ambulatory patients with relapsing and remitting MS. Immunosuppressants such as azathioprine may suppress the immune response.

During acute exacerbations, supportive care includes bed rest, comfort measures, prevention of fatigue and pressure ulcers, bowel and bladder training (if necessary), antibiotics for bladder infections, physical therapy, and counseling.

SPECIAL CONSIDERATIONS

• Patient comfort measures include massages and relaxing baths. Make sure the bath water isn't too hot because hot water may temporarily intensify some symptoms.
• Active, resistive, and stretching exercises help maintain muscle tone and joint mobility, decrease spasticity, and improve coordination.

PATHOPHYSIOLOGY

How MS affects the body

This transverse section of the cervical spine shows partial loss of myelin, which is characteristic of multiple sclerosis (MS). This degenerative process is called demyelination.

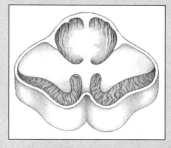

In the illustration below, demyelination is nearly complete. Signs and symptoms of MS depend on the extent of demyelination.

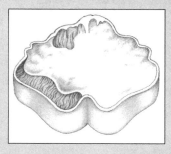

TEACHING TIP: Instruct the patient and family about the chronic course of MS; the need to avoid stress, infections, and fatigue; the importance of maintaining independence by developing new ways of performing daily activities; and the benefits of eating a nutritious, well-balanced diet with sufficient fiber.

Myasthenia gravis

Myasthenia gravis produces sporadic but progressive weakness and abnormal fatigability of skeletal muscles. These problems worsen with exercise and repeated movement but improve with anticholinesterase drugs. The disease follows an unpredictable course of periodic exacerbations and remissions.

Usually, myasthenia gravis affects muscles of the face, lips, tongue, neck, and throat, but it can affect any muscle group. When it involves the respiratory system, it may be life-threatening.

CAUSES

Myasthenia gravis is marked by failure in transmission of nerve impulses at the neuromuscular junction. Such impairment may result from an autoimmune response, ineffective acetylcholine release, or inadequate muscle fiber response to acetylcholine.

SIGNS AND SYMPTOMS

Onset may be sudden or insidious. Dominant symptoms are skeletal muscle weakness and fatigability — although in many patients, weak eye closure, ptosis, and diplopia appear first.

In early stages, the only symptom may be easy fatigability of certain muscles. Later, this symptom may be severe enough to cause paralysis. Typically, myasthenic muscles are strongest in the morning but weaken throughout the day, especially after exercise. Short rest periods temporarily restore muscle function.

Over time, more and more muscles become weak; eventually some muscles may lose function entirely. Resulting symptoms depend on the muscle group affected; they grow more intense during menses and after emotional stress, prolonged exposure to sunlight or cold, or infections.

Myasthenic patients typically have a blank, expressionless face and a nasal voice. They may regurgitate fluids nasally and have difficulty chewing and swallowing. Their eyelids droop, and they may have to tilt their heads back to see. Neck muscles may become too weak to support the head without bobbing.

Patients with weakened respiratory muscles may have difficulty breathing. Respiratory muscle weakness (*myasthenic crisis*) may be severe enough to require an emergency airway and mechanical ventilation.

DIAGNOSTIC TESTS

Muscle fatigability that improves with rest strongly suggests myasthenia gravis. Electromyography, with repeated neural stimulation, may help confirm this diagnosis.

Classic proof of myasthenia gravis is improved muscle function after I.V. injection of edrophonium or neostigmine. This test can differentiate a myasthenic crisis from a *cholinergic crisis* (caused by acetylcholine overactivity at the neuromuscular junction).

TREATMENT

There's no known cure for myasthenia gravis, so treatment is symptomatic. Drug therapy may improve the prognosis and allow the patient to lead a relatively normal life, except during exacerbations. Anticholinesterase drugs, such as neostigmine and pyridostigmine, counteract fatigue and muscle weakness and increase normal muscle function; however, these drugs become less effective as the disease worsens. Corticosteroids may relieve some symptoms.

Plasmapheresis is used in severe exacerbations. Acute exacerbations that produce severe respiratory distress necessitate emergency treatment. Tracheotomy, positive-pressure ventilation, and vigorous suctioning to remove secretions usually bring improvement in a few days.

Myasthenic crisis requires immediate hospitalization and vigorous respiratory support.

Helping patients cope with myasthenia gravis

Thorough patient teaching can help patients with myasthenia gravis cope with this condition. Provide the following instructions.

Getting plenty of rest
● Advise the patient to plan daily activities to coincide with energy peaks.
● Instruct him to take frequent rest periods throughout the day.

Reporting adverse effects
Tell the patient to call the doctor if he experiences adverse effects of anticholinesterase or corticosteroids or signs or symptoms of toxicity. (Ask the doctor or nurse which symptoms he should report.)

Other advice
● Instruct the patient to avoid strenuous exercise, stress, infection, and needless exposure to the sun or cold weather.
● Make sure he knows that periodic remissions, exacerbations, and day-to-day fluctuations are common.
● If the patient has double vision, wearing an eye patch or glasses with one frosted lens may help.

Where to get more help
For more information and an opportunity to meet myasthenic patients who lead full, productive lives, advise the patient to contact the Myasthenia Gravis Foundation.

SPECIAL CONSIDERATIONS

● Signs and symptoms of an impending crisis are increased muscle weakness, respiratory distress, and difficulty talking or chewing.
● If swallowing is difficult, the patient should eat soft, solid foods to lessen the risk of choking.
● Exercise, meals, care, and other patient activities should be planned to make the most of the patient's energy peaks. (See *Helping patients cope with myasthenia gravis.*)

Myelitis and acute transverse myelitis

Myelitis, or inflammation of the spinal cord, can result from several diseases. *Poliomyelitis* affects the cord's gray matter and produces motor dysfunction. *Leukomyelitis* affects only the white matter and causes sensory dysfunction. *Acute transverse myelitis,* which affects the entire thickness of the cord, produces both motor and sensory dysfunctions. This form of myelitis is the most devastating.

Prognosis depends on the severity of cord damage and prevention of complications. With spinal cord necrosis, the prognosis for complete recovery is poor. Even without necrosis, residual neurologic deficits usually persist after recovery.

CAUSES

Acute transverse myelitis results from infection or numerous other causes. (See *Understanding the causes of acute transverse myelitis,* page 210.)

Other forms of myelitis may result from poliovirus, herpes zoster, herpesvirus B, or rabies virus; disorders that cause meningeal inflammation, such as syphilis and tuberculosis; smallpox or polio vaccination; parasitic and fungal infections; and chronic adhesive arachnoiditis.

SIGNS AND SYMPTOMS

In acute transverse myelitis, onset is rapid; motor and sensory dysfunctions below the level of spinal cord damage appear in 1 to 2 days. Patients develop flaccid paralysis of the legs with loss of sensory and sphincter functions. Such sensory loss may follow pain in the legs or trunk. Reflexes disappear in the early stages but may reappear later.

The extent of damage depends on which level of the spinal cord is af-

Understanding the causes of acute transverse myelitis

Infection, demyelinating disease, certain spinal cord disorders, and toxic agents may lead to acute transverse myelitis.

Acute infection
Acute transverse myelitis often follows an acute infectious disease, such as measles or pneumonia (inflammation occurs after the infection subsides). It may also result from a primary infection of the spinal cord itself, such as syphilis or acute disseminated encephalomyelitis.

Other precipitating conditions
Sometimes, acute transverse myelitis accompanies a demyelinating disease such as acute multiple sclerosis or an inflammatory and necrotizing disorder of the spinal cord such as hematomyelia.

Certain toxic agents (carbon monoxide, lead, and arsenic) can cause a type of myelitis in which acute inflammation destroys the entire circumference of the spinal cord.

fected; transverse myelitis rarely involves the arms. If spinal cord damage is severe, it may cause shock.

DIAGNOSTIC TESTS
Paraplegia of rapid onset usually suggests acute transverse myelitis. In such patients, neurologic examination confirms paraplegia or neurologic deficit below the level of the spinal cord lesion, with absent or, later, hyperactive reflexes. Cerebrospinal fluid may be normal or show increased lymphocyte or protein levels.

Diagnostic evaluation must rule out a spinal cord tumor and identify the cause of any underlying infection.

TREATMENT
No effective treatment exists for acute transverse myelitis. However, underlying infection must be treated. Some patients with postinfectious or multiple sclerosis–induced myelitis have received steroid therapy, but its benefits aren't clear.

SPECIAL CONSIDERATIONS
• Range-of-motion exercises and proper alignment can help prevent contractures.
• Meticulous skin care helps to prevent skin infections and pressure ulcers. Pressure points should be checked often and the skin should be kept clean and dry. A water bed or another pressure-relieving device may increase patient comfort.

Myocardial infarction

In myocardial infarction (MI), commonly called heart attack, reduced blood flow through one of the coronary arteries leads to myocardial ischemia and necrosis.

Mortality from MI is high when treatment is delayed; almost half of sudden deaths due to an MI occur before hospitalization, within 1 hour of symptom onset. Typically, death stems from severe tissue damage or from complications. (See *Complications of MI*.) The prognosis improves if vigorous treatment begins immediately.

CAUSES
Predisposing factors for cardiovascular disease (the most common underlying cause of MI) include:
• positive family history
• hypertension
• smoking
• elevated serum triglyceride, total cholesterol, and low-density lipoprotein levels
• diabetes mellitus

• obesity or excessive intake of saturated fats, carbohydrates, or salt
• sedentary lifestyle
• aging
• stress or a Type A personality (aggressive, ambitious, competitive, addicted to work, chronically impatient).

SIGNS AND SYMPTOMS
The cardinal symptom of MI is persistent, crushing substernal pain that may spread to the left arm, jaw, neck, or shoulder blade. However, in some patients, pain may not occur; in others, it may be mild and confused with indigestion.

Other clinical effects of MI include a feeling of impending doom, fatigue, nausea, vomiting, shortness of breath, cool extremities, perspiration, anxiety, and restlessness. Some patients have no symptoms ("silent MI").

DIAGNOSTIC TESTS
Persistent chest pain, ST-segment changes on electrocardiography (ECG), and elevated levels of total creatine kinase (CK) and the CK-MB isoenzyme over a 72-hour period usually confirm MI.

When clinical features aren't clear-cut, the doctor assumes the patient has had an MI until tests rule it out. Diagnostic tests typically include a serial 12-lead ECG, echocardiography, and technetium scans.

TREATMENT
Treatment goals are to relieve chest pain, stabilize the heart rhythm, reduce the cardiac workload, revascularize the blocked coronary artery, and preserve myocardial tissue.

Arrhythmias — the predominant problem during the first 48 hours after MI — may require antiarrhythmics, possibly a pacemaker and, rarely, cardioversion.

To preserve myocardial tissue, I.V. thrombolytic therapy (streptokinase, alteplase, or urokinase) should be started within 6 hours after symptom onset. Percutaneous transluminal coronary angioplasty may be another option.

Complications of MI

The most common complications of myocardial infarction (MI) are:
• recurrent or persistent chest pain
• arrhythmias
• left-sided heart failure
• cardiogenic shock.
Rare but potentially lethal complications include thromboembolism, papillary muscle dysfunction or rupture, rupture of the myocardium or ventricular septum, and ventricular aneurysm.

Delayed complication
Up to several months after MI, some patients experience Dressler's syndrome — pericarditis accompanied by pericardial friction rub, chest pain, fever, and possibly lung inflammation.

Other treatments consist of:
• lidocaine or other drugs for ventricular arrhythmias
• atropine I.V. or a temporary pacemaker for heart block or bradycardia
• nitroglycerin, calcium channel blockers, or isosorbide dinitrate to relieve pain
• heparin I.V.
• morphine I.V. for pain and sedation
• bed rest
• oxygen administration at a modest flow rate
• drugs to increase myocardial contractility or blood pressure
• beta-adrenergic blockers (after acute MI to help prevent reinfarction)
• aspirin to inhibit platelet aggregation
• pulmonary artery catheterization to detect ventricular failure and to monitor response to treatment.

SPECIAL CONSIDERATIONS
• Patient care and other activities should be scheduled to allow periods of uninterrupted rest.

● Stool softeners may be used to prevent straining during defecation, which causes vagal stimulation and may slow the heart rate.

● Range-of-motion exercises should be performed, if possible. If the patient is completely immobilized by a severe MI, frequent turning is used instead.

 TEACHING TIP: Before discharge, the patient should learn about the importance of complying with therapy, how to recognize adverse reactions to drugs, dietary and sexual activity restrictions, symptoms to report, and participation in a cardiac rehabilitation program.

Myocarditis

Myocarditis is a focal or diffuse inflammation of the cardiac muscle (myocardium). It may be acute or chronic and can occur at any age.

In many cases, this disease doesn't cause specific cardiovascular symptoms or electrocardiogram abnormalities. Recovery usually is spontaneous, without residual defects. Occasionally, it's complicated by congestive heart failure.

CAUSES

Myocarditis may result from:
● viral infections, such as coxsackievirus A and B strains and, possibly, polio, influenza, measles, German measles, adenoviruses, and echoviruses
● bacterial infections, such as diphtheria, tuberculosis, typhoid fever, tetanus, staphylococcal, pneumococcal, and gonococcal infections
● hypersensitive immune reactions such as acute rheumatic fever
● radiation therapy involving large doses of radiation to the chest
● chemical poisons, as in chronic alcoholism
● parasitic infections, especially South American trypanosomiasis (Chagas' disease) in infants and immunosuppressed adults, and toxoplasmosis

● infections caused by parasitic worms such as trichinosis.

SIGNS AND SYMPTOMS

Myocarditis usually causes nonspecific symptoms (such as fatigue, shortness of breath, palpitations, and fever) that reflect the accompanying infection. Occasionally, it may cause mild, continuous pressure or soreness in the chest.

DIAGNOSTIC TESTS

The patient history commonly reveals recent febrile upper respiratory tract infection, viral pharyngitis, or tonsillitis. Physical examination detects abnormal heart sounds and possibly a murmur. An electrocardiogram typically shows arrhythmias. Stool and throat cultures may identify bacteria.

TREATMENT

Treatment includes antibiotics for bacterial infection, modified bed rest to decrease the cardiac workload, and careful management of complications.

Heart failure calls for restricted physical activity to minimize myocardial oxygen consumption, supplemental oxygen therapy, restricted salt intake, diuretics to decrease fluid retention, and digoxin to increase myocardial contractility. (Digoxin must be used cautiously because some patients may be sensitive to even small doses.) Arrhythmias require prompt, cautious administration of antiarrhythmic drugs.

SPECIAL CONSIDERATIONS

● The patient taking digitalis glycosides is observed for signs and symptoms of digitalis toxicity: anorexia, nausea, vomiting, blurred vision, and arrhythmias.
● Reassure the patient that activity limitations are temporary.

Nasal polyps

Benign and edematous growths, nasal polyps usually are multiple, mobile, and bilateral. They may become large and numerous enough to cause nasal distention and enlargement of the bony framework, possibly blocking the airway. Nasal polyps tend to recur.

CAUSES
Nasal polyps usually stem from the continuous pressure caused by a chronic allergy that leads to prolonged swelling of the mucous membrane in the nose and sinuses. Other predisposing factors include chronic sinusitis, chronic rhinitis, and recurrent nasal infections.

SIGNS AND SYMPTOMS
Nasal obstruction is the primary sign of nasal polyps. Such obstruction causes an impaired sense of smell, a sensation of fullness in the face, nasal discharge, headache, and shortness of breath. Associated clinical features usually resemble those of allergic rhinitis.

DIAGNOSTIC TESTS
Diagnosis of nasal polyps is determined by the presence of soft-tissue shadows over the affected areas visible on X-ray and a dry, red surface, with clear or gray growths visible on examination. Large growths may resemble tumors. Children require further testing to rule out cystic fibrosis and Peutz-Jeghers syndrome.

TREATMENT
Generally, treatment consists of corticosteroids (by direct injection into the polyps or by local spray) to temporarily reduce them.

Treatment of the underlying cause may include antihistamines to control allergy, and antibiotic therapy if infection is present. Local application of an astringent shrinks hypertrophied tissue. However, medical management alone is rarely effective.

Consequently, the treatment of choice is polypectomy. The use of surgical lasers is growing more popular. Continued recurrence may require surgical opening of the ethmoid and maxillary sinuses and evacuation of diseased tissue.

SPECIAL CONSIDERATIONS
● After surgery, elevating the head of the bed, applying ice compresses, and changing dressings as needed increase patient comfort.
● To control nasal bleeding, which may occur after packing is removed, the patient should sit upright and the outside of the nose should be compressed against the septum for 10 to 15 minutes. He should be advised not to swallow blood.

 PREVENTION TIP: To help prevent nasal polyps, instruct patients with allergies to avoid exposure to allergens, to take antihistamines at the first sign of an allergic reaction, and to avoid overuse of nose drops and sprays.

Nephrotic syndrome

Nephrotic syndrome is characterized by marked proteinuria, hypoalbuminemia, hyperlipemia, and edema. Not a disease itself, this syndrome results from a specific glomerular defect and reflects renal damage. (See *What happens in nephrotic syndrome,* page 214.)

Prognosis varies greatly, depending on the underlying cause. Some forms of nephrotic syndrome may progress to end-stage renal failure.

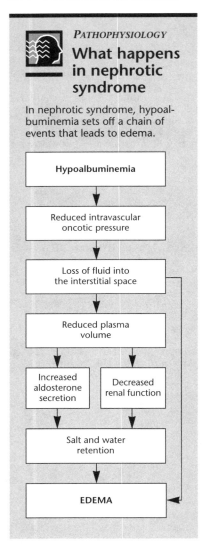

PATHOPHYSIOLOGY

What happens in nephrotic syndrome

In nephrotic syndrome, hypoalbuminemia sets off a chain of events that leads to edema.

| Hypoalbuminemia |
| Reduced intravascular oncotic pressure |
| Loss of fluid into the interstitial space |
| Reduced plasma volume |
| Increased aldosterone secretion | Decreased renal function |
| Salt and water retention |
| EDEMA |

CAUSES
About 75% of cases result from primary (idiopathic) glomerulonephritis. Classifications of nephrotic syndrome include the following:
● In *lipid nephrosis (nil lesions),* the glomeruli appear normal by light microscopy. Some tubules may contain increased lipid deposits.

● *Membranous glomerulonephritis* is characterized by uniform thickening of the glomerular basement membrane containing dense deposits. It eventually progresses to renal failure.
● *Focal glomerulosclerosis* can develop spontaneously at any age, follow kidney transplantation, or result from heroin abuse. Glomerular lesions generally cause slowly progressive deterioration of renal function.
● In *membranoproliferative glomerulonephritis,* slowly progressive lesions develop in the subendothelial region of the basement membrane. These lesions may follow infection.

Other causes of nephrotic syndrome include metabolic diseases such as diabetes mellitus; collagenvascular disorders such as systemic lupus erythematosus; circulatory diseases, such as heart failure and sickle cell anemia; nephrotoxins, such as mercury and gold; allergic reactions; and infections such as tuberculosis.

SIGNS AND SYMPTOMS
The dominant clinical feature of nephrotic syndrome is mild to severe dependent edema of the ankles or sacrum, or periorbital edema. Such edema may lead to ascites, pleural effusion, and swollen external genitalia.

Accompanying signs and symptoms may include orthostatic hypotension, lethargy, anorexia, depression, and pallor. Major complications are malnutrition, infection, coagulation disorders, thromboembolic vascular occlusion, and accelerated atherosclerosis.

DIAGNOSTIC TESTS
Consistent proteinuria in excess of 3.5 g/24 hours strongly suggests nephrotic syndrome; urine examination also reveals an increased number of hyaline, granular, and waxy fatty casts and oval fat bodies.

TREATMENT
The underlying cause is treated, if possible. Supportive treatment consists of protein replacement with a diet of 1.5 g protein/kg of body weight, with restricted sodium in-

take; diuretics for edema; and antibiotics for infection.

Some patients respond to an 8-week course of corticosteroid therapy, followed by a maintenance dose. Others respond better to a combination course of prednisone and azathioprine or cyclophosphamide.

SPECIAL CONSIDERATIONS
• After a kidney biopsy, the patient is observed for bleeding and shock.
• Adverse reactions to drug therapy include bone marrow toxicity from cytotoxic immunosuppressives and cushingoid symptoms (muscle weakness, mental changes, acne, moon face, hirsutism, girdle obesity, purple striae, amenorrhea) from long-term steroid therapy.
• Steroids also may mask infections and cause increased susceptibility to infections, ulcers, GI bleeding, and diabetes. GI complications can be eased by giving steroids with an antacid or with cimetidine.

Neuritis, peripheral

Peripheral neuritis is the degeneration of peripheral nerves supplying mainly the distal muscles of the extremities. It is associated with noninflammatory degeneration of the axon and myelin sheaths. The condition leads to muscle weakness with sensory loss and atrophy, and decreased or absent deep tendon reflexes.

Because onset is usually insidious, patients may compensate by overusing unaffected muscles; however, onset is rapid with severe infection and chronic alcohol intoxication. If the cause can be identified and eliminated, the prognosis is good.

CAUSES
Causes of peripheral neuritis include:
• chronic intoxication (ethyl alcohol, arsenic, lead, carbon disulfide, benzene, phosphorus, and sulfonamides)
• infectious diseases (meningitis, diphtheria, syphilis, tuberculosis, pneumonia, mumps, and Guillain-Barré syndrome)
• metabolic and inflammatory disor-

ders (gout, diabetes mellitus, rheumatoid arthritis, polyarteritis nodosa, systemic lupus erythematosus)
• nutritive diseases (beriberi and other vitamin deficiencies and cachectic states).

SIGNS AND SYMPTOMS
Clinical effects of peripheral neuritis develop slowly, and the disease usually affects motor and sensory nerve fibers. Neuritis typically produces flaccid paralysis, wasting, loss of reflexes, pain, inability to perceive vibratory sensations, and paresthesia, hyperesthesia, or anesthesia in the hands and feet.

Deep tendon reflexes are diminished or absent, and atrophied muscles are tender or hypersensitive to pressure or palpation. Footdrop may be present. The skin may become glossy and red, and sweating may diminish.

DIAGNOSTIC TESTS
The patient history and physical findings suggest the typical distribution of motor and sensory deficits. Electromyography may show a delayed action potential if motor nerve function is impaired.

TREATMENT
Effective treatment consists of supportive measures to relieve pain, adequate bed rest, and physical therapy as needed. Most important, the underlying cause must be identified and corrected. For instance, it's essential to identify and remove the toxic agent, correct nutritional and vitamin deficiencies, or counsel the patient to avoid alcohol.

SPECIAL CONSIDERATIONS
• Pain can be relieved with correct patient positioning, analgesics, or possibly phenytoin. Resting and refraining from using the affected extremity enhance patient comfort.
• A foot cradle is used to prevent pressure ulcers. Splints, boards, braces, or other orthopedic appliances help prevent contractures.
• After pain subsides, passive range-

Features of brain infection

If nocardiosis spreads through the bloodstream to the brain, abscesses form. The patient then may exhibit the following signs and symptoms:
- confusion
- disorientation
- dizziness
- headache
- nausea
- seizures.

Rupture of a brain abscess may cause purulent meningitis.

of-motion exercises or massage may be beneficial.

 TEACHING TIP: Instruct the patient to maintain a high-calorie diet rich in vitamins, especially B complex.

Nocardiosis

A bacterial infection, nocardiosis is caused by a gram-positive species of the genus *Nocardia* — usually *Nocardia asteroides*. If the infection enters the brain, mortality exceeds 80%. With other forms of nocardiosis, mortality is 50%, even with appropriate therapy.

CAUSES

Nocardia organisms are aerobic, gram-positive bacteria with branching filaments. Normally found in soil, these organisms cause occasional sporadic disease in humans and animals throughout the world. The incubation period is probably several weeks.

The usual transmission mode is inhalation of organisms suspended in dust. Less commonly, transmission occurs by direct inoculation through puncture wounds or abrasions.

SIGNS AND SYMPTOMS

Nocardiosis originates as a pulmonary infection and causes a cough that produces thick, tenacious, purulent or mucopurulent and, possibly, blood-tinged sputum. It may also produce a fever as high as 105° F (40.6° C), chills, night sweats, anorexia, malaise, and weight loss.

This infection may lead to pleurisy, intrapleural effusions, and empyema. Other effects may include tracheitis, bronchitis, pericarditis, endocarditis, peritonitis, mediastinitis, septic arthritis, and keratoconjunctivitis.

Nocardiosis that spreads to the brain can cause serious neurologic signs and symptoms. (See *Features of brain infection.*)

DIAGNOSTIC TESTS

Identification of *Nocardia* by culture of sputum or discharge is difficult. Diagnosis may hinge on special staining techniques, in conjunction with a typical clinical picture.

TREATMENT

Nocardiosis requires 12 to 18 months of treatment, preferably with cotrimoxazole or high doses of sulfonamides. Patients who don't respond to sulfonamides may receive other drugs, such as ampicillin or erythromycin.

Treatment also includes surgical drainage of abscesses and excision of necrotic tissue. The acute phase requires complete bed rest; as the patient improves, activity can increase.

SPECIAL CONSIDERATIONS

- Nocardiosis isn't transmitted from person to person and doesn't require isolation.
- Fever can be reduced with tepid sponge baths and antipyretics.
- In patients with pulmonary infection, chest physiotherapy should be administered.
- In patients with brain infection, neurologic function must be assessed regularly.

 TEACHING TIP: Before discharge, the patient should be instructed to continue taking prescribed drugs even after symptoms subside, and to get frequent follow-up examinations.

Optic atrophy

Degeneration of the optic nerve, or optic atrophy, can develop spontaneously (primary) or can follow inflammation or edema of the nerve head (secondary). Some forms of this condition may subside without treatment, but degeneration of the optic nerve is irreversible.

CAUSES

Optic atrophy usually results from central nervous system disorders, such as:
• pressure on the optic nerve from aneurysms or intraorbital or intracranial tumors
• optic neuritis, in multiple sclerosis, retrobulbar neuritis, and tabes. (For other causative conditions, see *Less common causes of optic atrophy,* page 218.)

SIGNS AND SYMPTOMS

Optic atrophy causes abrupt or gradual, painless loss of the visual field or visual acuity, with subtle changes in color vision.

DIAGNOSTIC TESTS

Slit-lamp examination usually reveals a pupil that reacts sluggishly to direct light stimulation. Ophthalmoscopy may reveal pallor of the nerve head from loss of microvascular circulation in the disk and deposition of fibrous or glial tissue. Visual field testing reveals a scotoma and, possibly, major visual field impairment.

TREATMENT

Optic atrophy is irreversible, so treatment aims to correct the underlying cause and prevent further vision loss. Steroids may be given to decrease inflammation and swelling, if a space-occupying lesion is the cause. In multiple sclerosis, optic neuritis often subsides spontaneously but may recur and subside.

SPECIAL CONSIDERATIONS

• Offer emotional support to help the patient deal with vision loss.
• As appropriate, assist the visually compromised patient to perform activities of daily living.

Osteoarthritis

The most common form of arthritis, osteoarthritis is a chronic disorder marked by deterioration of the joint cartilage and formation of reactive new bone at the joint margins and subchondral areas. Degeneration results from breakdown of chondrocytes.

The degree of disability depends on the site and severity of involvement; it can range from minor finger limitation to severe disability in hip or knee involvement. The progression rate varies; joints may remain stable for years in an early stage of deterioration.

CAUSES

Primary osteoarthritis, a normal part of aging, results from many conditions, including metabolic, genetic, chemical, and mechanical factors. Secondary osteoarthritis usually follows an identifiable predisposing event — most commonly trauma, congenital deformity, or obesity — and leads to degenerative changes.

SIGNS AND SYMPTOMS

The most common symptom is deep, aching joint pain, particularly after exercise or weight-bearing, which is usually relieved by rest. Other signs and symptoms include:
• stiffness in the morning and after exercise (relieved by rest)

Less common causes of optic atrophy

Although optic atrophy usually results from a neurologic disorder, it sometimes stems from one of the following conditions:
• retinitis pigmentosa
• chronic papilledema and papillitis
• congenital syphilis
• glaucoma
• central retinal artery or vein occlusion that interrupts the blood supply to the optic nerve, causing degeneration of ganglion cells
• trauma
• ingestion of toxins, such as methanol and quinine
• deficiencies of vitamin B_{12}, amino acids, and zinc.

• aching during weather changes
• "grating" of the joint during motion
• altered gait contractures
• limited movement.

These symptoms worsen with poor posture, obesity, and occupational stress.

Osteoarthritis of the interphalangeal joints produces irreversible changes in the distal joints (Heberden's nodes) and proximal joints (Bouchard's nodes). These nodes may be painless at first but eventually become red, swollen, and tender, causing numbness and dexterity loss. (See *Viewing osteoarthritis*.)

DIAGNOSTIC TESTS
A thorough physical examination confirms typical signs and symptoms; absence of systemic findings rules out an inflammatory joint disorder. X-rays of the affected joint help confirm diagnosis (although they may be normal in early stages). Typically, X-rays show narrowing of the joint space or margin, joint deformity, and other characteristic find-

ings. No laboratory test is specific for osteoarthritis.

TREATMENT
Treatment aims to relieve pain, maintain or improve mobility, and minimize disability. Medications include aspirin or other nonnarcotic analgesics, phenylbutazone, indomethacin, fenoprofen, ibuprofen, propoxyphene and, in some cases, intraarticular corticosteroid injections. Such injections, given every 4 to 6 months, may delay the development of nodes in the hands.

Effective treatment also reduces stress by supporting or stabilizing the joint with crutches, braces, a cane, a walker, a cervical collar, or traction. Other supportive measures include massage, moist heat, paraffin dips for hands, protective techniques to prevent undue stress on the joints, adequate rest and, occasionally, exercise when the knees are affected.

Surgical treatment, reserved for patients with severe disability or uncontrollable pain, may involve:
• *arthroplasty* (partial or total): replacement of the deteriorated joint portion with a prosthetic appliance
• *arthrodesis:* surgical fusion of bones; used primarily in the spine (laminectomy)
• *osteoplasty:* scraping and lavage of deteriorated bone from the joint
• *osteotomy:* change in bone alignment to relieve stress by excising a wedge of bone or by cutting bone.

SPECIAL CONSIDERATIONS
• Encourage the patient to avoid fatigue through adequate rest, pacing of activities, and restful sleep. Help him maintain mobility through use of gentle, isometric range-of-motion exercises.

 TEACHING TIP: Instruct the patient to wear well-fitting supportive shoes, install safety devices in the home, maintain proper weight to lessen strain on joints, and avoid activities that involve repeated impact on joints.

PATHOPHYSIOLOGY

Viewing osteoarthritis

Involvement of the interphalangeal joints causes irreversible changes in the distal joints (Heberden's nodes) and the proximal joints (Bouchard's nodes). These nodes may be painless initially, with gradual progression to or sudden flare-up of redness, swelling, tenderness, and impaired sensation and dexterity.

Heberden's nodes

Bouchard's nodes

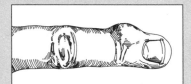

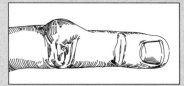

Osteomyelitis

A pyogenic bone infection, osteomyelitis may be chronic or acute. It commonly results from a combination of local trauma and an acute infection arising elsewhere in the body. Although osteomyelitis may remain localized, it can spread through the bone to the marrow, cortex, and periosteum.

Acute osteomyelitis is usually a blood-borne disease, most often affecting rapidly growing children. Chronic osteomyelitis (rare) is marked by multiple draining sinus tracts and metastatic lesions.

With prompt treatment, the prognosis for acute osteomyelitis is good; for chronic osteomyelitis, the prognosis is poor.

CAUSES

The most common pyogenic organism in osteomyelitis is *Staphylococcus aureus*. Typically, this organism finds a culture site in a hematoma from recent trauma or in a weakened area, such as the site of local infection, and then spreads directly to bone. (See *The road to chronic osteomyelitis,* page 220.)

SIGNS AND SYMPTOMS

Acute osteomyelitis has a rapid onset, with sudden pain in the affected bone and tenderness, heat, swelling, and restricted movement over it. Associated systemic symptoms may include tachycardia, sudden fever, nausea, and malaise.

Generally, chronic and acute osteomyelitis have similar clinical features, except that chronic infection can persist intermittently for years, flaring up spontaneously after minor trauma. Sometimes, however, chronic infection causes only persistent drainage of pus from an old pocket in a sinus tract.

DIAGNOSTIC TESTS

Patient history, physical examination, white blood cell count, erythrocyte sedimentation rate, and blood cultures help to confirm osteomyelitis.

X-rays may not show bone involvement until the disease has been active for some time, usually 2 to 3 weeks. Bone scans can detect early infection. Diagnosis must rule out poliomyelitis, rheumatic fever, myositis, and bone fractures.

PATHOPHYSIOLOGY

The road to chronic osteomyelitis

Osteomyelitis begins when pathogenic organisms — typically *Staphylococcus aureus* — find a culture site in the body and then spread to the bone.

Clogged canals
As the organisms grow and form pus within the bone, tension builds in the rigid medullary cavity, forcing pus through the haversian canals.

Abscess formation
This leads to formation of a subperiosteal abscess. The abscess deprives the bone of its blood supply and eventually may cause necrosis.

In turn, necrosis stimulates the periosteum to create new bone. The old bone (sequestrum) detaches and works its way out through an abscess or the sinuses. By the time sequestrum forms, osteomyelitis is chronic.

TREATMENT
Treatment varies for acute and chronic osteomyelitis.

Acute osteomyelitis
Acute osteomyelitis should be treated before definitive diagnosis. Treatment includes large doses of I.V. antibiotics; early surgical drainage to relieve pressure buildup and old bone formation; immobilization of the affected bone by plaster cast, traction, or bed rest; and supportive measures, such as analgesics and I.V. fluids.

Abscesses must be incised and drained. Antibiotic therapy may include systemic antibiotics; intracavitary instillation of antibiotics through closed-system continuous irrigation with low intermittent suction; limited irrigation with blood drainage system with suction (Hemovac); or local application of packed, wet, antibiotic-soaked dressings.

Chronic osteomyelitis
For chronic osteomyelitis, surgery is usually done to remove dead bone and to promote drainage. The prognosis is poor even after surgery. Patients are often in great pain and require prolonged hospitalization. Resistant chronic osteomyelitis in an arm or leg may necessitate amputation.

Other treatments used in some centers include hyperbaric oxygen, free tissue transfers, and local muscle flaps.

SPECIAL CONSIDERATIONS
• The affected limb should be supported with firm pillows and kept level with the body.
• To reduce the risk of injury, advise the patient to move slowly and deliberately. Point out that mishaps, such as from jerky movements and falls, may threaten bone integrity.

Osteoporosis
Osteoporosis is a metabolic bone disorder in which the rate of bone resorption accelerates while the rate of bone formation slows, causing loss of bone mass. Bones affected by this disease lose calcium and phosphate salts, becoming porous, brittle, and abnormally vulnerable to fracture. Osteoporosis primarily affects the weight-bearing vertebrae.

Osteoporosis may be primary or secondary to an underlying disease. Primary osteoporosis is often called postmenopausal osteoporosis because it most commonly develops in elderly, postmenopausal women.

CAUSES

The cause of primary osteoporosis is unknown; however, a mild but prolonged negative calcium balance resulting from inadequate dietary intake of calcium may be an important contributing factor — as may declining gonadal adrenal function, faulty protein metabolism due to estrogen deficiency, and a sedentary lifestyle. (See *Preventing osteoporosis*.)

Causes of secondary osteoporosis include prolonged therapy with steroids or heparin, total immobilization or disuse of a bone, alcoholism, malnutrition, malabsorption, lactose intolerance, hyperthyroidism, and osteogenesis imperfecta.

SIGNS AND SYMPTOMS

Osteoporosis is usually discovered when an elderly person bends to lift something, hears a snapping sound, then feels a sudden pain in the lower back. Vertebral collapse may cause a backache with pain that radiates around the trunk. Movement or jarring worsens the backache.

In another common pattern, osteoporosis develops gradually, with increasing deformity, kyphosis, height loss, and a markedly aged appearance. As vertebral bodies weaken, spontaneous wedge fractures, pathologic fractures of the neck and femur, Colles' fractures after a minor fall, and hip fractures are common.

DIAGNOSTIC TESTS

Diagnosis rests on patient history and ruling out other causes of bone-depleting disease. Diagnostic procedures include:
• X-rays, which show typical degeneration in lower-back vertebrae
• dual or single photon absorptiometry, which measures bone mass
• blood tests, which may reveal elevated parathyroid hormone levels
• bone biopsy, which may reveal thin, porous, but otherwise normal-looking bone.

TREATMENT

Effective treatment aims to prevent fractures and control pain. A physical

---

Preventing osteoporosis

Adequate intake of dietary calcium and regular exercise may reduce the risk for postmenopausal osteoporosis. Hormonal and fluoride treatments may also offer some preventive benefit.

Secondary osteoporosis can be prevented through effective treatment of the underlying disease as well as through steroid therapy, early mobilization after surgery or trauma, decreased alcohol consumption, careful observation for signs of malabsorption, and prompt treatment of hyperthyroidism.

---

therapy program, emphasizing gentle exercise and activity, plays an important role. Estrogen, to be started within 3 years after menopause, may be given to slow bone resorption; sodium fluoride, to stimulate bone formation; and calcium and vitamin D, to support normal bone metabolism. However, drug therapy merely arrests osteoporosis and doesn't cure it.

Weakened vertebrae should be supported, usually with a back brace. Surgery can correct pathologic fractures of the femur by open reduction and internal fixation.

SPECIAL CONSIDERATIONS

• Explain how easily the patient's bones can fracture. Stress the importance of taking safety measures to prevent injury.
• Instruct the patient to report new pain sites immediately, especially after trauma, no matter how slight.
• A balanced diet high in vitamin D, calcium, and protein supports bone metabolism.

 TEACHING TIP: Instruct the patient to sleep on a firm mattress, avoid excessive bed rest, stoop correctly when lifting ob-

PATHOPHYSIOLOGY

Site of otitis externa

In the illustration below, the shaded area indicates the parts of the ear that become inflamed in otitis externa.

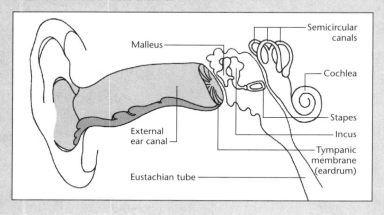

jects, and avoid bending and twisting motions.
• Advise the female patient taking estrogen on how to perform a breast self-examination. Tell her to do this examination at least once a month and to report lumps immediately.

Otitis externa

Also known as swimmer's ear, otitis externa is an inflammation of the skin of the external ear canal and auricle. (See *Site of otitis externa.*) It may be acute or chronic. With treatment, acute otitis externa usually subsides within 7 days. However, it tends to recur.

CAUSES
Otitis externa usually results from bacterial infection with an organism, such as *Pseudomonas, Proteus vulgaris,* streptococci, or *Staphylococcus aureus.* Sometimes it stems from a fungus, such as *Aspergillus niger* or *Candida albicans.* Predisposing factors include:
• swimming in contaminated water

• cleaning the ear canal with a cotton swab, bobby pin, finger, or other foreign object
• exposure to dust, hair care products, or other irritants
• regular use of earphones, earplugs, or earmuffs
• chronic drainage from a perforated tympanic membrane.

SIGNS AND SYMPTOMS
Acute otitis externa typically produces moderate to severe pain. Other effects may include fever, foul-smelling ear discharge, regional cellulitis, and partial hearing loss.
Fungal otitis externa may be asymptomatic. Chronic otitis externa is marked by pruritus, which may lead to scaling and skin thickening. An ear discharge may appear.

DIAGNOSTIC TESTS
Physical examination confirms otitis externa. With acute otitis externa, otoscopy reveals a swollen external ear canal and tender nodes in front of the tragus, behind the ear, or in

the upper neck. In fungal otitis externa, removal of growth shows a thick, red epithelium. In chronic otitis externa, epithelium in the ear canal is thick and red. Further tests identify the causative organism and determine antibiotic selection.

TREATMENT
Treatment varies with the type of otitis externa.

Acute otitis externa
To relieve pain, treatment includes heat therapy (heat lamp; hot, damp compresses; heating pad), aspirin or acetaminophen, and codeine. Use of antibiotic eardrops follows ear cleaning and removal of debris. If fever persists or regional cellulitis develops, a systemic antibiotic is necessary.

Fungal otitis externa
The ear is carefully cleaned. A keratolytic or 2% salicylic acid in cream containing nystatin may help treat otitis externa resulting from candidal organisms. Instilling slightly acidic eardrops creates an unfavorable environment in the ear canal for most fungi as well as for *Pseudomonas*.

Chronic otitis externa
The ear is cleaned and debris removed. Supplemental therapy includes antibiotic eardrops or antibiotic ointment or cream (neomycin, bacitracin, or polymyxin, possibly combined with hydrocortisone).

For mild chronic otitis externa, treatment may include instilling antibiotic eardrops once or twice weekly and wearing specially fitted earplugs while showering, shampooing, or swimming.

SPECIAL CONSIDERATIONS
 TEACHING TIP: Instruct an adult to instill eardrops by pulling the pinna upward and backward. To ensure that the drops reach the epithelium, tell him to insert a wisp of cotton moistened with eardrops.

 PREVENTION: To help prevent otitis externa, advise using lamb's wool earplugs coated with petroleum jelly, keeping water out of the ears when showering or shampooing, wearing earplugs or keeping the head above water when swimming, and avoiding use of cotton swabs or other objects for cleaning the ear.

Otitis media
Otitis media is an inflammation of the middle ear. (See *Site of otitis media*, page 224.) The condition may be suppurative or secretory, acute or chronic. Acute otitis media is common in children.

CAUSES
Otitis media results from disruption of eustachian tube patency.

Suppurative otitis media
The suppurative form is caused by conditions that allow nasopharyngeal flora to reflux through the eustachian tube and colonize the middle ear, such as respiratory tract infection and allergic reaction. Suppurative otitis media usually results from infection with pneumococci, *Haemophilus influenzae*, and certain other organisms.

Predisposing factors include the normally wider, shorter, more horizontal eustachian tubes in children as well as anatomic anomalies. Chronic suppurative otitis media results from inadequate treatment of acute otitis episodes or from infection by resistant strains of bacteria.

Secretory otitis media
Obstruction of the eustachian tube causes buildup of negative pressure in the middle ear, promoting transudation of serous fluid from blood vessels in the middle ear. Such effusion may result from eustachian tube dysfunction due to viral infection or allergy, rapid aircraft descent in a person with an upper respiratory tract

PATHOPHYSIOLOGY

Site of otitis media

In otitis media, the parts of the ear shaded in the illustration below become inflamed.

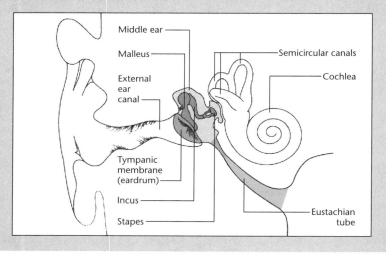

infection, or rapid underwater ascent in scuba diving.

Chronic secretory otitis media follows persistent eustachian tube dysfunction from mechanical obstruction, edema, or inadequate treatment of acute suppurative otitis media.

SIGNS AND SYMPTOMS
Clinical features vary with the specific type of the disorder.

Suppurative otitis media
Many patients are asymptomatic. Some patients have severe, deep, throbbing pain, signs of upper respiratory tract infection, mild to very high fever, mild hearing loss, dizziness, nausea, and vomiting.

Secretory otitis media
Severe conductive hearing loss occurs, possibly accompanied by a sensation of fullness in the ear and popping, crackling, or clicking sounds on swallowing or with jaw movement. The patient may hear an echo when he speaks and may report a vague feeling of top-heaviness.

Chronic otitis media
Over time, chronic otitis media leads to thickening and scarring of the tympanic membrane, decreased or absent tympanic membrane mobility, cholesteatoma (a cystlike mass in the middle ear) and, in chronic suppurative otitis media, a painless, purulent discharge. Conductive hearing loss is also typical.

DIAGNOSTIC TESTS
Patient history and physical findings are important in diagnosis. Findings vary with the type of infection present. In some cases, pneumatic otoscopy may be used to detect decreased eardrum movement.

TREATMENT
The type of otitis media dictates treatment.

Suppurative otitis media
Antibiotic therapy includes ampicillin, amoxicillin, or amoxicillin/clavulanate potassium; patients allergic to penicillin derivatives may receive cefaclor or co-trimoxazole. Severe, painful bulging of the tympanic membrane usually warrants myringotomy.

Secretory otitis media
Inflating the eustachian tube by performing Valsalva's maneuver several times a day may be the only treatment required. Otherwise, nasopharyngeal decongestant therapy may be helpful.

If decongestant therapy fails, myringotomy and aspiration of middle ear fluid are necessary, followed by insertion of a polyethylene tube into the tympanic membrane; the tube falls out spontaneously after 9 to 12 months.

Chronic otitis media
Treatment includes broad-spectrum antibiotics for exacerbations of acute otitis media, eliminating eustachian tube obstruction, treating otitis externa, myringoplasty and tympanoplasty to reconstruct middle ear structures when thickening and scarring are present and, possibly, mastoidectomy. Cholesteatoma requires excision.

SPECIAL CONSIDERATIONS
• After tympanoplasty, warn the patient against blowing his nose or getting the ear wet when bathing.

 PREVENTION: Teach parents ways to prevent otitis media in infants, such as by avoiding placing the infant in a supine position for feeding or putting him to bed with a bottle.

Ovarian cancer
After cancer of the lung, breast, and colon, primary ovarian cancer ranks as the most common cause of cancer deaths among American women. In women with previously treated breast cancer, metastatic ovarian cancer is more common than cancer at any other site.

The prognosis varies with the histologic type and disease stage but is generally poor because ovarian tumors produce few early signs and are usually advanced at diagnosis. (See *Types of ovarian cancer,* page 226.)

CAUSES
Exactly what causes ovarian cancer isn't known, but its incidence is higher in women of upper socioeconomic levels between ages 20 and 54. However, it can occur during childhood. Other contributing factors include age at menopause, infertility, celibacy, high-fat diet, nulliparity, familial tendency, history of breast or uterine cancer, and exposure to asbestos, talc, and industrial pollutants.

SIGNS AND SYMPTOMS
Findings vary with tumor size. Occasionally, early-stage ovarian cancer causes vague abdominal discomfort, dyspepsia, and other mild GI disturbances. As it progresses, it causes urinary frequency, constipation, pelvic discomfort, abdominal distention, and weight loss.

Tumor rupture, torsion, or infection may cause pain. Granulosa cell tumors have feminizing effects; arrhenoblastomas have virilizing effects. Advanced ovarian cancer causes ascites, signs and symptoms relating to metastatic sites and, rarely, postmenopausal bleeding and pain.

DIAGNOSTIC TESTS
Diagnosis typically involves a pelvic examination, a complete history, and a Pap smear (although this is rarely positive). The doctor may also order abdominal ultrasonography, a computed tomography scan, X-rays, and lymphangiography. Usually, a surgeon performs exploratory surgery, taking cell and tissue samples for analysis.

PATHOPHYSIOLOGY

Types of ovarian cancer

Three main types of ovarian cancer occur.

Primary epithelial tumors
These tumors, which account for 90% of ovarian cancers, include serous cystadenocarcinoma, mucinous cystadenocarcinoma, and endometrioid and mesonephric malignancies.

Germ cell tumors
Types of germ cell tumors include endodermal sinus cancer, embryonal carcinoma (a rare cancer that occurs in children), immature teratoma, and dysgerminoma.

Sex cord (stromal) tumors
Besides granulosa-theca cell tumors, sex cord tumors include:
• granulosa cell tumors, which produce estrogen and may have feminizing effects
• arrhenoblastomas, rare tumors that produce androgen and have virilizing effects.

TREATMENT
Depending on the disease stage and the patient's age, the doctor may order varying combinations of surgery, chemotherapy and, in some cases, radiation.

Occasionally, in girls or young women with a unilateral encapsulated tumor who wish to maintain fertility, a conservative approach, such as resection of the involved ovary and biopsies of the omentum and uninvolved ovary, may be appropriate.

Usually, though, ovarian cancer requires more aggressive treatment, including total abdominal hysterectomy and bilateral salpingo-oophorectomy with tumor resection, omentectomy, appendectomy, lymph node biopsies with lymphadenectomy, tissue biopsies, and peritoneal washings.

Chemotherapy extends survival time in most patients. It's largely palliative in advanced disease, but prolonged remissions are being achieved in some patients.

Other treatments
Radioisotopes have been used as adjuvant therapy. I.V. administration of biological response modifiers — interleukin-2, interferon, and monoclonal antibodies — is being investigated.

SPECIAL CONSIDERATIONS
• Inform a patient who will undergo bilateral oophorectomy that this surgery induces early menopause. Tell her she may experience hot flashes, headaches, palpitations, insomnia, depression, and excessive perspiration.
• If the patient is a young woman who grieves for her lost fertility, she and her family may need to overcome feelings that "there's nothing else to live for."

Ovarian cysts

Most ovarian cysts are nonneoplastic sacs on an ovary that contain fluid or semisolid material. Although typically small and asymptomatic, they require thorough investigation as possible sites of cancerous changes.

Common types of ovarian cysts include follicular cysts, lutein cysts (granulosa-lutein and theca-lutein cysts), and polycystic ovarian disease. Ovarian cysts can develop any time between puberty and menopause. For nonneoplastic cysts, the prognosis is excellent.

CAUSES

Follicular cysts generally arise from follicles that overdistend instead of going through the atretic stage of the menstrual cycle. When such cysts persist into menopause, they secrete excessive amounts of estrogen. (See *Viewing a follicular cyst.*)

Granulosa-lutein cysts, which occur within the corpus luteum, are functional, nonneoplastic enlargements of the ovaries, caused by excessive blood accumulation during the hemorrhagic phase of the menstrual cycle.

Theca-lutein cysts are commonly bilateral and filled with clear, straw-colored fluid. They are often associated with hydatidiform moles, choriocarcinomas, or certain types of hormone therapy.

Polycystic ovarian disease, part of Stein-Leventhal syndrome, stems from endocrine abnormalities.

SIGNS AND SYMPTOMS

Small ovarian cysts usually don't produce symptoms unless torsion or rupture causes abdominal tenderness, distention, and rigidity. Large or multiple cysts may induce mild pelvic discomfort, low back pain, dyspareunia, or abnormal uterine bleeding. Ovarian cysts with torsion cause acute abdominal pain.

Granulosa-lutein cysts appearing early in pregnancy may cause unilateral pelvic discomfort and, if rupture occurs, massive intraperitoneal hemorrhage. In nonpregnant women, these cysts may cause delayed menses followed by prolonged or irregular bleeding. Polycystic ovarian disease may also produce secondary amenorrhea, oligomenorrhea, or infertility.

DIAGNOSTIC TESTS

Diagnosis hinges on signs and symptoms. Physical examination and laboratory tests may also help detect certain types of cysts. Visualization of the ovary through ultrasound, la-

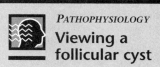

PATHOPHYSIOLOGY

Viewing a follicular cyst

A common type of ovarian cyst, a follicular cyst is usually small, semitransparent, and overdistended with watery fluid that's visible through its thin walls.

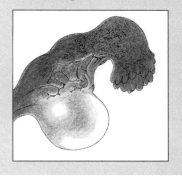

paroscopy, or surgery confirms ovarian cyst.

TREATMENT

The type of cyst dictates treatment.

Follicular cyst

This cyst usually doesn't require treatment because it tends to disappear on its own within 60 days. However, if it interferes with daily activities, oral clomiphene citrate or I.M. progesterone are given for 5 days to reestablish the ovarian hormonal cycle. Oral contraceptives may also speed involution of functional cysts.

Granulosa-lutein and theca-lutein cysts

If granulosa-lutein cysts occur during pregnancy, treatment is symptomatic because they diminish during the third trimester and rarely require surgery. Theca-lutein cysts disappear spontaneously after elimination of the hydatidiform mole, destruction of choriocarcinoma, or discontinuation of hormone therapy.

Polycystic ovarian disease

Treatment may include such drugs as clomiphene citrate to induce ovulation, medroxyprogesterone acetate for 10 days a month for the patient who does not want to become pregnant, or low-dose oral contraceptives for the patient who needs reliable contraception.

Surgery (laparoscopy or exploratory laparotomy with possible ovarian cystectomy or oophorectomy) may become necessary if an ovarian cyst persists or is suspicious.

SPECIAL CONSIDERATIONS

• Provide emotional support and offer appropriate reassurance if the patient fears cancer or infertility.

 TEACHING TIP: Advise the postoperative patient to increase her activities at home gradually and to abstain from intercourse and from using tampons and douches during this period.

Paget's disease

Paget's disease is a slowly progressive metabolic bone disease marked by an initial phase of excessive bone resorption (osteoclastic phase), followed by a reactive phase of excessive abnormal bone formation (osteoblastic phase). The new bone structure, which is chaotic, fragile, and weak, causes painful deformities of both external contour and internal structure.

Paget's disease usually localizes in one or several areas of the skeleton, but occasionally, skeletal deformity is widely distributed. In about 5% of patients, involved bone undergoes malignant changes. Paget's disease can even be fatal.

CAUSES
Although the cause of Paget's disease is unknown, one theory holds that early viral infection causes a dormant skeletal infection that erupts many years later as Paget's disease.

SIGNS AND SYMPTOMS
Clinical effects of Paget's disease vary.

Pain
Early stages may be asymptomatic, but when pain does develop, it's usually severe and persistent and may coexist with impaired movement caused by impingement of abnormal bone on the spinal cord or sensory nerve root. Weight-bearing intensifies pain.

Other features
The patient with skull involvement shows cranial enlargement over frontal and occipital areas and may complain of headaches. Other deformities include kyphosis (spinal curvature), a barrel-shaped chest, and asymmetric bowing of the tibia and femur. Pagetic sites are warm and tender and susceptible to pathologic fractures after minor trauma. Pagetic fractures heal slowly and many of them incompletely.

DIAGNOSTIC TESTS
X-rays may show increased bone expansion and density. A bone scan clearly shows early so-called pagetic lesions. Bone biopsy reveals a characteristic mosaic pattern. Blood tests and other laboratory tests aid early diagnosis.

TREATMENT
An asymptomatic patient doesn't require treatment. The patient with signs and symptoms requires drug therapy, which may include:
• *calcitonin* (a hormone) and *etidronate* to retard bone resorption and reduce serum alkaline phosphate and urinary hydroxyproline secretion. Calcitonin brings noticeable improvement after the first few weeks; etidronate, after 1 to 3 months.
• *mithramycin,* a cytotoxic antibiotic. This drug produces symptom remission within 2 weeks and biochemical improvement in 1 to 2 months. However, it may destroy platelets or compromise renal function.

Self-administration of calcitonin and etidronate helps patients lead near-normal lives. Nevertheless, they may need surgery to reduce or prevent pathologic fractures, correct secondary deformities, and relieve neurologic impairment. (See *Complications of Paget's disease,* page 230.)

Other treatments depend on the patient's symptoms. Aspirin, indomethacin, or ibuprofen usually controls pain.

SPECIAL CONSIDERATIONS
• Pain levels are assessed daily to evaluate analgesic effectiveness. New areas of pain or restricted move-

Complications of Paget's disease

Complications of Paget's disease may include:
● bony impingement on the cranial nerves, which may cause blindness and hearing loss with tinnitus and vertigo
● hypertension
● renal calculi
● hypercalcemia
● gout
● congestive heart failure
● a waddling gait (from softening of pelvic bones).

ments may indicate new fracture sites.

● The patient may benefit from frequent repositioning, wearing high-topped sneakers to prevent footdrop and, possibly, using a flotation mattress.

● Encourage the patient to maintain adequate fluid intake to minimize kidney stone formation.

● Advise the patient receiving etidronate to take this medication with fruit juice 2 hours before or after meals and to watch for and report stomach cramps, diarrhea, fractures, and increasing or new bone pain.

● To help ensure safety, advise the patient to remove throw rugs and other small obstacles from the home.

 TEACHING TIP: To help the patient adjust to lifestyle changes imposed by this disease, recommend pacing activities, using assistive devices, following a recommended exercise program that avoids immobilization and excessive activity, and using a firm mattress or a bedboard.

Pancreatic cancer

A deadly GI cancer, pancreatic cancer progresses rapidly. Pancreatic tumors are almost always adenocarcinomas and usually arise in the head of the pancreas. Rarer tumors are those of the body and tail of the pancreas and islet cell tumors.

CAUSES
Evidence links pancreatic cancer to inhalation or absorption of the following carcinogens, which are then excreted by the pancreas:
● cigarette smoke
● foods high in fat and protein
● food additives
● industrial chemicals, such as beta-naphthalene, benzidine, and urea.

Possible predisposing factors are chronic pancreatitis, diabetes mellitus, and chronic alcohol abuse.

SIGNS AND SYMPTOMS
The most common features of pancreatic cancer are weight loss, abdominal or low back pain, jaundice, and diarrhea. Other generalized effects include fever, skin lesions, and emotional disturbances, such as depression, anxiety, and premonition of fatal illness.

DIAGNOSTIC TESTS
Confirming the diagnosis involves exploratory surgery and biopsy. Additional laboratory tests of blood, urine, and stools help confirm the diagnosis. Other diagnostic studies may include:
● ultrasonography, to identify an abdominal mass
● computed tomography scan, which shows greater detail than ultrasound
● angiography, to determine the tumor's blood supply
● endoscopic retrograde cholangiopancreatography, which permits visual inspection and specimen biopsy
● magnetic resonance imaging, to help determine tumor size and location.

TREATMENT
Treatment rarely succeeds because the disease has usually metastasized widely by the time of diagnosis. Therapy consists of surgery and, possibly, radiation and chemotherapy. (See *Understanding surgery for pancreatic cancer.*)

Although pancreatic cancer generally responds poorly to chemotherapy, recent studies using combinations of fluorouracil, streptozocin, ifosfamide, and doxorubicin show a trend toward longer survival. Other medications used to relieve disease effects include antibiotics, anticholinergics, antacids, diuretics, insulin (to provide adequate exogenous insulin supply after pancreatic resection), narcotics (but only after analgesics fail to relieve pain because narcotics can lead to biliary tract spasm and increase common bile duct pressure), and pancreatic enzymes.

SPECIAL CONSIDERATIONS

• Explain any ordered dietary restrictions, such as a low-sodium, fluid-retention, or reduced-calorie diet. The doctor may prescribe an oral pancreatic enzyme to be taken at mealtimes and antacids to prevent stress ulcers.
• To ensure adequate nutrition, advise the patient to eat small, frequent, nutritious meals.

 TEACHING TIP: Instruct the patient about measures prescribed to prevent constipation, such as using laxatives, stool softeners, and cathartics, modifying the diet, and increasing fluid intake.
• Advise the patient to balance exercise with rest. Range-of-motion and isometric exercises in particular promote health.
• To prevent excoriation in a pruritic patient, suggest that he clip his nails and wear cotton gloves.

Pancreatitis

Pancreatitis, or inflammation of the pancreas, occurs in acute and chronic forms. It may result from edema, necrosis, or hemorrhage. The prognosis is good when pancreatitis follows biliary tract disease but poor when it follows alcoholism.

CAUSES

The most common causes of pancreatitis are biliary tract disease and alcoholism. Other causes include pancreatic cancer, trauma, and certain drugs (such as glucocorticoids, sul-

---

Understanding surgery for pancreatic cancer

Surgery has brought small advances in the survival rate of patients with pancreatic cancer. Surgical procedures for this disease include:
• total pancreatectomy, which may increase survival time by resecting a localized tumor or by controlling postoperative gastric ulceration
• cholecystojejunostomy, choledochoduodenostomy, and choledochojejunostomy, which have partially replaced radical resection to bypass obstructing common bile duct extensions
• Whipple's operation, which removes the head of the pancreas, the duodenum, and portions of the body and tail of the pancreas, stomach, jejunum, pancreatic duct, and distal portion of the bile duct. This rarely used procedure has a high mortality but can produce wide lymphatic clearance with some pancreatic tumors.
• gastrojejunostomy, performed if radical resection isn't indicated and duodenal obstruction is expected to develop later.

---

fonamides, chlorothiazide, and azathioprine).

The disease may also arise as a complication of peptic ulcer, mumps, or hypothermia. Rarer causes are stenosis or obstruction of Oddi's sphincter, hyperlipemia, metabolic endocrine disorders, vasculitis or vascular disease, viral infections, mycoplasmal pneumonia, and pregnancy.

Afro-Asian syndrome (diabetes, pancreatic insufficiency, and calcification) occurs in young people, probably from malnutrition and alcoholism, and leads to pancreatic atrophy. Regardless of the cause, pancreatitis involves autodigestion: Enzymes normally excreted by the pancreas digest pancreatic tissue.

SIGNS AND SYMPTOMS
In many patients, the first and only symptom of mild pancreatitis is steady epigastric pain near the umbilicus, unrelieved by vomiting. However, a severe attack causes extreme pain, persistent vomiting, abdominal rigidity, diminished bowel activity, crackles at lung bases, and left pleural effusion.

Severe pancreatitis may produce extreme malaise and restlessness, with mottled skin, tachycardia, low-grade fever (100° to 102° F [37.8° to 38.9° C]), and cold, sweaty extremities. Proximity of the inflamed pancreas to the bowel may cause ileus.

If pancreatitis damages the islets of Langerhans, complications may include diabetes mellitus. Fulminant pancreatitis causes massive hemorrhage and total destruction of the pancreas, resulting in diabetic acidosis, shock, or coma.

DIAGNOSTIC TESTS
Diagnosis depends on patient history, especially diet and alcohol consumption, along with physical examination. Blood tests and analysis of urine and other fluids help distinguish pancreatitis from other disorders. Electrocardiograms can identify chemical imbalances caused by pancreatitis. X-rays reveal calcification of the pancreas or lung changes. A GI series measures gastric pressure. Ultrasonography determines the extent of damage to the pancreas.

TREATMENT
The goal of therapy is to maintain circulation and fluid volume. Treatment measures must also relieve pain and decrease pancreatic secretions.

Emergency measures
Emergency treatment for shock (the most common cause of death in early-stage pancreatitis) consists of vigorous I.V. replacement of electrolytes and proteins.

Metabolic acidosis (secondary to hypovolemia and impaired cellular perfusion) requires vigorous fluid volume replacement. Drug therapy may include morphine sulfate for pain; diazepam for restlessness and agitation; and antibiotics, such as gentamicin, clindamycin, or chloramphenicol, for bacterial infection.

After the emergency
After the emergency phase, continuing I.V. therapy should provide adequate electrolytes and protein solutions that don't stimulate the pancreas for 5 to 7 days.

If the patient isn't ready to resume oral feedings by then, hyperalimentation may be necessary. In extreme cases, laparotomy to drain the pancreatic bed, 95% pancreatectomy, or a combination of cholecystostomy-gastrostomy, feeding jejunostomy, and drainage may be necessary.

SPECIAL CONSIDERATIONS
 ACTION STAT: Get medical help right away if the patient suddenly has muscle twitching, sharp wrist and ankle flexion, cramps, or seizures. These are signs and symptoms of calcium deficiency.

Parkinson's disease
Parkinson's disease (also known as parkinsonism) produces progressive muscle rigidity, akinesia (slow movement), and involuntary tremor. Deterioration progresses for an average of 10 years, at which time death usually results from aspiration pneumonia or some other infection.

CAUSES
Although the cause of Parkinson's disease is unknown, researchers have established that a dopamine deficiency prevents affected brain cells from performing their normal inhibitory function.

SIGNS AND SYMPTOMS
The hallmarks of Parkinson's disease are muscle rigidity and akinesia, along with an insidious tremor that

begins in the fingers (unilateral pill-rolling tremor), worsens with stress or anxiety, and decreases with purposeful movement and sleep.

Muscle rigidity leads to resistance to passive muscle stretching, which may be uniform or jerky. Akinesia causes the patient to walk with difficulty.

Parkinson's disease also produces a high-pitched, monotone voice; drooling; a masklike facial expression; loss of posture control (the patient walks with body bent forward); and difficulty speaking or swallowing, or both. Occasionally, akinesia may cause oculogyric crises (eyes that are fixed upward, with involuntary tonic movements) or blepharospasm (eyelids that are completely closed).

DIAGNOSTIC TESTS
Laboratory tests rarely help identify Parkinson's disease, so diagnosis hinges on the patient's age, history, and clinical features. However, urinalysis may support the diagnosis by revealing decreased dopamine levels. Diagnosis is confirmed only after other disorders with similar clinical features are ruled out.

TREATMENT
Because there's no cure, treatment for Parkinson's disease aims to relieve symptoms and keep the patient functional as long as possible. Therapeutic measures include drug therapy, physical therapy, and surgery. (See *Drug therapy for Parkinson's disease.*)

Physical therapy
Individually planned physical therapy complements drug treatment and neurosurgery to maintain normal muscle tone and function. Physical therapy includes both active and passive range-of-motion exercises along with activities of daily living, walking, and baths and massage to help relax muscles.

Surgery
In severe disease unresponsive to drugs, stereotactic neurosurgery may be an alternative. In this procedure, electrical coagulation, freezing, ra-

---

Drug therapy for Parkinson's disease

Typically, drug therapy for patients with Parkinson's disease includes levodopa, a dopamine replacement. Most effective during early disease stages, levodopa is given in increasing doses until symptoms are relieved or adverse effects appear. Because adverse effects can be serious, levodopa is commonly given in combination with carbidopa.

When levodopa proves ineffective or too toxic, alternative drug therapy includes anticholinergics such as trihexyphenidyl, antihistamines such as diphenhydramine, and amantadine, an antiviral agent. Selegiline, an enzyme-inhibiting agent, enhances the therapeutic effect of levodopa.

---

dioactivity, or ultrasound destroys part of the thalamus to prevent involuntary movement. This is most effective in young, otherwise healthy patients with unilateral tremor or muscle rigidity.

SPECIAL CONSIDERATIONS
● To minimize fatigue and ensure adequate rest, thereby reducing feelings of helplessness, help the patient manage his activities.

 TEACHING TIP: Teach the patient about techniques to help overcome limitations and promote overall health. Such methods include using the arms of a chair to steady the body; eating small, frequent meals to ensure adequate caloric intake while reducing fatigue and frustration; establishing a regular bowel routine; drinking at least 2 qt (2 L) of liquids every day; consuming plenty of high-bulk foods; and using an elevated toilet seat to make returning to a standing position easier.

• Inform the patient and his family of the dietary restrictions levodopa imposes, and explain household safety measures to prevent accidents.

Pelvic inflammatory disease

Pelvic inflammatory disease (PID) is any acute, subacute, recurrent, or chronic infection of the oviducts and ovaries, with adjacent tissue involvement. It includes inflammation of the cervix (cervicitis), uterus (endometritis), fallopian tubes (salpingitis), and ovaries (oophoritis), which can extend to the connective tissue lying between the broad ligaments (parametritis). (See *Forms of pelvic inflammatory disease.*)

Early diagnosis and treatment prevents damage to the reproductive system. Untreated PID may cause infertility and lead to potentially fatal septicemia, pulmonary emboli, and shock.

CAUSES

PID may result from infection with aerobic or anaerobic organisms. Conditions or procedures that alter or destroy cervical mucus impair the protective mechanism of cervical secretions, allowing bacteria in the cervix or vagina to ascend into the uterine cavity.

Uterine infection can also follow transfer of contaminated cervical mucus into the endometrial cavity by instrumentation. Consequently, PID can follow insertion of an intrauterine device, use of a biopsy curet or an irrigation catheter, or tubal insufflation. Other predisposing factors include abortion, pelvic surgery, and infection during or after pregnancy.

Bacteria may also enter the uterine cavity through the bloodstream or from drainage from a chronically infected fallopian tube, pelvic abscess, ruptured appendix, diverticulitis of the sigmoid colon, or other infectious foci.

SIGNS AND SYMPTOMS

Clinical features vary with the affected area but generally include a profuse, purulent vaginal discharge, sometimes accompanied by low-grade fever and malaise. The patient experiences lower abdomen pain; movement of the cervix or palpation of the adnexa may be extremely painful.

DIAGNOSTIC TESTS

Diagnosis comes from patient history and results of the following diagnostic tests:

• Gram stain of secretions from the endocervix or cul-de-sac (Culture and sensitivity testing aids selection of the appropriate antibiotic. Urethral and rectal secretions may also be cultured.)
• ultrasonography to identify an adnexal or uterine mass (X-rays seldom identify pelvic masses.)
• culdocentesis to obtain peritoneal fluid or pus for culture and sensitivity testing.

TREATMENT

To prevent progression of PID, antibiotic therapy begins immediately after culture specimens are obtained. Such therapy may be reevaluated as soon as laboratory results are available. Infection may become chronic if treated inadequately.

Guidelines of the Centers for Disease Control and Prevention (CDC) for outpatient treatment include a single dose of cefoxitin plus probenecid given concurrently or a single dose of ceftriaxone. Each regimen is given with doxycycline for 14 days. CDC guidelines for inpatient treatment include doxycycline alone or a combination of clindamycin and gentamicin.

Development of a pelvic abscess necessitates drainage. A ruptured abscess is life-threatening and may warrant a total abdominal hysterectomy with bilateral salpingo-oophorectomy.

SPECIAL CONSIDERATIONS

 PREVENTION: To help prevent recurrence, emphasize the seriousness of PID, compliance with treatment, and the need for sex-

PATHOPHYSIOLOGY

Forms of pelvic inflammatory disease

Pelvic inflammatory disease may affect the cervix, uterus, fallopian tubes, or ovaries, causing inflammation at the sites shown here.

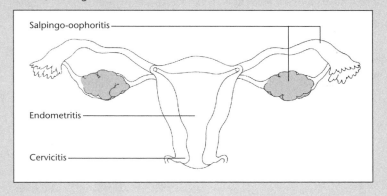

ual partners to be examined and, if necessary, treated for infection.

Peptic ulcers

Peptic ulcers are circumscribed lesions in the mucosal membrane of the lower esophagus, stomach, pylorus, duodenum, or jejunum. About 80% of peptic ulcers are duodenal ulcers, which affect the proximal part of the small intestine. Gastric ulcers, in contrast, affect the stomach mucosa.

Duodenal ulcers usually follow a chronic course, with remissions and exacerbations. Roughly 5% to 10% of patients develop complications that necessitate surgery.

CAUSES

Researchers recognize three major causes of peptic ulcer disease: infection with *Helicobacter pylori*, use of nonsteroidal anti-inflammatory drugs (NSAIDs), and pathologic hypersecretory states such as Zollinger-Ellison syndrome.

How *H. pylori* produces an ulcer isn't clear, but the disorder can be cured. Gastric acid, once considered a primary cause, now appears mainly to contribute to the consequences of infection. Ongoing studies should soon unveil the full mechanism of ulcer formation.

Also, certain conditions can predispose a person to peptic ulcers. (See *Who's at risk for peptic ulcers?* page 236.)

SIGNS AND SYMPTOMS

Clinical features vary with the area affected. With gastric ulcers, heartburn and indigestion usually signal onset of a gastric ulcer attack. Eating food stretches the gastric wall and may cause or, in some cases, relieve pain and a feeling of fullness and distention. Other typical effects include weight loss and repeated episodes of massive GI bleeding.

Duodenal ulcers produce heartburn, well-localized midepigastric pain (relieved by food), weight gain (because the patient eats to relieve discomfort), and a sensation of hot water bubbling in the back of the throat. Attacks usually occur about 2

Who's at risk for peptic ulcers?

Besides peptic ulcers' main causes (infection with *Helicobacter pylori*, use of nonsteroidal anti-inflammatory drugs, and pathologic hypersecretory states), several predisposing factors are acknowledged. They include:
• blood type — gastric ulcers tend to strike people with type A blood; duodenal ulcers tend to afflict people with type O blood — and other genetic factors
• exposure to irritants, such as alcohol and tobacco, which may accelerate gastric acid emptying and promote mucosal breakdown
• physical trauma
• emotional stress
• normal aging.

hours after meals, whenever the stomach is empty, or after consumption of orange juice, caffeine, aspirin, or alcohol.

Complications

Both types of ulcers may be asymptomatic or may penetrate the pancreas and cause severe back pain. Other complications of peptic ulcers include perforation, hemorrhage, and pyloric obstruction.

DIAGNOSTIC TESTS

Upper GI tract X-rays show abnormalities in the mucus lining. Analysis of stomach secretions or visualization of the GI tract confirms diagnosis. Stools may test positive for traces of blood.

TREATMENT

Current recommendations include treating every patient at least once to eradicate *H. pylori*. Initial treatment includes tetracycline, bismuth subsalicylate, and metronidazole. Amoxicillin may be used as an alternative.

Patients taking NSAIDs may receive a prostaglandin analogue (misoprostol) to suppress ulceration. Histamine$_2$-receptor antagonists (cimetidine or nizatidine) or omeprazole may reduce acid secretion. A coating agent may be administered to patients with duodenal ulcers.

GI bleeding necessitates emergency treatment: insertion of a nasogastric tube to allow for iced saline lavage and gastroscopy to visualize the bleeding site and allow coagulation by laser or cautery to control bleeding. Such therapy allows postponement of surgery until the patient's condition stabilizes.

Surgery is indicated for perforation, unresponsiveness to conservative treatment and for suspected cancer. Surgical procedures include vagotomy with pyloroplasty and distal subtotal gastrectomy.

SPECIAL CONSIDERATIONS

• If the doctor prescribes antacids, advise patients with a history of heart disease and those on a sodium-restricted diet to take only those antacids with a low sodium content.

 TEACHING TIP: Inform the patient that steroids, NSAIDs, coffee, alcoholic beverages, and smoking all irritate the gastric mucosa. Stress also worsens peptic ulcer disease.

Pericarditis

Pericarditis is an inflammation of the pericardium — the fibroserous sac that envelops, supports, and protects the heart. The condition can be acute or chronic. Acute pericarditis can be fibrinous or effusive, with purulent, serous, or hemorrhagic exudate; chronic constrictive pericarditis is marked by dense fibrous pericardial thickening.

The prognosis depends on the underlying cause but is generally good in acute pericarditis, unless constriction occurs.

CAUSES

Common causes of pericarditis include:

- bacterial, fungal, or viral infection (infectious pericarditis)
- neoplasms (primary or metastases from the lungs, breasts, or other organs)
- high-dose radiation to the chest
- uremia
- hypersensitivity or autoimmune disease, such as acute rheumatic fever, systemic lupus erythematosus, or rheumatoid arthritis
- postcardiac injury, such as myocardial infarction (MI), which later causes an autoimmune reaction (Dressler's syndrome) in the pericardium; trauma; or surgery that causes blood to leak into the pericardial cavity
- drugs such as hydralazine or procainamide
- idiopathic factors.

SIGNS AND SYMPTOMS

Clinical features of the acute and chronic forms vary. (See *Comparing acute and chronic pericarditis.*)

DIAGNOSTIC TESTS

Diagnosis depends on typical signs and symptoms and elimination of other possible causes. Auscultation may reveal a pericardial friction rub. If acute inflammation has caused fluid to build up in the pericardial sac, the patient may have increased cardiac dullness, diminished or absent apical impulse, and distant heart sounds.

Laboratory tests, such as white blood cell count and measurement of cardiac enzymes, may help confirm inflammation and identify its cause. Open surgical drainage or cardiocentesis may be done to obtain a culture of pericardial fluid. Culturing may help identify a causative organism in bacterial or fungal inflammation. An electrocardiogram may show changes in heart rate and rhythm brought on by acute inflammation.

TREATMENT

The goal of treatment is to relieve symptoms and manage underlying systemic disease.

Comparing acute and chronic pericarditis

Signs and symptoms depend on which type of pericarditis the patient has.

Acute pericarditis

Typically, the patient experiences:

- a sharp and commonly sudden pain, which usually starts over the sternum and radiates to the neck, shoulders, back, and arms
- pericardial pain, which worsens with deep inspiration and eases when the patient sits up and leans forward
- pericardial effusion, the major complication of acute pericarditis, which may produce signs and symptoms of heart failure as well as ill-defined substernal chest pain and a feeling of fullness in the chest.

Chronic pericarditis

Chronic constrictive pericarditis causes a gradual increase in systemic venous pressure and produces signs similar to those of chronic right-sided heart failure — fluid retention, ascites, and an enlarged liver.

Bed rest and drug therapy

In acute idiopathic pericarditis, post-MI pericarditis, and postthoracotomy pericarditis, treatment consists of bed rest as long as fever and pain persist, along with nonsteroidal anti-inflammatory drugs, such as aspirin and indomethacin, to relieve pain and inflammation. If these drugs are ineffective, corticosteroids may be used.

Infectious pericarditis that results from disease of the left pleural space, mediastinal abscesses, or septicemia requires antibiotics, surgical drainage,

Pathophysiology

How abscesses form in peritonitis

In both chemical and bacterial inflammation, accumulated fluids containing protein and electrolytes make the transparent peritoneum opaque, red, inflamed, and edematous. Because the peritoneal cavity is so resistant to contamination, such infection is commonly localized as an abscess instead of disseminated as a generalized infection.

or both. Cardiac tamponade may warrant pericardiocentesis.

Pericardiectomy

Recurrent pericarditis may necessitate partial pericardiectomy, which creates a "window" that allows fluid to drain into the pleural space. In constrictive pericarditis, total pericardiectomy may be necessary. Treatment must also include management of any underlying disorder.

SPECIAL CONSIDERATIONS

• The patient requires complete bed rest.

• Reassure the patient with acute pericarditis that the condition is temporary and treatable.

Peritonitis

Peritonitis is an acute or chronic inflammation of the peritoneum — the membrane that lines the abdominal cavity and covers the visceral organs. Inflammation may extend throughout the peritoneum or may be localized as an abscess.

Peritonitis commonly decreases intestinal motility and causes intestinal distention with gas. Mortality is 10%, with death usually resulting from bowel obstruction.

CAUSES

In peritonitis, bacteria invade the normally sterile peritoneum. Generally, such infection results from inflammation and perforation of the GI tract. Common causes include appendicitis, diverticulitis, peptic ulcer, ulcerative colitis, volvulus, strangulated obstruction, abdominal neoplasms, and stab wounds.

Peritonitis may also result from chemical inflammation, as in bladder or fallopian tube rupture, gastric ulcer perforation, or released pancreatic enzymes. Such inflammation may lead to abscesses. (See *How abscesses form in peritonitis*.)

SIGNS AND SYMPTOMS

The key symptom of peritonitis is sudden, severe, diffuse abdominal pain. Many patients display weakness, pallor, excessive sweating, and cold skin from excessive loss of fluid, electrolytes, and protein into the abdominal cavity.

The effect of bacterial toxins on the intestinal muscles may lead to decreased intestinal motility and paralytic ileus. Intestinal obstruction causes nausea, vomiting, and abdominal rigidity.

Other clinical features

Typical features include hypotension, tachycardia, signs and symptoms of dehydration (oliguria, thirst, dry swollen tongue, pinched skin), acutely tender abdomen associated with rebound tenderness, temperature of 103° F (39.4° C) or higher, and hypokalemia.

Abdominal distention and upward displacement of the diaphragm may decrease respiratory capacity. To minimize pain, the patient tends to breathe shallowly and move as little as possible.

DIAGNOSTIC TESTS

Severe abdominal pain in a patient with tenderness suggests peritonitis. Abdominal X-rays confirm distention of the small and large intestines. With perforation of a visceral organ, X-rays show air in the abdominal cavity. Other helpful tests may include chest X-ray, blood studies, paracentesis, and laparotomy.

TREATMENT
Early treatment for GI inflammatory conditions and preoperative and postoperative antibiotic therapy helps prevent peritonitis. Once peritonitis develops, emergency treatment must combat infection, restore intestinal motility, and replace fluids and electrolytes.

Antibiotics and supplementary treatment
Massive antibiotic therapy is given, with antibiotic selection based on the infecting organism. The patient receives nothing by mouth; supportive fluids and electrolytes are given parenterally.

Other supplementary measures include preoperative and postoperative analgesics, nasogastric intubation to decompress the bowel and, possibly, use of a rectal tube to ease passage of flatus.

Surgery
When peritonitis results from perforation, surgery is done as soon as the patient can tolerate it. Surgery eliminates the source of infection by evacuating the spilled contents and inserting drains. Occasionally, abdominocentesis may be done to remove accumulated fluid.

SPECIAL CONSIDERATIONS
• Placing the patient in semi-Fowler's position helps him to breathe deeply with less pain and may prevent pulmonary complications.

Pernicious anemia
A megaloblastic anemia, pernicious anemia is marked by decreased gastric production of hydrochloric acid and deficiency of intrinsic factor (IF) — a substance normally secreted by the parietal cells of the gastric mucosa that is crucial for vitamin B_{12} absorption. The resulting vitamin B_{12} deficiency causes serious neurologic and

GI abnormalities. Untreated pernicious anemia may lead to permanent neurologic disability and death.

CAUSES
Familial incidence of pernicious anemia suggests a genetic predisposition. Significantly higher incidence in patients with immunologically related diseases, such as thyroiditis, myxedema, and Graves' disease, seems to support a widely held theory that an inherited autoimmune response causes gastric mucosal atrophy and, therefore, deficiency of hydrochloric acid and IF.

SIGNS AND SYMPTOMS
Typically, pernicious anemia has a gradual onset, but eventually it causes an unmistakable triad of symptoms: weakness, sore tongue, and numbness and tingling in the extremities. The lips, gums, and tongue appear markedly bloodless. The patient may also have faintly jaundiced sclera and pale to bright yellow skin, and may become highly susceptible to infection, especially of the genitourinary tract.

Pernicious anemia also has characteristic effects on the GI, central nervous, and cardiovascular systems. (See *Widespread effects of pernicious anemia*, page 240.)

DIAGNOSTIC TESTS
A positive family history and results of blood studies, bone marrow aspiration, gastric analysis, and the Schilling test establish the diagnosis. The doctor must rule out other anemias with similar symptoms, such as folic acid deficiency anemia, as well as vitamin B_{12} deficiency resulting from malabsorption caused by stomach disorders, gastric surgery, radiation, or drug therapy.

TREATMENT
Early parenteral vitamin B_{12} replacement can reverse pernicious anemia, minimize complications and, possibly, prevent permanent neurologic damage.

Widespread effects of pernicious anemia

Besides its hallmark symptoms (weakness, sore tongue, and numbness and tingling in the extremities), pernicious anemia can lead to GI, neurologic, and cardiovascular changes.

GI effects

Gastric mucosal atrophy and decreased hydrochloric acid production disturb digestion and lead to nausea, vomiting, anorexia, weight loss, flatulence, diarrhea, and constipation. Gingival bleeding and tongue inflammation may hinder eating and intensify anorexia.

Neurologic effects

Demyelination caused by vitamin B_{12} deficiency initially affects the peripheral nerves but gradually extends to the spinal cord. Consequently, neurologic effects of pernicious anemia may include neuritis, weakness in extremities, peripheral numbness and paresthesias, disturbed position sense, poor coordi-

nation, ataxia, impaired fine finger movements, positive Babinski's and Romberg's signs, light-headedness, optic muscle atrophy, loss of bowel and bladder control, impotence (in males), and altered vision (double or blurred vision), taste, and hearing (tinnitus).

The effects of pernicious anemia on the nervous system may also produce irritability, poor memory, headache, depression, and delirium.

Cardiovascular effects

Increasingly fragile cell membranes induce widespread destruction of red blood cells, resulting in low hemoglobin levels. The blood's impaired oxygen-carrying capacity leads to weakness, fatigue, and light-headedness. A compensatory increase in cardiac output cause palpitations, wide pulse pressure, dyspnea, orthopnea, tachycardia, premature beats and, eventually, heart failure.

An initial high dose of parenteral vitamin B_{12} causes rapid red blood cell regeneration. Concomitant iron and folic acid replacement is necessary to prevent iron deficiency anemia. Once the patient's condition improves, vitamin B_{12} dosage can be lowered to maintenance levels and given monthly.

Other measures

If anemia causes extreme fatigue, the patient may require bed rest until his hemoglobin level rises. A patient with dangerously low hemoglobin may need blood transfusions, digoxin, a diuretic, and a low-sodium diet for heart failure. Most important is vitamin B_{12} replacement to control the condition that led to this failure. Antibiotics help combat accompanying infections.

SPECIAL CONSIDERATIONS

• Because vitamin B_{12} injections must continue for life, the patient must learn self-administration.

• If the patient's sore mouth and tongue impair communication, he may need to use alternative methods such as writing.

• Diluted mouthwash or, with severe conditions, tap water or warm saline solution may ease mouth pain.

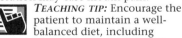 *TEACHING TIP:* Encourage the patient to maintain a well-balanced diet, including foods high in vitamin B_{12} (meat, liver, fish, eggs, and milk). Recommend eating between-meal snacks and favorite foods to help ensure adequate nutrition. Instruct him to avoid foods that worsen mouth and tongue soreness. Advise the patient to guard

against infection, and tell him to report signs of infection promptly.

Pertussis

Also called whooping cough, pertussis is a highly contagious infection. Typically, it causes an irritating cough that commonly ends in a high-pitched, inspiratory whoop.

Endemic throughout the world, pertussis usually occurs in early spring and late winter. About half the time, it strikes nonimmunized children under age 2.

Since the 1940s, immunization and aggressive diagnosis and treatment have significantly reduced mortality from pertussis in the United States. In children under age 1, death usually results from complications. (See *Complications of pertussis*.)

CAUSES
Pertussis usually results from the nonmotile, gram-negative coccobacillus *Bordetella pertussis*. It's usually transmitted by direct inhalation of contaminated droplets from a patient in the acute stage. It also may spread indirectly through soiled linen and other articles contaminated by respiratory secretions.

SIGNS AND SYMPTOMS
The patient's history may reveal lack of immunization coupled with exposure to pertussis during the previous 3 weeks. Pertussis follows a classic 6-week course that includes three 2-week stages with varying symptoms.
• During the first (catarrhal) stage, the patient experiences anorexia, sneezing, lacrimation, rhinorrhea, and a hacking, nocturnal cough.
• The second (paroxysmal) stage brings spasmodic, recurrent coughing that may expel tenacious mucus. Each cough typically ends in a loud, crowing, inspiratory whoop. Choking on mucus may cause vomiting.
• In the third (convalescent) stage, paroxysmal coughing and vomiting gradually subside. However, for

---

Complications of pertussis

The coughing spells that pertussis causes may lead to the following complications:
• increased venous pressure
• nosebleed
• periorbital edema
• conjunctival hemorrhage
• hemorrhage of the eye's anterior chamber
• detached retina and blindness
• rectal prolapse
• inguinal or umbilical hernia
• seizures
• atelectasis
• pneumonitis.

In infants, choking spells may cause apnea, anoxia, and disturbed acid-base balance. Residual mental retardation or learning disabilities may result. During the paroxysmal stage of pertussis, patients also are highly vulnerable to fatal secondary bacterial or viral infections.

---

months afterward, even a mild upper respiratory tract infection may trigger paroxysmal coughing.

DIAGNOSTIC TESTS
Pertussis is suspected in anyone with classic symptoms — especially during the paroxysmal stage — and confirmed by laboratory tests. Nose and throat swabs and sputum cultures show *B. pertussis* only in early disease stages. The white blood cell count is usually increased.

TREATMENT
Infants usually require hospitalization and vigorous supportive therapy with fluid and electrolyte replacement. Other measures include adequate nutrition, oxygen therapy as needed, antitussives, and antibiotics, as ordered.

SPECIAL CONSIDERATIONS
• Pertussis calls for respiratory isolation (masks only) for 5 to 7 days after antibiotic therapy begins.
• A quiet environment decreases coughing stimulation.
• Small, frequent meals are easier for the patient to manage.
• Encourage the patient (or parents) to urge close contacts to see a doctor promptly.

 PREVENTION: Infant immunization — usually with the diphtheria, tetanus toxoids, and pertussis vaccines — should take place at age 6 months and ages 2 and 4. Boosters follow at 18 months and at 4 to 6 years. Although the vaccine can cause nervous system damage and other complications, the risk of whooping cough is greater than the risk of these complications. The vaccine shouldn't be given to children over age 6 because it can cause a severe fever.

Pharyngitis
The most common throat disorder, pharyngitis is an acute or chronic inflammation of the pharynx. The condition is widespread among adults who live or work in dusty or dry environments, use their voices excessively, habitually use tobacco or alcohol, or suffer from chronic sinusitis, persistent coughs, or allergies. Uncomplicated pharyngitis usually subsides in 3 to 10 days.

CAUSES
Pharyngitis usually results from a virus. The most common bacterial cause is group A beta-hemolytic streptococci. Other causative organisms include *Mycoplasma* and *Chlamydia.*

SIGNS AND SYMPTOMS
Pharyngitis produces a sore throat and slight difficulty in swallowing. The patient may also report a sensation of a lump in the throat as well as a constant, aggravating urge to swallow. Associated features may include mild fever, headache, muscle and joint pain, inflammation of the nasal mucous membranes, and runny nose.

DIAGNOSTIC TESTS
Physical examination of the pharynx reveals generalized redness and inflammation. Bacterial sore throat usually produces a large amount of drainage. A throat culture may identify the causative bacterial organism.

TREATMENT
Treatment for acute and chronic pharyngitis differs.

Acute pharyngitis
Treatment is usually symptomatic, consisting mainly of rest, warm saline gargles, throat lozenges containing a mild anesthetic, plenty of fluids, and analgesics as needed. A patient who can't swallow fluids may need to be hospitalized for I.V. hydration.

Suspected bacterial pharyngitis requires rigorous treatment with penicillin or another broad-spectrum antibiotic. Antibiotic therapy should continue for 48 hours until culture results return.

If the culture (or a rapid strep test) is positive for group A beta-hemolytic streptococci or bacterial infection is suspected despite negative culture results, penicillin therapy continues for 10 days to prevent acute rheumatic fever.

Chronic pharyngitis
Treatment requires the same supportive measures used for acute pharyngitis, but with greater emphasis on eliminating the underlying cause such as an allergen. Preventive measures include adequate humidification and avoiding excessive exposure to air conditioning. Also, the patient who smokes should be urged to stop.

SPECIAL CONSIDERATIONS
• Comfort measures include administering analgesics and warm saline gargles, encouraging high fluid intake, providing meticulous mouth care, and maintaining a restful environment.

TEACHING TIP: Emphasize the importance of completing the full course of antibiotic therapy.

Pheochromocytoma

A pheochromocytoma is a chromaffin-cell tumor of the adrenal medulla that secretes an excessive amount of epinephrine and norepinephrine. Oversecretion of these catecholamines leads to severe hypertension, increased metabolism, and hyperglycemia.

The disorder is potentially fatal, but the prognosis is generally good with treatment. Pheochromocytoma-induced kidney damage, however, is irreversible.

CAUSES
A pheochromocytoma may result from an inherited autosomal dominant trait.

SIGNS AND SYMPTOMS
The cardinal sign of pheochromocytoma is persistent or episodic hypertension. Common clinical effects include palpitations, tachycardia, headache, diaphoresis, pallor, warmth or flushing, paresthesia, tremor, excitation, fright, nervousness, feelings of impending doom, abdominal pain, tachypnea, nausea, and vomiting.

Symptomatic episodes may recur as seldom as once every 2 months or as often as 25 times a day. They may occur spontaneously or follow triggering events, such as postural change, exercise, laughing, smoking, anesthesia induction, urination, a change in environmental or body temperature, or pregnancy. (See *Pheochromocytoma in pregnancy.*)

DIAGNOSTIC TESTS
Diagnosis rests on patient history, physical examination, and laboratory test results. Pheochromocytoma is suspected in a patient with a history of acute episodes of high blood pressure, headache, sweating, and palpitations, especially if the patient also

Pheochromocytoma in pregnancy

Pheochromocytoma sometimes is diagnosed during pregnancy, when uterine pressure on the tumor induces more frequent attacks. Such attacks can prove fatal to both the mother and fetus as a result of cerebrovascular accident, acute pulmonary edema, cardiac arrhythmias, or hypoxia.

In such women, the risk of spontaneous abortion is high, but most fetal deaths occur during labor or immediately after birth.

has high blood or urine glucose or hypermetabolism. In rare cases, the tumor is palpable.

Diagnosis is confirmed by a test of urine collected over a 24-hour period showing elevated catecholamine levels. Angiography reveals an adrenal medullary tumor. Various kidney function studies, adrenal venography, or computed tomography scan helps localize the tumor.

TREATMENT
Surgical tumor removal is the treatment of choice. To decrease blood pressure, metyrosine or alpha-adrenergic blockers are given 1 to 2 weeks before surgery. A beta-adrenergic blocker (propranolol) may be used after achieving alpha blockade.

Postoperatively, I.V. fluids, plasma volume expanders, vasopressors and, possibly, transfusions may be required to treat hypotension. Persistent hypertension may immediately follow surgery.

If surgery isn't feasible, alpha- and beta-adrenergic blockers (such as phenoxybenzamine and propranolol, respectively) may help control catecholamine effects and prevent attacks.

An acute attack or hypertensive crisis calls for I.V. phentolamine or nitroprusside to normalize blood pressure.

SPECIAL CONSIDERATIONS

• Instruct the patient to report headaches, palpitations, nervousness, and other symptoms of an acute hypertensive attack.

• If autosomal dominant transmission of pheochromocytoma is suspected, the patient's family should be evaluated for this condition.

Pituitary tumors

Constituting 10% of intracranial neoplasms, pituitary tumors most commonly arise in the anterior pituitary. The three tissue types of pituitary tumors are chromophobe adenoma (90%), basophil adenoma, and eosinophil adenoma.

Pituitary tumors aren't malignant, but because their growth is invasive, they're considered neoplastic. The prognosis is fair to good, depending on the extent of tumor spread.

CAUSES

Although the cause is unknown, a predisposition to pituitary tumors may be inherited.

Chromophobe adenoma may be associated with production of corticotropin, melanocyte-stimulating hormone, growth hormone, and prolactin; basophil adenoma, with evidence of excess corticotropin production and, consequently, with signs of Cushing's syndrome; eosinophil adenoma, with excessive growth hormone.

SIGNS AND SYMPTOMS

As pituitary adenomas grow, pressure on adjacent intracranial structures produces typical clinical manifestations.

Neurologic features

Typically, the patient has a frontal headache and visual symptoms. Cranial nerve involvement results in strabismus, double vision, conjugate deviation of gaze, nystagmus, lid ptosis, and limited eye movements.

Personality changes or dementia may occur if the tumor breaks through to the frontal lobes. Other features may include seizures and runny nose.

Endocrine features

Adenoma typically causes hypopituitarism, with such signs and symptoms as amenorrhea, decreased libido and impotence in men, skin changes (waxy appearance, decreased wrinkles, and pigmentation), loss of axillary and pubic hair, lethargy, weakness, increased fatigability, cold intolerance, and constipation.

Addisonian crisis may be triggered by stress and may lead to nausea, vomiting, hypoglycemia, hypotension, and circulatory collapse.

DIAGNOSTIC TESTS

Skull X-rays with tomography reveal enlargement of the sella turcica or erosion of its floor. If growth hormone secretion predominates, X-rays show enlarged paranasal sinuses and mandible, thickened cranial bones, and separated teeth.

Carotid angiography shows displacement of the anterior cerebral and internal carotid arteries if the tumor mass is enlarging; it also rules out intracerebral aneurysm. Computed tomography scan may confirm an adenoma and depict its size. Cerebrospinal fluid analysis may reveal increased protein levels. Endocrine function tests sometimes yield helpful information.

TREATMENT

Surgical options include transfrontal removal of a large tumor impinging on the optic apparatus and transsphenoidal resection for a smaller tumor confined to the pituitary fossa. (See *Transsphenoidal pituitary surgery*.)

Radiation is the primary treatment for small, nonsecretory tumors that don't extend beyond the sella turcica and for patients who may be poor postoperative risks; otherwise, it's an adjunct to surgery.

Postoperative treatment includes cortisone, thyroid, and sex hormone replacement; correction of electrolyte imbalance; and, as necessary, insulin therapy.

Drug therapy may include bromocriptine and cyproheptadine. Adjuvant radiotherapy is used when only partial removal of the tumor is possible. Cryohypophysectomy (freezing the area with a probe inserted by the transsphenoidal route) is a promising alternative to surgical tumor dissection.

SPECIAL CONSIDERATIONS
• Help the patient understand that he needs lifelong evaluations and, possibly, lifelong hormone replacement.
• Inform the patient that he will lose the sense of smell, but reassure him that he will probably recover his sight.
• Advise him to wear a medical identification bracelet or necklace that identifies his hormone deficiencies and their proper treatment.

Pleural effusion and empyema

Pleural effusion is an excess of fluid in the pleural space. Normally, this space contains a small amount of extracellular fluid that lubricates the pleural surfaces. Increased production or inadequate removal of the fluid results in pleural effusion.

Empyema is the accumulation of pus and necrotic tissue in the pleural space. Blood (hemothorax) and chyle (chylothorax) may also collect in this space.

CAUSES
Various conditions lead to pleural effusion and empyema. (See *Understanding the causes of pleural effusion and empyema*, page 246.)

SIGNS AND SYMPTOMS
Patients with pleural effusion typically have signs and symptoms relating to the underlying condition. Most patients with large effusions complain of dyspnea. Pleuritic chest pain accompanies effusions associated with pleurisy. Other clinical features depend on the cause of the effusion. Patients with empyema also develop fever and malaise.

Transsphenoidal pituitary surgery

In pituitary gland removal, a bivalve speculum and rongeur are placed as depicted here.

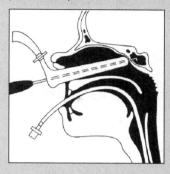

DIAGNOSTIC TESTS
Diagnosis rests on physical examination and chest X-ray. However, diagnosis also requires other tests to distinguish transudative from exudative effusions and to help pinpoint the underlying disorder. The most useful test is thoracentesis — removal and analysis of a sample of pleural fluid.

TREATMENT
Depending on the amount of fluid present, symptomatic effusion may call for thoracentesis to remove fluid or careful monitoring of the patient's own fluid reabsorption. Hemothorax warrants drainage to prevent fibrothorax formation.

Treatment for empyema requires insertion of one or more chest tubes after thoracentesis to allow drainage of purulent material and possibly decortication (surgical removal of the thick coating over the lung) or rib resection to allow open drainage and lung expansion. Empyema also requires parenteral antibiotics. Associated hypoxia necessitates oxygen administration.

PATHOPHYSIOLOGY

Understanding the causes of pleural effusion and empyema

Transudative pleural effusions commonly result from conditions in which excessive hydrostatic pressure or decreased osmotic pressure in parietal pleural capillaries allows excessive fluid to pass across intact capillaries. Such conditions include heart failure, hepatic disease with ascites, peritoneal dialysis, hypoalbuminemia, and disorders resulting in overexpanded intravascular volume.

Exudative pleural effusions occur with conditions in which increased capillary permeability allows protein-rich fluid to leak into the pleural space. These conditions include tuberculosis, subphrenic abscess, pancreatitis, bacterial or fungal pneumonitis or empyema, cancer, pulmonary embolism with or without infarction, collagen disease (lupus erythematosus and rheumatoid arthritis), myxedema, and chest trauma.

Empyema
Usually associated with infection in the pleural space, empyema may be idiopathic or may be related to pneumonitis, carcinoma, perforation, or esophageal rupture.

SPECIAL CONSIDERATIONS
● Encourage the patient to practice deep breathing exercises to expand the lungs and to use an incentive spirometer to promote deep breathing.

 PREVENTION: If pleural effusion arose as a complication of pneumonia or influenza, advise the patient to seek prompt medical attention for chest colds.

Pleurisy
Also known as pleuritis, pleurisy refers to inflammation of the visceral and parietal pleurae that line the inside of the thoracic cage and envelop the lungs.

CAUSES
Pleurisy develops as a complication of pneumonia, tuberculosis, viruses, systemic lupus erythematosus, rheumatoid arthritis, uremia, Dressler's syndrome, cancer, pulmonary infarction, and chest trauma.

Pleuritic pain results from inflammation or irritation of sensory nerve endings in the parietal pleura. As the lungs inflate and deflate, the visceral pleura covering them moves against the fixed parietal pleura lining the pleural space, causing pain. This disorder usually begins suddenly.

SIGNS AND SYMPTOMS
Sharp, stabbing pain that worsens with respiration may be severe enough to limit movement on the affected side during breathing. Dyspnea also occurs. Other signs and symptoms vary with the underlying pathologic process.

DIAGNOSTIC TESTS
Chest auscultation typically reveals a pleural friction rub — a coarse, creaky sound during late inspiration and early expiration, directly over the area of pleural inflammation. Palpation over the affected area may reveal coarse vibration.

TREATMENT
Generally symptomatic treatment includes anti-inflammatory agents, analgesics, and bed rest. Severe pain may call for an intercostal nerve block. Pleurisy with pleural effusion

calls for thoracentesis as both a thera-peutic and a diagnostic measure.

SPECIAL CONSIDERATIONS
● Bed rest is vital to recovery. Be sure to plan care activities so the patient gets as much uninterrupted rest as possible.
● If the patient needs a narcotic anal-gesic for pain, warn him to avoid overuse because such medication de-presses coughing and respiration.

Pneumocystis carinii pneumonia

Pneumocystis carinii pneumonia (PCP) is an opportunistic infection. Because of its association with human im-munodeficiency virus (HIV) infection, the incidence of PCP has increased since the 1980s. Before the advent of PCP prophylaxis, this disease was the first clue in about 60% of patients that HIV infection was present.

Up to 90% of HIV-infected patients in the United States get PCP at some point during their lifetime. Dissemi-nated infection doesn't occur.

PCP is also associated with other immunocompromising conditions, including organ transplantation, leukemia, and lymphoma.

CAUSES
P. carinii, the cause of PCP, usually is classified as a protozoan. Part of the normal flora in most healthy people, *P. carinii* becomes an aggressive patho-gen in the immunocompromised pa-tient. The organism invades the lungs bilaterally and multiplies extracellular-ly. As the infestation grows, alveoli fill with organisms and exudate, impair-ing gas exchange. Progressive alveolar enlargement and thickening eventual-ly lead to extensive consolidation.

The primary transmission route seems to be air, although the organ-ism is already resident in most people.

SIGNS AND SYMPTOMS
The patient typically has a history of an immunocompromising condition (such as HIV infection, leukemia, or lymphoma) or procedure (such as or-gan transplantation).

PCP begins gradually with increas-ing shortness of breath and a nonpro-ductive cough. Anorexia, generalized fatigue, and weight loss may follow. Some patients don't have significant symptoms but develop a low-grade, intermittent fever.

Other signs and symptoms include tachypnea, dyspnea, accessory mus-cle use for breathing, crackles, and decreased breath sounds.

DIAGNOSTIC TESTS
Tissue studies confirm *P. carinii* pneu-monia. In patients with HIV infec-tion, initial examination of a sputum specimen may be sufficient.

Fiberoptic bronchoscopy is the most commonly used study to con-firm PCP. In a small number of cases, invasive procedures are done.

TREATMENT
PCP may respond to co-trimoxazole or pentamidine isethionate. However, many patients who also have HIV ex-perience severe adverse reactions to such drug therapy. These reactions include bone marrow suppression, thrush, fever, hepatotoxicity, and anaphylaxis. Nausea, vomiting, and rashes are common. Diphenhy-dramine may be prescribed to treat the latter effects and leucovorin may reduce bone marrow suppression.

Pentamidine may be administered I.V. or in aerosol form. I.V. pentami-dine is associated with a high inci-dence of severe toxic effects. The in-haled form usually is well tolerated but may not effectively reach the lung apices.

Supportive measures, such as oxy-gen therapy, mechanical ventilation, adequate nutrition, and fluid bal-ance, are also important. Oral mor-phine sulfate solution may reduce the respiratory rate and anxiety, en-hancing oxygenation.

SPECIAL CONSIDERATIONS
● Use universal precautions to pre-vent contagion.
● Encourage the patient to perform

Predisposing factors for pneumonia

Conditions that increase the risk of bacterial and viral pneumonia include:
- chronic illness and debilitation
- cancer (particularly lung cancer)
- abdominal and thoracic surgery
- atelectasis
- common colds and other viral respiratory infections
- chronic respiratory disease (chronic obstructive pulmonary disease, asthma, bronchiectasis, cystic fibrosis)
- influenza
- smoking
- malnutrition
- alcoholism
- sickle cell disease
- tracheostomy
- exposure to noxious gases
- aspiration
- immunosuppressant therapy.

Aspiration pneumonia

Predisposing factors for aspiration pneumonia include old age, debilitation, nasogastric tube feedings, impaired gag reflex, poor oral hygiene, and decreased level of consciousness.

---

deep-breathing exercises and incentive spirometry to promote gas exchange.

- Because the patient is easily fatigued, plan care activities to allow adequate rest between procedures. A relaxing environment without excessive stimuli promotes rest and reduces fatigue.
- Encourage the patient to eat a high-calorie, protein-rich diet.

Pneumonia

An acute infection of the lung parenchyma, pneumonia commonly impairs gas exchange. The prognosis is generally good for patients who have normal lungs and adequate host defenses before pneumonia onset. However, pneumonia is the sixth leading cause of death in the United States.

CAUSES

Pneumonia can be classified in several ways:

Microbiological etiology — Pneumonia can be viral, bacterial, fungal, protozoal, mycobacterial, mycoplasmal, or rickettsial in origin.

Location — Bronchopneumonia involves distal airways and alveoli; lobular pneumonia involves part of a lobe; and lobar pneumonia involves an entire lobe.

Type — Primary pneumonia results from inhaling or aspirating a pathogen; it includes pneumococcal and viral pneumonia. Secondary pneumonia may follow initial lung damage from a noxious chemical or other insult (superinfection) or may result from hematogenous spread of bacteria from a distant focus.

Factors that can predispose a person to pneumonia range from chronic lung disease and cancer to smoking and alcoholism. (See *Predisposing factors for pneumonia*.)

SIGNS AND SYMPTOMS

The five cardinal signs and symptoms of early bacterial pneumonia are coughing, sputum production, pleuritic chest pain, shaking, chills, and fever. Physical signs vary widely.

DIAGNOSTIC TESTS

Typical clinical features and physical examination results, along with a chest X-ray showing pulmonary infiltrates and sputum containing acute inflammatory cells, are general indicators of pneumonia. If the patient has pleural effusions, fluid from the effusions is analyzed to detect infection. Occasionally, bronchoscopy is done to obtain materials for smear and culture. The patient's response to antibiotics also provides important clues to the presence of pneumonia.

TREATMENT

Antimicrobial therapy varies with the causative agent and is reevaluated early in the course of treatment.

Supportive measures include humidified oxygen therapy for hypoxia, mechanical ventilation for respiratory failure, a high-calorie diet and adequate fluid intake, bed rest, and an analgesic to relieve pleuritic chest pain. Patients with severe pneumonia on mechanical ventilation may require positive end-expiratory pressure to promote adequate oxygenation.

SPECIAL CONSIDERATIONS

• Encourage the patient to perform coughing and deep-breathing exercises frequently.
• A high-calorie, high-protein diet consisting of soft, easy-to-eat foods usually ensures adequate nutrition.
• Encourage family visits. Provide diversionary activities appropriate to the patient's age.

 PREVENTION: To help prevent pneumonia, advise patients to avoid taking antibiotics indiscriminately during minor viral infections. Encourage annual influenza vaccination and Pneumovax 23 for high-risk patients, such as those with chronic obstructive pulmonary disease, chronic heart disease, or sickle cell disease.

Polycystic kidney disease

Polycystic kidney disease is characterized by multiple, bilateral, grapelike clusters of fluid-filled cysts that grossly enlarge the kidneys. These cysts compress and eventually replace functioning renal tissue. (See *Viewing a polycystic kidney.*)

The disease appears in two distinct forms. The *infantile* form causes still-

PATHOPHYSIOLOGY

Viewing a polycystic kidney

In polycystic kidney disease, clusters of fluid-filled cysts cause kidney enlargement.

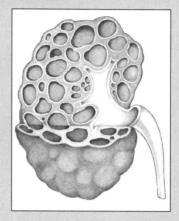

birth or early neonatal death. A few infants with this disease survive for 2 years and then develop fatal renal, heart, or respiratory failure.

The *adult* form begins gradually but usually becomes obvious between ages 30 and 50; rarely, it causes no symptoms until the patient is in his seventies. Renal deterioration is gradual but progresses relentlessly to fatal uremia.

The prognosis in adults is extremely variable. Progression may be slow. However, once uremic symptoms develop, polycystic kidney disease is usually fatal within 4 years unless the patient receives dialysis, a kidney transplant, or both.

CAUSES

Both types of polycystic kidney disease are inherited. However, the incidence in two distinct age-groups and

Two types of polycystic kidney disease

The infantile and adult forms of polycystic kidney disease produce different signs and symptoms.

Infantile form

The newborn with the disease often has pronounced epicanthal folds, a pointed nose, a small chin, and floppy, low-set ears. At birth, he has huge bilateral masses on the flanks that are symmetrical and tense. Typically, he shows signs of respiratory distress, heart failure and, eventually, uremia and renal failure.

Adult form

Adult polycystic kidney disease is commonly asymptomatic while the patient is in his thirties and forties.

However, it may produce nonspecific symptoms, such as hypertension, polyuria, and urinary tract infection. Later, the patient develops overt symptoms related to the enlarging kidney mass, such as lumbar pain, widening girth, and a swollen or tender abdomen.

In advanced stages, the disease may cause recurrent hematuria, life-threatening retroperitoneal bleeding resulting from a ruptured cyst, proteinuria, and colicky abdominal pain from ureteral passage of clots or calculi. Generally, about 10 years after symptoms appear, progressive compression of kidney structures by the enlarging mass causes renal failure and uremia.

different inheritance patterns suggest two unrelated disorders.

SIGNS AND SYMPTOMS

Clinical features vary with the disease form. (See *Two types of polycystic kidney disease*.)

DIAGNOSTIC TESTS

Family history, clinical features, and physical examination revealing large, irregular masses on both flanks identify the disease. In advanced cases, enlarged kidneys are palpable. Additional diagnostic tests include urinalysis, creatinine clearance tests, scans with intravenous dye, ultrasound, and computed tomography.

TREATMENT

Polycystic kidney disease can't be cured. The primary treatment goal is to preserve the renal parenchyma and prevent infectious complications. Managing secondary hypertension helps prevent rapid deterioration in function. Progressive renal failure requires treatment similar to that for other types of renal disease,

including dialysis or, rarely, a kidney transplant.

Asymptomatic stage

Asymptomatic adult polycystic kidney disease calls for careful monitoring, including urine cultures and creatinine clearance tests every 6 months. When a urine culture detects infection, prompt and vigorous antibiotic treatment is needed.

Progressive renal impairment

As renal impairment progresses, selected patients may undergo dialysis, transplantation, or both. Cystic abscess or retroperitoneal bleeding may warrant surgical drainage; intractable pain may also require surgery. However, because this disease affects both kidneys, nephrectomy usually isn't recommended because it increases the risk of infection in the remaining kidney.

SPECIAL CONSIDERATIONS

• The young adult patient or the parents of an infant with polycystic kidney disease should be referred for genetic counseling.

Polycythemia, secondary

Also known as reactive polycythemia, secondary polycythemia is characterized by excessive production of circulating red blood cells (RBCs). It occurs in approximately 2 out of every 100,000 people living at or near sea level; incidence rises among persons living at high altitudes.

CAUSES

Secondary polycythemia may result from increased production of erythropoietin. This hormone, which is possibly produced and secreted in the kidneys, stimulates bone marrow production of RBCs. Increased production may be a compensatory response to hypoxemia, which can result from:

• chronic obstructive pulmonary disease

• hemoglobin abnormalities (such as carboxyhemoglobinemia, seen in heavy smokers)

• heart failure (causing a decreased ventilation-perfusion ratio)

• right-to-left shunting of blood in the heart (as in transposition of the great vessels)

• central or peripheral alveolar hypoventilation (as in barbiturate intoxication or pickwickian syndrome)

• low oxygen content at high altitudes.

Increased erythropoietin production may also be an inappropriate response to renal disease (such as renal vascular impairment, renal cysts, and hydronephrosis), central nervous system disease (such as encephalitis and parkinsonism), neoplasms (such as renal tumors, uterine myomas, and cerebellar hemangiomas), or endocrine disorders (such as Cushing's syndrome, Bartter's syndrome, and pheochromocytomas).

Rarely, secondary polycythemia results from a recessive genetic trait.

SIGNS AND SYMPTOMS

In the hypoxic patient, suggestive physical findings include ruddy cyanotic skin, emphysema, hypoxemia without hepatosplenomegaly, and hypertension. Finger clubbing may occur with an underlying cardiovascular disease. When secondary polycythemia isn't caused by hypoxemia, it's usually found incidentally during treatment for an underlying disease.

DIAGNOSTIC TESTS

Laboratory values include an increased RBC mass (increased hematocrit, hemoglobin level, mean corpuscular volume, and mean corpuscular hemoglobin), urinary erythropoietin, and blood histamine, with decreased or normal arterial oxygen saturation (SaO_2). Bone marrow biopsy reveals hyperplasia confined to the erythroid series.

TREATMENT

The goal of treatment is to correct the underlying condition. Generally, secondary polycythemia disappears when the primary disease is corrected.

In severe secondary polycythemia where altitude is a contributing factor, relocation may be advisable. If secondary polycythemia has produced hazardous hyperviscosity or if the patient doesn't respond to treatment for the primary disease, reduction of blood volume by phlebotomy or pheresis may be effective.

Emergency phlebotomy is indicated to prevent impending vascular occlusion or before emergency surgery.

SPECIAL CONSIDERATIONS

• Inform the patient that maintaining a high level of activity decreases the risk of thrombosis from increased blood viscosity. Also tell him that reducing his caloric and sodium intake may combat the tendency to experience hypertension.

• Emphasize the importance of regular blood studies (every 2 to 3 months), even after the disease is controlled.

• Teach the patient and family about the underlying disorder. Help them understand its relationship to polycythemia and the measures needed to control both.

PATHOPHYSIOLOGY

Understanding the causes of spurious polycythemia

Dehydration, hemoconcentration brought on by stress, and a high red blood cell (RBC) mass with low-normal plasma volume can result in spurious polycythemia.

Dehydration

Conditions that promote severe fluid loss decrease plasma levels and lead to hemoconcentration. Such conditions include:
- persistent vomiting or diarrhea, burns
- adrenocortical insufficiency
- aggressive diuretic therapy
- decreased fluid intake
- diabetic acidosis
- renal disease.

Hemoconcentration due to stress

Nervous stress leads to hemoconcentration by an unknown mechanism. This is particularly common in middle-aged men who are chronic smokers and have type A personalities (tense, hard-driving, anxious).

High-normal RBC mass and low-normal plasma volume

In many patients, an increased hematocrit merely reflects a normally high RBC mass and low plasma volume. This is especially common in patients who are nonsmokers, are not obese, and lack a history of hypertension.

Polycythemia, spurious

Spurious polycythemia has many other names, including stress polycythemia, benign polycythemia, and pseudopolycythemia. The condition is characterized by increased hematocrit and normal or decreased red blood cell (RBC) total mass resulting from decreasing plasma volume and subsequent hemoconcentration.

CAUSES

The three possible causes of spurious polycythemia are dehydration, hemoconcentration due to stress, and high-normal RBC mass and low normal plasma volume. (See *Understanding the causes of spurious polycythemia.*)

SIGNS AND SYMPTOMS

The patient usually has no specific symptoms but may have vague complaints, such as headaches, dizziness, and fatigue. Less commonly, he may develop diaphoresis, dyspnea, and claudication.

Typically, the patient has a ruddy appearance, a short neck, slight hypertension, and a tendency to hypoventilate when recumbent. He shows no associated spleen or liver enlargement but may have cardiac or pulmonary disease.

DIAGNOSTIC TESTS

Hemoglobin level, hematocrit, and RBC count are typically elevated; RBC mass, SaO_2, and bone marrow are normal. Plasma volume may be decreased or normal. Hypercholesterolemia, hyperlipemia, or hyperuricemia may be present.

Spurious polycythemia is distinguishable from polycythemia vera by its normal RBC mass, elevated hematocrit, and absence of leukocytosis.

TREATMENT

The principal treatment goals are to correct dehydration and to prevent life-threatening thromboembolism. Rehydration with appropriate fluids and electrolytes is the primary therapy for spurious polycythemia secondary to dehydration. Therapy also includes appropriate measures to prevent continuing fluid loss.

SPECIAL CONSIDERATIONS

 TEACHING TIP: Inform the patient that complying with prescribed treatment can control symptoms. Advise him to get regular exercise and eat a low-cholesterol diet to help prevent thromboemboli. Urge an obese patient to reduce his caloric intake.

● When appropriate, suggest counseling about the patient's work habits and lack of relaxation. If the patient smokes, stress the importance of stopping smoking.

Polycythemia vera

Polycythemia vera is a chronic myeloproliferative disorder marked by increased red blood cell (RBC) mass, leukocytosis, thrombocytosis, and increased hemoglobin levels; plasma volume is normal or increased. The condition usually occurs between ages 40 and 60, most commonly among males of Jewish ancestry. It rarely affects children or blacks.

The prognosis depends on age at diagnosis, treatment used, and complications. Mortality is high if polycythemia goes untreated or is associated with leukemia or myeloid metaplasia.

CAUSES

Uncontrolled cellular activity (rapid reproduction and maturation, causing proliferation or hyperplasia of all bone marrow cells) occurs for an unknown reason.

SIGNS AND SYMPTOMS

Increased RBC mass results in hyperviscosity and inhibits blood flow to the microcirculation. Subsequently, increased viscosity, diminished velocity, and thrombocytosis promote in-

---

> ## Progressive features of polycythemia vera
>
> In early stages, polycythemia vera usually produces no symptoms. However, as altered circulation (secondary to increased red blood cell mass) causes hypervolemia and hyperviscosity, the patient may complain of a feeling of fullness in the head, headache, dizziness, and other symptoms, depending on the body system affected. Hyperviscosity may lead to thrombosis of smaller vessels, with ruddy cyanosis of the nose and clubbing of fingers and toes.

travascular thrombosis. (See *Progressive features of polycythemia vera.*)

Complications

Paradoxically, hemorrhage is a complication of polycythemia vera. It may result from defective platelet function or from hyperviscosity and the local effects of excess RBCs exerting pressure on distended venous and capillary walls.

DIAGNOSTIC TESTS

Laboratory studies confirm polycythemia vera by showing increased RBC mass and other characteristic findings. Bone marrow biopsy reveals increased levels of all bone marrow components.

TREATMENT

Phlebotomy can reduce RBC mass promptly. Typically, 350 to 500 ml of blood can be removed every other day until the hematocrit falls to the low-normal range.

After repeated phlebotomies, the patient develops iron deficiency, which stabilizes RBC production and reduces the need for phlebotomy. Pheresis returns plasma to the patient, diluting the blood and reducing hypovolemic symptoms.

Severe symptoms may warrant myelosuppressive therapy. In the past, radioactive phosphorus (^{32}P) or chemotherapeutic agents, such as melphalan, busulfan, or chlorambucil, could usually control the disease. But these agents may cause leukemia and should be reserved for older patients and those with problems uncontrolled by phlebotomy.

The currently preferred myelosuppressive agent is hydroxyurea, which is not associated with leukemia. Patients who have had previous thrombotic problems should be considered for myelosuppressive therapy.

SPECIAL CONSIDERATIONS

• Reassure the patient who requires phlebotomy that the procedure will relieve distressing symptoms. Instruct him to watch for and report signs and symptoms of iron deficiency — pale skin, weight loss, lack of energy, and a swollen, painful tongue.

 PREVENTION: Advise the patient to stay active to prevent thrombosis. If bed rest is absolutely necessary, a daily program of active and passive range-of-motion exercises can reduce the risk of thrombosis.

 TEACHING TIP: Emphasize the importance of regular examinations for bleeding. Instruct the patient to perform periodic self-examination of the most common bleeding sites (such as the nose, gingiva, and skin) and to report any abnormal bleeding promptly.

Premenstrual syndrome

Premenstrual syndrome (PMS) refers to a complex of signs and symptoms that appear 7 to 14 days before menses and usually subside with its onset. PMS effects range from minimal discomfort to severe, disruptive symptoms and can include nervousness, irritability, depression, and multiple somatic complaints.

Researchers believe that 70% to 90% of women experience PMS at some time during their childbearing years.

CAUSES

Biological theories offered to explain the cause of PMS include such conditions as a progesterone deficiency in the luteal phase of the menstrual cycle and vitamin deficiencies. Failure to identify a specific disorder with a specific mechanism suggests that PMS represents various manifestations triggered by normal physiologic hormonal changes.

SIGNS AND SYMPTOMS

Clinical effects of PMS vary widely among patients and may include any combination of the following:
• *behavioral* — mild to severe personality changes, nervousness, hostility, irritability, agitation, sleep disturbances, fatigue, lethargy, and depression
• *somatic* — breast tenderness or swelling, abdominal tenderness or bloating, joint pain, headache, edema, diarrhea or constipation, worsening of skin problems (such as acne or rashes), respiratory problems (such as asthma), or neurologic problems (such as seizures).

DIAGNOSTIC TESTS

The patient's history shows typical symptoms related to the menstrual cycle. Before PMS is diagnosed, the patient may be asked to record her menstrual symptoms and body temperature on a calendar for 2 to 3 months. Evaluating estrogen and progesterone levels helps rule out hormonal imbalance. A psychological evaluation may be done to rule out or detect an underlying psychiatric disorder.

TREATMENT

Education and reassurance that PMS is a real physiologic syndrome are important aspects of treatment. Because treatment is predominantly symptomatic, each patient must learn to cope with her own individual set of symptoms.

Treatment may include diuretics, antidepressants, vitamins such as B complex, progestins, prostaglandin inhibitors, and nonsteroidal anti-inflammatory drugs. For effective treatment, the patient may have to maintain a diet low in simple sugars, caffeine, and salt.

SPECIAL CONSIDERATIONS
• A complete patient history can help identify emotional problems that may contribute to PMS. If necessary, the patient may be referred for psychological counseling.
• Inform the patient that self-help groups exist for women with PMS; if appropriate, help her to contact such a group.

 TEACHING TIP: Inform the patient of lifestyle changes that may promote comfort, such as modifying the diet and avoiding stimulants and alcohol. Tell her that she may need to seek further medical help if her symptoms are severe and interfere with her lifestyle.

Prostatic cancer

Prostatic cancer — cancer of the prostate — is the second most common neoplasm in men over age 50. Adenocarcinoma is its most common form; sarcoma occurs rarely. Most prostatic carcinomas originate in the posterior prostate gland; the rest originate near the urethra.

When primary prostatic lesions metastasize, they typically invade the prostatic capsule and spread along the ejaculatory ducts in the space between the seminal vesicles or perivesicular fascia.

CAUSES
Although androgens regulate prostate growth and function and may also speed tumor growth, no definite link between increased androgen levels and prostatic cancer has been found.

SIGNS AND SYMPTOMS
Prostatic cancer seldom causes symptoms until it's advanced. Indications include difficulty initiating a urinary stream, dribbling, urine retention, unexplained cystitis and, rarely, hematuria.

DIAGNOSTIC TESTS
A digital rectal examination may reveal a small, hard mass, or nodule. The American Cancer Society recommends a yearly rectal examination for men over age 40, a yearly blood test to detect prostate-specific antigen in men over age 50, and ultrasonography if results are abnormal.

Biopsy confirms the diagnosis. Magnetic resonance imaging, computed tomography scan, and excretory urography may aid diagnosis.

TREATMENT
Management of prostatic cancer depends on clinical assessment, the patient's tolerance of therapy, his expected life span, and the disease stage.

Therapy varies with each disease stage. Generally, it includes radiation, prostatectomy, orchiectomy to reduce androgen production, and hormone therapy with synthetic estrogen (diethylstilbestrol) and antiandrogens such as cyproterone, megestrol, and flutamide. Radical prostatectomy is usually effective for localized lesions.

Radiation therapy may be used in an effort to cure some locally invasive lesions and relieve pain from metastatic bone involvement. A single injection of the radionuclide strontium-89 may be given to treat pain caused by bone metastasis.

If hormone therapy, surgery, and radiation therapy aren't feasible or successful, chemotherapy (using combinations of cyclophosphamide, doxorubicin, fluorouracil, cisplatin, etoposide, and vindesine) may be tried. However, current drug therapy offers limited benefit. Combining several treatment methods may be most effective.

SPECIAL CONSIDERATIONS
• Before prostatectomy, explain the expected aftereffects of surgery, such as impotence and incontinence.

Teaching tip: Encourage the patient to perform perineal exercises by squeezing his buttocks together, holding this position for a few seconds, and then relaxing. Tell him to repeat the exercises 1 to 10 times an hour.

• After perineal prostatectomy, avoid taking a rectal temperature or inserting any kind of rectal tube.

Prostatitis

An inflammation of the prostate gland, prostatitis may be acute or chronic. Acute prostatitis most commonly results from gram-negative bacteria and is easily recognized and treated. Chronic prostatitis, the most common cause of recurrent urinary tract infection (UTI) in men, is harder to recognize. As many as 35% of men over age 50 have chronic prostatitis.

CAUSES
About 80% of bacterial prostatitis cases result from infection by *Escherichia coli;* the rest, from infection by *Klebsiella, Enterobacter, Proteus, Pseudomonas, Streptococcus,* or *Staphylococcus.* (See *How microorganisms spread to the prostate.*)

SIGNS AND SYMPTOMS
Acute prostatitis begins with fever, chills, low back pain, myalgia, perineal fullness, and arthralgia. Urination is frequent and urgent. Dysuria, nocturia, and urinary obstruction may also occur. The urine may appear cloudy. When palpated rectally, the prostate is tender, indurated, swollen, firm, and warm.

Chronic bacterial prostatitis sometimes produces no symptoms but usually elicits the same urinary symptoms as the acute form, although to a lesser degree. UTI is a common complication. Other possible signs include painful ejaculation, hemospermia, persistent urethral discharge, and sexual dysfunction.

DIAGNOSTIC TESTS
Urine cultures identify the causative bacteria. In some patients, swelling is palpable through the rectum. Diagnosis is confirmed by analysis of a four-stage specimen — three samples taken as the person urinates and then one secretion pressed from the prostate gland. A significantly increased bacteria count in the prostatic specimen confirms prostate inflammation.

TREATMENT
Appropriate treatment includes drug therapy and supportive measures. Surgery may be necessary if drug therapy fails.

Drug therapy
Systemic antibiotic therapy is the treatment of choice for acute prostatitis. Co-trimoxazole is given orally and, if the pathogen is sensitive to it, continued for about 30 days. If sepsis is likely, I.V. co-trimoxazole or I.V. gentamicin plus ampicillin may be given until sensitivity test results are known.

If test results and clinical response are favorable, parenteral therapy continues for 48 hours to 1 week; then an oral agent is substituted for 30 more days. In chronic prostatitis due to *E. coli,* co-trimoxazole is usually given for at least 6 weeks.

Supportive measures
Supportive therapy includes bed rest, adequate hydration, and administration of analgesics, antipyretics, sitz baths, and stool softeners as necessary. In symptomatic chronic prostatitis, regular prostate massage is most effective. Regular ejaculation may promote drainage of prostatic secretions. Anticholinergics and analgesics may relieve nonbacterial prostatitis symptoms. Alpha-adrenergic blockers and muscle relaxants may relieve prostatic pain.

Surgery
If drug therapy fails, treatment may include transurethral resection of the prostate, which removes all infected tissue. However, this procedure usually isn't performed on young adults because it may cause retrograde ejaculation and sterility. Total prostatec-

PATHOPHYSIOLOGY

How microorganisms spread to the prostate

The organisms that cause prostatitis — most commonly *Escherichia coli* — probably spread to the prostate by the bloodstream or in one of the following ways:
● ascending urethral infection
● invasion of rectal bacteria by way of lymphatics
● reflux of infected bladder urine into prostate ducts
● infrequent or excessive sexual intercourse or such procedures as cystoscopy or catheterization.
   Chronic prostatitis usually results from bacterial invasion from the urethra.

---

tomy is curative but may cause impotence and incontinence.

SPECIAL CONSIDERATIONS
● Ensure bed rest and adequate hydration, and help administer sitz baths.
● Emphasize the need for strict adherence to the prescribed regimen. Instruct the patient to drink at least 8 glasses of water daily. Tell him to report adverse drug reactions (rash, nausea, vomiting, fever, chills, and GI upset).

Pseudomembranous enterocolitis

Pseudomembranous enterocolitis refers to acute inflammation and necrosis of the small and large intestines. It usually affects the mucosa but may extend into the submucosa and, rarely, other layers. Necrotized mucosa is replaced by a pseudomembrane filled with staphylococci, leukocytes, mucus, fibrin, and inflammatory cells.
   Marked by severe diarrhea, this rare condition is generally fatal in 1 to 7 days from severe dehydration and from toxicity, peritonitis, or perforation.

CAUSES
The cause of pseudomembranous enterocolitis is unknown. However, *Clostridium difficile* is thought to produce a toxin that may play a role in its development.
   Pseudomembranous enterocolitis has occurred postoperatively in debilitated patients who have undergone abdominal surgery and in patients who have received broad-spectrum antibiotics.

SIGNS AND SYMPTOMS
Pseudomembranous enterocolitis begins suddenly with copious watery or bloody diarrhea, abdominal pain, and fever. Serious complications associated with this disorder include severe dehydration, electrolyte imbalance, hypotension, shock, and colonic perforation.

DIAGNOSTIC TESTS
Diagnosis sometimes poses a problem because enterocolitis comes on suddenly and creates an emergency situation. Patient history supports the diagnosis, but confirmation requires a rectal biopsy. Stool cultures can identify *C. difficile*.

TREATMENT
If the patient is receiving broad-spectrum antibiotic therapy, antibiotics are discontinued immediately. Effective treatment usually includes metronidazole. Vancomycin is usually reserved for severe or resistant cases.
   A patient with mild pseudomembranous enterocolitis may receive anion exchange resins, such as cholestyra-

Hospitals and *Pseudomonas* infections

Like many other infections, *Pseudomonas* infections may be acquired during a hospital stay. That's because the organisms that cause *Pseudomonas* infections (*P. aeruginosa* and various other species of *Pseudomonas*) are commonly found in hospital liquids that have been allowed to stand for a long time. These liquids include benzalkonium chloride, hexachlorophene soap, saline solution, penicillin, water in flower vases, and fluids in incubators, humidifiers, and respiratory therapy equipment.

mine, to bind the toxin produced by *C. difficile.* Supportive treatment must maintain fluid and electrolyte balance and combat hypotension and shock with pressors, such as dopamine and levarterenol.

SPECIAL CONSIDERATIONS
• The patient is monitored for dehydration, hypokalemia, hypotension, and shock.

Pseudomonas infections

Pseudomonas is a small, gram-negative bacillus that causes hospital-acquired infections, superinfections of various parts of the body, and a rare disease called melioidosis. This bacillus is also associated with bacteremia, endocarditis, and osteomyelitis in drug addicts.

In local *Pseudomonas* infections, treatment is usually successful and complications rare. However, in patients with poor immunologic resistance — premature infants, the elderly, and those with debilitating disease, burns, or wounds — septicemic

Pseudomonas infections are serious and sometimes fatal.

CAUSES
The most common species of *Pseudomonas* is *P. aeruginosa.* Other species that typically cause disease in humans include *P. maltophilia, P. cepacia, P. fluorescens, P. testosteroni, P. acidovorans, P. alcaligenes, P. stutzeri, P. putrefaciens,* and *P. putida.* (See *Hospitals and Pseudomonas infections.*)

In elderly patients, *Pseudomonas* infection usually enters through the genitourinary tract; in infants, through the umbilical cord, skin, and GI tract.

SIGNS AND SYMPTOMS
The most common infections associated with *Pseudomonas* include skin infections (such as burns and decubitus ulcers), urinary tract infections (UTIs), infant epidemic diarrhea and other diarrheal illnesses, bronchitis, pneumonia, bronchiectasis, meningitis, corneal ulcers, mastoiditis, otitis externa, otitis media, endocarditis, and bacteremia.

Drainage in these infections has a distinct, sickly sweet odor and a greenish blue pus that forms a crust on wounds. Other signs and symptoms depend on the infection site. For example, when it invades the lungs, *Pseudomonas* causes pneumonia with fever, chills, and a productive cough.

DIAGNOSTIC TESTS
Diagnosis requires isolation of the *Pseudomonas* organism in blood, spinal fluid, urine, exudate, or sputum culture.

TREATMENT
In the debilitated or otherwise vulnerable patient with clinical evidence of *Pseudomonas* infection, treatment should begin immediately, without waiting for laboratory test results. Antibiotic treatment includes aminoglycosides, such as gentamicin or tobramycin, combined with a *Pseudomonas*-sensitive penicillin, such as carbenicillin disodium or ticarcillin.

Such combination therapy is necessary because *Pseudomonas* quickly grows resistant to carbenicillin alone.

In UTIs, carbenicillin indanyl sodium can be used alone if the organism is susceptible and the infection doesn't produce systemic effects; it's excreted in the urine and builds up high urine levels that prevent resistance.

Local *Pseudomonas* infections and septicemia secondary to wound infection call for 1% acetic acid irrigation, topical application of colistimethate and polymyxin B, and debridement or drainage of the infected wound.

SPECIAL CONSIDERATIONS

 PREVENTION: Measures to help prevent *Pseudomonas* infection include maintaining proper endotracheal and tracheostomy suctioning technique. For instance, strict sterile technique must be used when caring for I.V. lines, catheters, and other tubes.

Pulmonary edema

In pulmonary edema, fluid accumulates in the extravascular spaces of the lung. In cardiogenic pulmonary edema, fluid accumulation results from elevations in pulmonary venous and capillary hydrostatic pressures.

A common complication of cardiac disorders, pulmonary edema can occur as a chronic condition or develop quickly and rapidly become fatal.

CAUSES

Pulmonary edema usually results from left-sided heart failure due to arteriosclerotic, hypertensive, cardiomyopathic, or valvular heart disease. In such disorders, the compromised left ventricle requires increased filling pressures to maintain adequate output; these pressures are transmitted to the left atrium, pulmonary veins, and pulmonary capillary bed.

This increased pulmonary capillary hydrostatic force promotes transudation of intravascular fluids into the pulmonary interstitium, decreasing lung compliance and impeding gas exchange. Other factors may also predispose a person to pulmonary edema. (See *Predisposing factors for pulmonary edema*, page 260.)

SIGNS AND SYMPTOMS

Clinical features vary with the stage of pulmonary edema. Early signs and symptoms of pulmonary edema reflect interstitial fluid buildup and diminished lung compliance: dyspnea on exertion, paroxysmal nocturnal dyspnea, orthopnea, and coughing. Clinical features include tachycardia, tachypnea, dependent crackles, and neck vein distention.

In severe pulmonary edema, alveoli and bronchioles may fill with fluid and intensify early symptoms. Respiration becomes rapid and labored, with more diffuse crackles and coughing that produces frothy, bloody sputum. Tachycardia increases and arrhythmias may occur. Skin becomes cold, clammy, diaphoretic, and cyanotic. Blood pressure falls and pulse becomes thready as cardiac output falls.

DIAGNOSTIC TESTS

A working diagnosis rests on clinical evidence. Arterial blood gas (ABG) analysis usually shows decreased oxygen with a variable carbon dioxide level. ABG results may also reveal a metabolic disturbance, such as respiratory acidosis or alkalosis or metabolic acidosis. Chest X-rays typically reveal diffuse haziness in the lungs and, in many cases, an enlarged heart and abnormal fluid buildup in the lungs.

Pulmonary artery catheterization may be done to help confirm left-sided heart failure and rule out adult respiratory distress syndrome, which causes similar symptoms.

TREATMENT

Treatment focuses on reducing extravascular fluid, improving gas exchange and myocardial function and,

Predisposing factors for pulmonary edema

Pulmonary edema doesn't always result from cardiovascular disease. Other factors that can predispose a person to this condition include:
● infusion of excessive volumes of I.V. fluids
● decreased serum colloid osmotic pressure as a result of nephrosis, protein-losing enteropathy, extensive burns, hepatic disease, or nutritional deficiency
● impaired lung lymphatic drainage from Hodgkin's disease or obliterative lymphangitis after radiation
● pulmonary veno-occlusive disease.

if possible, correcting the underlying disorder.

To improve oxygen delivery to tissues and correct acid-base disturbances, the patient typically receives high concentrations of oxygen by cannula, by face mask or, if necessary, by assisted ventilation. Diuretics (for instance, furosemide and bumetanide) promote diuresis, which in turn helps to mobilize extravascular fluid.

Treatment for heart dysfunction includes a digitalis glycoside or pressor agents to increase cardiac contractility, antiarrhythmics and, occasionally, arterial vasodilators (such as nitroprusside).

Other treatment may include morphine to reduce anxiety and dyspnea and to promote blood flow from the pulmonary circulation to the periphery.

SPECIAL CONSIDERATIONS
● Be aware that patients receiving digitalis glycosides are at risk for arrhythmias, while those receiving

morphine may experience marked respiratory depression.
● Reassure the patient, who will be frightened by decreased respiratory capability, in a calm voice and explain all procedures. Provide emotional support to the family as well.

Pulmonary embolism and infarction

Pulmonary embolism is an obstruction of the pulmonary arterial bed by a dislodged thrombus or foreign substance. It strikes an estimated 6 million adults each year in the United States, resulting in 100,000 deaths. Massive embolism and infarction can be rapidly fatal.

CAUSES
Pulmonary embolism generally results from dislodged thrombi that originate in the leg veins. More than half of these thrombi arise in deep veins of the legs and are usually multiple.

Thrombus formation results directly from vascular wall damage, venostasis, or hypercoagulability of the blood. Certain conditions predispose a person to pulmonary embolism. (See *Risk factors for pulmonary embolism.*)

Rare causes
Rarely, emboli contain air, fat, amniotic fluid, talc (from oral drugs that are injected I.V. by addicts), or tumor cells. Thrombi may embolize spontaneously during clot dissolution or may be dislodged during trauma, sudden muscular action, or a change in peripheral blood flow. In a few patients, pulmonary infarction (tissue death) may evolve from pulmonary embolism.

SIGNS AND SYMPTOMS
Total blockage of the main pulmonary artery is rapidly fatal; smaller or fragmented emboli produce signs and symptoms that vary with emboli size, number, and location.

Usually, the first symptom is dyspnea, which may be accompanied by chest pain. Other clinical features include tachycardia, productive cough, low-grade fever, and pleural effusion. Less common signs include massive hemoptysis, chest splinting, leg edema, cyanosis, syncope, and distended neck veins.

DIAGNOSTIC TESTS

The patient history is explored for factors that predispose a person to pulmonary embolism. To confirm diagnosis, a physical examination is combined with one or more of the following tests: chest X-ray, lung scan, pulmonary angiography, electrocardiography, and arterial blood gas measurement.

TREATMENT

Treatment aims to maintain adequate cardiovascular and pulmonary function as the obstruction resolves and to prevent recurrence of embolic episodes.

Oxygen and anticoagulants

Because most emboli resolve within 10 to 14 days, treatment consists of oxygen therapy, as needed, and anticoagulation with heparin to inhibit new thrombus formation.

Drug therapy

Patients with massive pulmonary embolism and shock may need fibrinolytic therapy with urokinase, streptokinase, or alteplase. Emboli that cause hypotension may call for vasopressors. Treatment for septic emboli involves antibiotics and evaluation for the infection's source.

Surgery

Inferior vena cava interruption is used for patients who can't receive anticoagulants, who experience recurrent emboli during anticoagulant therapy, or who have been treated with thrombolytic agents or pulmonary thromboendarterectomy. Surgery consists of vena caval liga-

---

Risk factors for pulmonary embolism

Predisposing factors for pulmonary embolism include:
- long-term immobility
- chronic pulmonary disease
- heart failure or atrial fibrillation
- thrombophlebitis
- thrombocytosis
- polycythemia vera
- autoimmune hemolytic anemia
- sickle cell disease
- varicose veins and vascular injury
- recent surgery
- advanced age
- pregnancy
- lower extremity fractures or surgery
- burns
- obesity
- cancer
- use of oral contraceptives.

---

tion, plication, or insertion of an umbrella filter to filter blood returning to the heart and lungs.

SPECIAL CONSIDERATIONS

 ACTION STAT: If the patient's breathing becomes severely compromised, be prepared to assist with endotracheal intubation and assisted ventilation.

- *Never* massage the patient's legs.

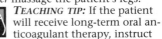 *TEACHING TIP:* If the patient will receive long-term oral anticoagulant therapy, instruct him to watch for signs of bleeding (bloody stools, blood in urine, large bruises), to take medication exactly as prescribed, and to avoid taking additional medications without consulting the doctor.

 PREVENTION: To help prevent pulmonary emboli, encourage early ambulation in patients at high risk for this condition.

Pulmonary hypertension

Pulmonary hypertension occurs when pulmonary artery pressure (PAP) rises above normal and is not attributable to the effects of aging or altitude. No definitive set of values is used to diagnose pulmonary hypertension, but the National Institutes of Health requires that the resting mean PAP measure 25 mm Hg or more.

Primary, or *idiopathic, pulmonary hypertension* is rare, occurring mostly in women between ages 20 and 40; pregnant women have the highest mortality. *Secondary pulmonary hypertension* results from existing cardiac or pulmonary disease. The prognosis depends on the severity of the underlying disorder.

CAUSES

Primary pulmonary hypertension begins as hypertrophy of the small pulmonary arteries. The muscle layers of these vessels thicken, decreasing distensibility and increasing resistance. The disorder then progresses to vascular sclerosis and obliteration of small vessels. Because this form of pulmonary hypertension is associated with collagen diseases, it's thought to result from altered immune mechanisms.

Usually, pulmonary hypertension arises secondary to hypoxemia from an underlying disease process, including:
• alveolar hypoventilation from chronic obstructive pulmonary disease, sarcoidosis, diffuse interstitial pneumonia, pulmonary metastasis, and certain other diseases such as scleroderma
• vascular obstruction from pulmonary embolism, vasculitis, and disorders that cause blockage of small or large pulmonary veins, such as left atrial myxoma, idiopathic venoocclusive disease, and mediastinal neoplasm
• primary cardiac disease, which may be congenital or acquired (Congenital defects that cause left-to-right shunting of blood, such as patent ductus arteriosus increase blood flow to the lungs and consequently raise pulmonary vascular pressure).

Acquired cardiac disease, such as rheumatic valvular disease and mitral stenosis, increases pulmonary venous pressure by restricting blood flow returning to the heart.

SIGNS AND SYMPTOMS

Most patients complain of increasing dyspnea on exertion, weakness, syncope, and fatigability. Many also show signs of right-sided heart failure, including peripheral edema, ascites, neck vein distention, and hepatomegaly. Other clinical effects vary with the underlying disorder.

DIAGNOSTIC TESTS

Diagnostic studies for pulmonary hypertension include arterial blood gas analysis, electrocardiography, cardiac catheterization (which shows increased PAP), pulmonary angiography, and pulmonary function tests.

TREATMENT

Treatment usually includes oxygen therapy to decrease hypoxemia and resulting pulmonary vascular resistance. For patients with right-sided heart failure, treatment also includes fluid restriction, digitalis glycosides to increase cardiac output, and diuretics to lower intravascular volume and extravascular fluid accumulation. The underling cause also must be corrected.

SPECIAL CONSIDERATIONS

 TEACHING TIP: Explain the limitations imposed by this disorder. Suggest ways for the patient to avoid overexertion such as frequent rest periods between activities. Provide instructions for obtaining and using special equipment such as oxygen equipment.

Pyelonephritis, acute

Acute pyelonephritis is a common inflammation caused by bacteria that primarily affects the interstitial area and the renal pelvis. With treatment

Who's at high risk for pyelonephritis?

Pyelonephritis occurs more commonly in females — probably because of a shorter urethra and proximity of the urinary meatus to the vagina and rectum. Both of these conditions allow bacteria to reach the bladder more easily. Also, females lack the antibacterial prostatic secretions produced by males.

Other high-risk groups

● Sexually active women are at increased risk due to bacterial contamination from intercourse.

● About 5% of pregnant women develop asymptomatic bacteriuria; if untreated, about 40% develop pyelonephritis.
● Diabetics with neurogenic bladder risk pyelonephritis because neurogenic bladder causes incomplete emptying and urinary stasis. Also, glycosuria may support bacterial growth in the urine.
● Patients with other renal diseases have an increased susceptibility because of compromised renal function.

and continued follow-up, the prognosis is good and extensive permanent damage is rare.

CAUSES

Acute pyelonephritis results from bacterial infection of the kidneys. Infecting bacteria usually are normal intestinal and fecal flora that grow readily in urine. The most common causative organism is *Escherichia coli.*

Typically, the infection spreads from the bladder to the ureters, then to the kidneys. Infection may also result from instrumentation (such as catheterization, cystoscopy, or urologic surgery), from a hematogenic infection (as in septicemia or endocarditis), or possibly from lymphatic infection.

Other causes of pyelonephritis include inability to empty the bladder (for example, from neurogenic bladder), urinary stasis, and urinary obstruction due to tumors, strictures, or benign prostatic hyperplasia.

Incidence of pyelonephritis increases with age and in certain groups. (See *Who's at high risk for pyelonephritis?*)

SIGNS AND SYMPTOMS

Typical clinical features include urgency, frequency, burning during urination, dysuria, nocturia, and hematuria. Urine may be cloudy, with a

fishy or ammonia-like odor. Other common signs and symptoms include a temperature of 102° F (38.9° C) or higher, shaking chills, flank pain, anorexia, and general fatigue.

Although these features may disappear within days, even without treatment, residual bacterial infection is likely and may cause later recurrence of symptoms.

DIAGNOSTIC TESTS

Diagnosis requires urinalysis and culture. Typical findings include pus, significant numbers of bacteria, a slightly alkaline urine pH and, possibly, some red blood cells.

A plain X-ray film of the kidneys, ureters, and bladder may reveal stones, tumors, or cysts in the kidneys and urinary tract. Excretory urography may show asymmetrical kidneys.

TREATMENT

Effective treatment centers on antibiotic therapy. When the infecting organism can't be identified, therapy usually consists of a broad-spectrum antibiotic, such as ampicillin or cephalexin. Urinary analgesics such as phenazopyridine are also appropriate.

Signs and symptoms may disappear after several days of antibiotic therapy. However, the course of such therapy is 10 to 14 days.

Follow-up treatment
Urine should be recultured 1 week after drug therapy stops, then periodically for the next year to detect residual or recurring infection. Most patients with uncomplicated infections respond well to therapy and don't suffer reinfection.

In infection from obstruction or vesicoureteral reflux, antibiotics may be less effective; surgery may then be necessary. Patients at high risk for recurring urinary tract and kidney infections require long-term follow-up.

SPECIAL CONSIDERATIONS
• Encourage high fluid intake to empty the bladder of contaminated urine. However, intake should not exceed 2 to 3 qt (2 to 3 L) because this may decrease antibiotic effectiveness.
• Stress the need to complete the entire course of antibiotic therapy, even after symptoms subside.

 TEACHING TIP: Teach patients with a history of urinary tract infections to recognize signs and symptoms of infection, such as cloudy urine, burning on urination, urgency, and frequency.

 PREVENTION: To prevent bacterial contamination, instruct females to wipe the perineum from front to back after defecation.

Raynaud's disease

Raynaud's disease is marked by episodic vasospasms in the small peripheral arteries and arterioles, brought on by exposure to cold or stress. The condition occurs bilaterally and usually affects the hands or, less commonly, the feet.

Raynaud's disease is most prevalent in women, particularly between puberty and age 40. A benign condition, it requires no specific treatment and has no serious consequences. In contrast, a different condition with a similar name — *Raynaud's phenomenon* — takes a progressive course. (See *Understanding Raynaud's phenomenon,* page 266.)

CAUSES

Although the cause of Raynaud's disease is unknown, several theories account for the reduced digital blood flow: intrinsic vascular wall hyperactivity to cold, increased vasomotor tone resulting from sympathetic stimulation, and antigen-antibody immune response.

SIGNS AND SYMPTOMS

After exposure to cold or stress, the skin on the fingers typically blanches, then becomes cyanotic before changing to red and before changing from cold to normal temperature. Numbness and tingling may also occur. Warmth relieves these symptoms.

In longstanding disease, trophic changes, such as sclerodactyly, ulcerations, or chronic paronychia, may occur. Although it's extremely uncommon, minimal cutaneous gangrene necessitates amputation of one or more phalanges.

DIAGNOSTIC TESTS

Signs and symptoms that establish Raynaud's disease include skin color changes on both hands or feet induced by cold or stress, normal arterial pulses, and a history of symptoms lasting longer than 2 years.

TREATMENT

Initially, treatment consists of avoidance of mechanical, chemical, or cold injury; smoking cessation; and reassurance that the condition is benign.

Because adverse drug effects may be more bothersome than the disease itself, drug therapy is reserved for patients with unusually severe symptoms. Such therapy may include phenoxybenzamine or reserpine.

When conservative treatment fails to prevent ischemic ulcers, sympathectomy may be helpful; fewer than one-quarter of all patients require this procedure.

SPECIAL CONSIDERATIONS

• Frequent skin inspections are important to prevent skin breakdown or infection.

 TEACHING TIP: Instruct the patient about ways to prevent discomfort, such as avoiding exposure to the cold, wearing mittens or gloves in cold weather or when handling cold items or defrosting the freezer, avoiding stressful situations, and stopping smoking.

Rectal polyps

Rectal polyps are masses of tissue that rise above the mucosal membrane and protrude into the GI tract. Types of rectal polyps include common polypoid adenomas, villous adenomas, hereditary polyposis, focal polypoid hyperplasia, and juvenile polyps (hamartomas).

Most rectal polyps are benign. However, villous and hereditary polyps show a marked inclination to be-

Understanding Raynaud's phenomenon

Don't confuse *Raynaud's disease* — a benign condition — with *Raynaud's phenomenon*. The latter is commonly associated with several connective tissue disorders, such as scleroderma, systemic lupus erythematosus, and polymyositis. What's more, it has a progressive course, leading to ischemia, gangrene, and amputation.

Differentiating the two disorders is difficult because some patients who experience mild symptoms of Raynaud's disease for several years may later develop overt connective tissue disease — most commonly scleroderma.

come malignant. Familial polyposis is commonly associated with rectosigmoid adenocarcinoma.

CAUSES
Predisposing factors for rectal polyps include heredity, age, infection, and diet. Polyp formation results from unrestrained cell growth in the upper epithelium.

SIGNS AND SYMPTOMS
Because rectal polyps usually don't cause symptoms, they are typically discovered incidentally during a digital examination or rectosigmoidoscopy. Rectal bleeding is a common sign: High rectal polyps leave a streak of blood on stools; low rectal polyps bleed freely.

Rectal polyps vary in appearance. (See *Comparing features of rectal polyps.*)

DIAGNOSTIC TESTS
Confirmation requires a colonoscopy and analysis of a biopsy specimen. A barium enema test can help identify polyps located high in the colon. Supportive laboratory findings include traces of blood in the stool, low hemoglobin level and low hematocrit (with anemia) and, possibly, serum electrolyte imbalances in patients with villous adenomas.

TREATMENT
Specific treatment varies with the type, size, and location of the polyps.

Common polypoid adenomas less than ⅜" (1 cm) in size require polypectomy, frequently by fulguration (destruction by high-frequency electricity) during endoscopy. For common polypoid adenomas over 1½" (4 cm) and all invasive villous adenomas, treatment usually consists of abdominoperineal resection or low anterior resection. A biopsy can obliterate focal polypoid hyperplasia.

Depending on GI involvement, hereditary polyps necessitate total abdominoperineal resection with a permanent ileostomy, subtotal colectomy with ileoproctostomy, or ileoanal anastomosis. Juvenile polyps are prone to autoamputation; if this doesn't occur, snare removal during colonoscopy is the treatment of choice.

SPECIAL CONSIDERATIONS
● After polyp removal, the patient should attempt to ambulate within 24 hours. Sitz baths can promote patient comfort.
● If the patient has benign polyps, stress the need for routine follow-up to check the polypoid growth rate.

Rectal prolapse

Rectal prolapse refers to the circumferential protrusion of one or more layers of the mucous membrane through the anus. Rectal prolapse may be complete (with anal sphincter displacement or bowel herniation) or partial (mucosal layer). (See *Two types of rectal prolapse,* page 268.)

The condition is most common in men under age 40, in women around age 45, and in children ages 1 to 3.

Comparing features of rectal polyps

The different types of rectal polyps vary in appearance.

Common polypoid adenomas

These small, multiple lesions are redder than normal mucosa. Typically attached to the rectal mucosa by a long, thin stalk, they have a red, lobular, or eroded surface.

Villous adenomas

These polyps are usually attached to the mucosa by a wide base. They vary in size from ¼" to 4¾" (0.5 to 12 cm). Soft, friable, and finely lobulated, they may grow large and cause painful defecation. However, because they're soft, they rarely cause bowel obstruction.

Sometimes adenomas prolapse outside the anus, expelling parts of the adenoma with the feces. These polyps may cause diarrhea, bloody stools, and subsequent fluid and electrolyte depletion, with hypotension and oliguria.

Hereditary polyposis

With this condition, rectal polyps resemble benign adenomas but occur as hundreds of small ¼" (0.5-cm) lesions carpeting the entire mucosal surface. Associated signs include diarrhea, bloody stools, and secondary anemia. In patients with hereditary polyposis, a change in bowel habits with abdominal pain usually signals rectosigmoid cancer.

Juvenile polyps

These large, inflammatory lesions commonly lack an epithelial covering. Mucus-filled cysts cover their usually smooth surface.

Focal polypoid hyperplasia

This condition produces small (less than ⅛" [3-mm]), granular, sessile lesions, similar in color to the colon, or gray or translucent. They usually occur at the rectosigmoid junction.

CAUSES

Several factors predispose a person to rectal prolapse, especially straining during defecation, which increases intra-abdominal pressure. Other predisposing factors include:
• conditions that affect the pelvic floor or rectum such as weak sphincter muscles
• weak longitudinal, rectal, or levator ani muscles resulting from neurologic disorders, injury, tumors, or aging
• chronic wasting diseases, such as tuberculosis and cystic fibrosis.

SIGNS AND SYMPTOMS

Protrusion of tissue from the rectum may occur during defecation or walking. Other indications include a persistent sensation of rectal fullness, bloody diarrhea, and pain in the lower abdomen (from ulceration). Hemorrhoids or rectal polyps may coexist with a prolapse.

DIAGNOSTIC TESTS

Clinical features and visual examination confirm the diagnosis. In complete prolapse, examination reveals the full thickness of the bowel wall and, possibly, the sphincter muscle protruding and mucosa falling into bulky, concentric folds.

In partial prolapse, examination reveals only partial mucosal protrusion and a smaller mass of radial mucosal folds. Straining during examination may disclose the full extent of prolapse.

TREATMENT

The underlying cause of rectal prolapse dictates treatment. Sometimes eliminating this condition is the only treatment necessary.

In a child, prolapsed tissue usually diminishes with age. In an older patient, injection of a sclerosing agent

PATHOPHYSIOLOGY

Two types of rectal prolapse

Partial rectal prolapse involves only the mucosa and a small mass of radial mucosal folds. However, in complete rectal prolapse, the full rectal wall, sphincter muscle, and a large mass of concentric mucosal folds protrude. Ulceration is possible after complete prolapse.

Partial prolapse

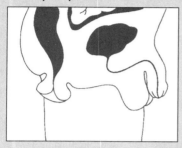

Complete prolapse

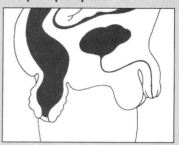

to cause a fibrotic reaction fixes the rectum in place.

Severe or chronic prolapse requires surgical repair by strengthening or tightening the sphincters with wire or by anterior or rectal resection of prolapsed tissue.

SPECIAL CONSIDERATIONS

• To prevent straining at defecation, which can lead to rectal prolapse, explain to the patient ways to avoid constipation, such as by eating a high-fiber diet, getting regular exercise, and using stool softeners.

• Advise the patient with severe prolapse and incontinence to wear a perineal pad.

TEACHING TIP: Teach the patient how to perform perineal strengthening exercises by lying down with his back flat on the mattress, and then pulling in the abdomen and squeezing while taking a deep breath. Or instruct him to repeatedly squeeze and relax his buttocks while sitting in a chair.

Renal calculi

Although renal calculi, or kidney stones, may form anywhere in the urinary tract, they usually develop in the renal pelvis or the calyces of the kidneys. Such formation follows precipitation of substances normally dissolved in the urine — calcium oxalate, calcium phosphate, magnesium ammonium phosphate or, occasionally, urate or cystine.

Renal calculi vary in size and may be solitary or multiple. They may remain in the renal pelvis or enter the ureter and damage the renal parenchyma; large calculi cause pressure necrosis. (See *Picturing renal calculi.*) In certain locations, calculi cause obstruction.

CAUSES

Although the cause of renal calculi is unknown, predisposing factors include dehydration, renal infection, urinary obstruction, and such metabolic factors as hyperparathyroidism, elevated uric acid, genetic defect in cystine metabolism, and excessive intake of vitamin D or dietary calcium.

SIGNS AND SYMPTOMS

Clinical effects vary with the size, location, and cause of the calculi. Pain, the key symptom, usually results from obstruction. Large, rough calculi block the ureter opening and increase the frequency and force of peristaltic contractions. The pain of classic renal colic travels from the costovertebral angle to the flank, to the suprapubic region and external genitalia.

Pain intensity fluctuates and may be excruciating at its peak. With calculi in the renal pelvis and calyces, pain may be more constant and dull. Nausea and vomiting usually accompany severe pain.

Other associated signs and symptoms include fever, chills, hematuria, abdominal distention, pyuria and, rarely, anuria.

DIAGNOSTIC TESTS

Diagnosis is based on clinical findings and various diagnostic tests. For instance, kidney-ureter-bladder X-rays reveal most kidney stones; kidney ultrasonography detects obstructions and changes.

Excretory urography confirms the diagnosis and determines calculi size and location. Calculus analysis shows the mineral content of calculi.

Urine culture of a midstream sample may indicate urinary tract infection. Urinalysis may be normal, or may show evidence of stone formation. A 24-hour urine collection may be evaluated to determine calcium, phosphorus, and uric acid excretion levels. Blood tests may show other imbalances and may indicate gout as the underlying cause.

TREATMENT

Treatment usually consists of measures to promote natural passage of calculi. Along with vigorous hydration, such treatment includes antimicrobial therapy for infection, analgesics such as meperidine for pain, and diuretics to prevent urinary stasis and further calculus formation.

PATHOPHYSIOLOGY
Picturing renal calculi

Multiple small calculi may vary in size. They may remain in the renal pelvis or pass down the ureter.

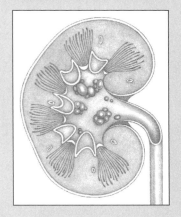

Calculi too large for natural passage may require surgical removal. For a calculus in the ureter, a cystoscope may be inserted through the urethra and the calculus manipulated with catheters or retrieval instruments. Extracting calculi from other areas may necessitate a flank or lower abdominal approach.

Percutaneous lithotripsy and extracorporeal shock wave lithotripsy shatter the calculus into fragments for removal by suction or natural passage.

SPECIAL CONSIDERATIONS

● To promote spontaneous passage of calculi, encourage the patient to walk, if possible. Also advise him to drink enough fluids to maintain a urine output of 3 to 4 qt (3 to 4 L)/day. Recommend fruit juices, particularly cranberry juice, to help acidify urine.

● Stress the importance of proper diet and compliance with therapy. For ex-

Understanding the causes of acute renal failure

Based on where the problem starts, acute renal failure is classified as prerenal, intrinsic, or postrenal.

Prerenal failure

Prerenal failure is caused by any condition that reduces blood flow to the kidneys. Such conditions include hypovolemia, shock, embolism, blood loss, sepsis, fluid pooling in ascites or burns, and cardiovascular disorders (such as heart failure, arrhythmias, and tamponade).

Intrinsic renal failure

Intrinsic renal failure results from damage to the kidneys themselves. The most common cause is acute

tubular necrosis. Such damage may also occur with acute poststreptococcal glomerulonephritis, systemic lupus erythematosus, periarteritis nodosa, vasculitis, sickle cell disease, bilateral renal vein thrombosis, nephrotoxins, ischemia, renal myeloma, and acute pyelonephritis.

Postrenal failure

Postrenal failure is caused by any condition that blocks urine flow from both kidneys. These conditions include kidney stones, blood clots, papillae from papillary necrosis, tumors, benign prostatic hyperplasia, strictures, and urethral edema from catheterization.

ample, if the patient's stone is caused by a hyperuricemic condition, advise him to avoid foods high in purine, such as sardines, herring, mussels, liver, kidney, and sweetbreads.

Renal failure, acute

Obstruction, reduced circulation, and renal parenchymal disease can all cause a sudden interruption in kidney function. Acute renal failure is usually reversible with medical treatment; otherwise, it may progress to end-stage renal disease, uremic syndrome, and death.

CAUSES

Acute renal failure can be classified as prerenal, intrinsic (or parenchymal), and postrenal. Each type has different causes. (See *Understanding the causes of acute renal failure.*)

SIGNS AND SYMPTOMS

Acute renal failure is a critical illness. Early signs are oliguria, azotemia and, rarely, anuria. Electrolyte imbalances, metabolic acidosis, and other severe effects follow as uremia worsens and

renal dysfunction disrupts other body systems:
- *GI* — anorexia, nausea, vomiting, diarrhea or constipation, stomatitis, bleeding, hematemesis, dry mucous membranes, uremic breath
- *Central nervous system (CNS)* — headache, drowsiness, irritability, confusion, peripheral neuropathy, seizures, coma
- *Skin* — dryness, pruritus, pallor, purpura, uremic frost (rare)
- *Cardiovascular* — early in the disease, hypotension; later, hypertension, arrhythmias, fluid overload, heart failure, systemic edema, anemia, altered clotting mechanisms
- *Respiratory* — Kussmaul's respirations, pulmonary edema.

Fever and chills indicate infection, a common complication.

DIAGNOSTIC TESTS

Diagnosis is based on patient history, with special attention to any previous disorders that might cause kidney failure. Blood and urine tests to check for specific evidence may confirm the diagnosis. Other studies include ultrasonography and X-ray studies of the kidneys, ureter, and bladder.

TREATMENT
Supportive measures include a diet high in calories and low in protein, sodium, and potassium, with supplemental vitamins and restricted fluids. Meticulous electrolyte monitoring is essential to detect hyperkalemia.

If hyperkalemia occurs, acute therapy may include dialysis, hypertonic glucose and insulin infusions, and sodium bicarbonate and sodium polystyrene sulfonate (to remove potassium from the body).

If these measures fail to control uremic symptoms, hemodialysis or peritoneal dialysis may be necessary.

SPECIAL CONSIDERATIONS
• Encourage the patient to adhere to the prescribed diet.
• A patient with acute renal failure is highly susceptible to infection. Personnel with upper respiratory tract infections shouldn't care for him.
• Add lubricating lotion to the patient's bath water to combat skin dryness.
• Provide good mouth care frequently for dry mucous membranes. If stomatitis occurs, the patient may need an antibiotic solution. Have him swish the solution around in his mouth before swallowing.
• If the patient requires hemodialysis, don't use the arm with the shunt or fistula for taking blood pressures or drawing blood.

Renal failure, chronic
Chronic renal failure usually results from a gradual loss of kidney function. Occasionally it follows rapid loss of kidney function. Few symptoms develop until more than 75% of the kidney's function is lost. Without treatment, unfiltered toxins in the blood damage all major organs.

CAUSES
Chronic renal failure may result from:
• chronic glomerular disease such as glomerulonephritis
• chronic infections, such as chronic pyelonephritis or tuberculosis
• congenital anomalies such as polycystic kidney disease
• vascular diseases, such as renal nephrosclerosis or hypertension
• obstructive processes such as renal calculi
• collagen diseases such as systemic lupus erythematosus
• nephrotoxic agents such as long-term aminoglycoside therapy
• endocrine diseases such as diabetic neuropathy.

These conditions gradually destroy the nephrons and eventually cause irreversible kidney failure. Similarly, acute renal failure that fails to respond to treatment becomes chronic renal failure.

SIGNS AND SYMPTOMS
Chronic renal failure affects all body systems. (See *Chronic renal failure: Effects on body systems,* page 272.)

DIAGNOSTIC TESTS
A history of chronic progressive debilitation and gradual deterioration of kidney function (as determined by creatinine clearance tests) leads to diagnosis of chronic renal failure. Blood studies, urine specific gravity, X-ray studies, and kidney biopsy aid diagnosis.

TREATMENT
Dietary therapy may correct specific signs and symptoms. A low-protein diet reduces production of end-products of protein metabolism that the kidneys can't excrete. (However, a patient on continuous peritoneal dialysis should maintain a high-protein diet.) The doctor also restricts dietary sodium and potassium.

Correction of fluid imbalance may be accomplished with fluid restriction and drugs that control blood pressure, swelling, nausea and vomiting, stomach irritation or constipation, and itchy skin. The patient may benefit from supplementary vitamins, especially B, D, and essential amino acids.

If the GI tract is affected, the patient may need regular stool analysis to detect blood and cleansing enemas

Chronic renal failure: Effects on body systems

The widespread effects of chronic renal failure include those described here.

Renal and urologic changes
- Hypotension, dry mouth, poor skin turgor, listlessness, fatigue, nausea and, later, somnolence and confusion
- Salt retention and overload
- Muscle irritability and, later, muscle weakness
- Fluid overload and metabolic acidosis
- Decreased urine output, with dilute urine containing casts and crystals

Cardiovascular changes
- Hypertension
- Arrhythmias
- Cardiomyopathy
- Uremic pericarditis
- Pericardial effusion with possible cardiac tamponade, heart failure, and peripheral edema

Respiratory changes
- Increased susceptibility to infection
- Pulmonary edema
- Pleuritic pain
- Pleural friction rub and effusions
- Uremic pleuritis and uremic lung

GI changes
- Inflammation and ulceration of GI mucosa causing stomatitis, gum ulceration and bleeding, esophagitis, gastritis, duodenal ulcers, bowel lesions, uremic colitis, pancreatitis, and proctitis
- Metallic taste in the mouth
- Ammonia breath odor
- Anorexia
- Nausea and vomiting

Cutaneous changes
- Pale, yellowish bronze, dry, scaly skin
- Severe itching
- Purpura
- Bruising
- Petechiae
- Uremic frost
- Thin, brittle fingernails with characteristic lines
- Dry, brittle hair that may change color and fall out easily

Neurologic changes
- Restless leg syndrome, leading to pain, burning, and itching in the legs and feet
- Muscle cramping and twitching
- Shortened memory and attention span
- Apathy, drowsiness, irritability, and confusion
- Coma
- Seizures
- Metabolic encephalopathy

Endocrine changes
- Stunted growth in children
- Infertility and decreased libido in both sexes
- Amenorrhea and cessation of menses in women
- Impotence and decreased sperm production in men
- Increased blood glucose levels

Hematopoietic changes
- Anemia and decreased red blood cell survival time
- Platelet defects
- Increased bleeding and clotting disorders

Skeletal changes
- Muscle and bone pain
- Bone loss
- Pathologic fractures
- Calcium deposits in the brain, eyes, gums, joints, myocardium, and blood vessels
- Arterial calcification, which may cause coronary artery disease
- Renal rickets in children

to remove blood. Anemia calls for iron and folate supplements; severe anemia may require transfusions. Hormone therapy may be used to increase red blood cell production.

Patients with end-stage renal failure may undergo hemodialysis or peritoneal dialysis to help control symptoms. However, anemia, nerve damage, and other complications may persist. Some patients with end-stage renal failure may eventually need a kidney transplant.

SPECIAL CONSIDERATIONS
• Good skin care and oral hygiene are important. Appropriate care may include daily baths using superfatted soaps, oatmeal baths, skin lotion to ease pruritus, padding of side rails to prevent ecchymoses, frequent turning, use of an egg-crate mattress, brushing the teeth often with a soft brush or sponge, and using mouthwash to minimize bad taste in the mouth.

 TEACHING TIP: Instruct the patient to eat high-calorie foods and avoid high-sodium and high-potassium foods. Suggest small, palatable meals. Emphasize the importance of adhering to fluid and protein restrictions.
• A patient undergoing dialysis is under a great deal of stress, as is his family. Refer them to appropriate counseling agencies.

Renal tubular acidosis

A syndrome of persistent dehydration, hyperchloremia, hypokalemia, metabolic acidosis, and nephrocalcinosis, renal tubular acidosis (RTA) results from the kidneys' inability to conserve bicarbonate. The disorder occurs as distal RTA (type 1, or classic RTA) or proximal RTA (type 2). The prognosis is usually good but depends on the severity of renal damage that precedes treatment.

CAUSES
Metabolic acidosis associated with RTA results from a defect in the kidneys' tubular acidification of urine.

Distal RTA
Type 1 RTA results from inability of the distal tubule to secrete hydrogen ions against established gradients across the tubular membrane. This results in decreased excretion of titratable acids and ammonium, increased loss of potassium and bicarbonate in the urine, and systemic acidosis.

Prolonged acidosis causes mobilization of calcium from bone and eventually hypercalciuria, setting the stage for renal calculi formation.

Distal RTA may be classified as primary or secondary. Primary distal RTA may occur sporadically or through a hereditary defect. Secondary distal RTA has been linked to many renal or systemic conditions, such as starvation, malnutrition, hepatic cirrhosis, and several genetically transmitted disorders.

Proximal RTA
Type 2 RTA results from defective bicarbonate reabsorption in the proximal tubule. This causes bicarbonate to flood the distal tubule and leads to impaired formation of titratable acids and ammonium for excretion. Ultimately, metabolic acidosis results.

SIGNS AND SYMPTOMS
In infants, RTA produces anorexia, vomiting, occasional fever, polyuria, dehydration, growth retardation, apathy, weakness, tissue wasting, constipation, nephrocalcinosis, and rickets.

In children and adults, RTA may lead to urinary tract infection, rickets, and growth problems. Possible complications include nephrocalcinosis and pyelonephritis.

DIAGNOSTIC TESTS
Demonstration of impaired urine acidification with systemic metabolic acidosis confirms distal RTA. Demonstration of bicarbonate wasting from impaired reabsorption confirms proximal RTA.

Other relevant laboratory test results show:
- decreased serum bicarbonate, pH, potassium, and phosphorus levels
- increased serum chloride and alkaline phosphatase levels
- alkaline pH; increased urinary bicarbonate and potassium levels, with low specific gravity.

In later stages, X-rays may show nephrocalcinosis.

TREATMENT

Supportive treatment involves replacement of substances being abnormally excreted, especially bicarbonate. It may include sodium bicarbonate tablets or Shohl's solution to control acidosis, oral potassium for dangerously low potassium levels, and vitamin D for bone disease. If pyelonephritis occurs, treatment may include antibiotics.

SPECIAL CONSIDERATIONS

 TEACHING TIP: Urge the patient to comply with all medication instructions. Teach him to report signs and symptoms of calculi (hematuria, low abdominal or flank pain) immediately.
- Advise the patient with low potassium levels to eat foods with a high potassium content, such as bananas, baked potatoes, and orange juice.
- Because RTA may be caused by a genetic defect, encourage family members to seek genetic counseling or screening for this disorder.

Renal vein thrombosis

Clotting in the renal vein results in renal congestion, engorgement and, possibly, infarction. Renal vein thrombosis may affect both kidneys and may occur in an acute or chronic form.

Chronic thrombosis usually impairs renal function, causing nephrotic syndrome. Abrupt onset of thrombosis that causes extensive damage may trigger rapidly fatal renal infarction.

If thrombosis affects both kidneys, the prognosis is poor. Less severe thrombosis that affects only one kidney or gradual progression that allows development of collateral circulation may preserve partial renal function.

CAUSES

Renal vein thrombosis commonly results from a tumor that blocks the renal vein. Other causes include thrombophlebitis of the inferior vena cava (such as from abdominal trauma) or of blood vessels of the legs, heart failure, and periarteritis. In infants, renal vein thrombosis usually follows diarrhea that causes severe dehydration.

Chronic renal vein thrombosis commonly arises as a complication of other glomerulopathic diseases, such as amyloidosis, systemic lupus erythematosus, diabetic nephropathy, and membranoproliferative glomerulonephritis.

SIGNS AND SYMPTOMS

Clinical features of renal vein thrombosis vary with the speed of onset.

Rapid onset of venous obstruction produces severe lumbar pain and tenderness in the epigastric region and costovertebral angle. Other typical features include fever, leukocytosis, pallor, hematuria, proteinuria, peripheral edema and, with bilateral obstruction, oliguria and other uremic signs. The kidneys enlarge and become easily palpable.

Gradual onset causes signs and symptoms of nephrotic syndrome. Pain is usually absent. Other clinical signs include proteinuria, hypoalbuminemia, and hyperlipemia.

Infants with this disease have enlarged kidneys, oliguria, and renal insufficiency that may progress to renal failure.

DIAGNOSTIC TESTS

Excretory urography provides reliable diagnostic evidence, showing enlarged kidneys with diminished excretory function. In chronic blockage, this study may show ureteral indentations. Renal arteriography and tissue biopsy confirm the diagnosis. Other tests may include urinalysis, blood studies, and venography.

TREATMENT

Gradual thrombosis that affects only one kidney responds best to treatment. Anticoagulant therapy may prove helpful.

Surgery must be performed within 24 hours of thrombosis, but even then has limited success because thrombi often extend into the small veins. Extensive intrarenal bleeding may necessitate nephrectomy.

Patients who survive abrupt thrombosis with extensive renal damage develop nephrotic syndrome and require treatment for renal failure, such as dialysis and, possibly, kidney transplantation. Some infants with renal vein thrombosis recover completely after heparin therapy or surgery; others suffer irreversible kidney damage.

SPECIAL CONSIDERATIONS

• During anticoagulant therapy, the patient is at risk for bleeding. Watch for such signs and symptoms as tachycardia, hypotension, hematuria, bleeding from the nose or gums, unusual bruises, petechiae, and black, tarry stools.
• Safety measures for the patient on maintenance warfarin therapy include using an electric razor and a soft toothbrush to avoid trauma; wearing a medical identification bracelet; and avoiding aspirin, which increases bleeding tendencies.

Renovascular hypertension

Renovascular hypertension refers to a rise in systemic blood pressure resulting from stenosis of the major renal arteries or their branches or from intrarenal atherosclerosis. The narrowing, or sclerosis, may be partial or complete; the resulting blood pressure elevation may be benign or malignant. (See *How renovascular hypertension develops,* page 276.)

Approximately 5% to 10% of patients with high blood pressure experience renovascular hypertension.

CAUSES

Atherosclerosis and fibromuscular diseases of the renal artery wall layers — are the primary causes in 95% of patients with renovascular hypertension. Other causes include arteritis, renal artery abnormalities, embolism, trauma, tumors, and dissecting aneurysm.

SIGNS AND SYMPTOMS

Besides elevated systemic blood pressure, renovascular hypertension usually produces signs and symptoms common to hypertensive states — headache, palpitations, tachycardia, anxiety, light-headedness, decreased tolerance of temperature extremes, retinopathy, and mental sluggishness.

Significant complications include heart failure, myocardial infarction, cerebrovascular accident and, occasionally, renal failure.

DIAGNOSTIC TESTS

Diagnosis requires a thorough patient history combined with isotopic renal blood flow scans and rapid-sequence excretory urography to identify abnormalities of renal blood flow and discrepancies of kidney size and shape.

Renal arteriography reveals the arterial stenosis or obstruction. Blood samples from the right and left renal veins are taken to compare plasma renin levels with those in the inferior vena cava. An increased renin level implicates the affected kidney and determines whether surgery can reverse hypertension.

TREATMENT

Surgery, the treatment of choice, aims to restore adequate circulation and control severe hypertension or severely impaired renal function. Procedures may include renal artery bypass, endarterectomy, arterioplasty or, as a last resort, nephrectomy.

Renal artery dilatation by balloon catheter is used in selected cases to correct renal artery stenosis without the risks of surgery. Symptomatic measures include antihypertensives, diuretics, and a sodium-restricted diet.

PATHOPHYSIOLOGY

How renovascular hypertension develops

In renovascular hypertension, stenosis or blockage of the renal artery stimulates the affected kidney to release the enzyme renin, which converts angiotensinogen — a plasma protein — to angiotensin I.

Fateful conversion
As angiotensin I circulates through the lungs and liver, it converts to angiotensin II. This causes peripheral vasoconstriction, increased arterial pressure and aldosterone secretion, and eventual hypertension.

SPECIAL CONSIDERATIONS

• Provide a quiet, stress-free environment, if possible. Urge the patient and family members to have regular blood pressure screenings.
• If a nephrectomy is necessary, reassure the patient that the remaining kidney is adequate for renal function.

TEACHING TIP: Educate the patient and family about the disorder and the importance of following prescribed treatment.

Respiratory acidosis

Respiratory acidosis is an acid-base disturbance marked by reduced alveolar ventilation and hypercapnia (partial pressure of arterial carbon dioxide [$PaCO_2$] greater than 45 mm Hg).

Respiratory acidosis can be acute (from a sudden failure in ventilation) or chronic (as in long-term pulmonary disease). The prognosis depends on the severity of the underlying disturbance and the patient's general clinical condition.

CAUSES

Several factors predispose a person to respiratory acidosis:
• Drugs, such as narcotics, anesthetics, hypnotics, and sedatives decrease sensitivity of the respiratory center.
• Central nervous system (CNS) trauma may impair ventilatory drive.
• In chronic metabolic alkalosis, the body attempts to normalize pH by decreasing alveolar ventilation.
• In some neuromuscular diseases (such as myasthenia gravis, Guillain-Barré syndrome, and poliomyelitis), weakened muscles make breathing more difficult, reducing alveolar ventilation.

In addition, respiratory acidosis can result from airway obstruction or parenchymal lung disease, which interferes with alveolar ventilation, or from chronic obstructive pulmonary disease (COPD), asthma, severe adult respiratory distress syndrome, chronic bronchitis, large pneumothorax, extensive pneumonia, or pulmonary edema.

Hypoventilation compromises excretion of carbon dioxide produced through metabolism. The retained carbon dioxide then combines with water to form an excess of carbonic acid, decreasing the blood pH. As a result, the concentration of hydrogen ions in body fluids, which directly reflects acidity, increases.

SIGNS AND SYMPTOMS

Acute respiratory acidosis produces CNS disturbances ranging from restlessness, confusion, and apprehension to somnolence, with a fine or flapping tremor (asterixis), or coma. The patient may complain of headaches and exhibit dyspnea and tachypnea with papilledema and depressed reflexes. Unless he's receiving oxygen, hypoxemia accompanies respiratory acidosis.

This disorder may also cause cardiovascular abnormalities, such as tachycardia, hypertension, arrhythmias and, in severe acidosis, hypotension with vasodilation (bounding pulses and warm periphery).

DIAGNOSTIC TESTS
The following arterial blood gas (ABG) levels confirm respiratory acidosis: a $PaCO_2$ above 45 mm Hg, pH usually below the normal range of 7.35 to 7.45, and a bicarbonate level that's normal in the acute stage but elevated in the chronic stage.

TREATMENT
Effective treatment aims to correct the underlying source of alveolar hypoventilation. Some patients may require mechanical ventilation until the underlying condition can be treated.

In COPD, treatment includes bronchodilators, oxygen, corticosteroids and, frequently, antibiotics. Drug therapy is used for conditions such as myasthenia gravis, antibiotics for pneumonia, and dialysis or charcoal to remove toxic drugs. Metabolic alkalosis is corrected.

SPECIAL CONSIDERATIONS
 PREVENTION: To help prevent respiratory acidosis, patients with COPD and chronic carbon dioxide retention should be monitored closely for evidence of acidosis. Also, a patient who has received general anesthetics should be instructed to turn, cough, and perform deep-breathing exercises frequently to prevent respiratory acidosis.

Respiratory alkalosis
Respiratory alkalosis is an acid-base disturbance caused by alveolar hyperventilation in which the partial pressure of arterial carbon dioxide ($PaCO_2$) drops below 35 mm Hg.

Uncomplicated respiratory alkalosis leads to a decrease in hydrogen ion concentration, which causes elevated blood pH. Hypocapnia occurs when the lungs eliminate carbon dioxide faster than cells produce it.

CAUSES
Respiratory alkalosis can result from pulmonary or nonpulmonary causes. Pulmonary causes include pneumonia, interstitial lung disease, pulmonary vascular disease, and acute asthma.

Nonpulmonary causes include anxiety, fever, aspirin toxicity, metabolic acidosis, central nervous system (CNS) disease (inflammation or tumor), sepsis, hepatic failure, and pregnancy.

SIGNS AND SYMPTOMS
The cardinal sign of respiratory alkalosis is deep, rapid breathing, possibly exceeding 40 breaths/minute. Such hyperventilation usually leads to CNS and neuromuscular disturbances, such as light-headedness or dizziness, agitation, circumoral and peripheral paresthesias, carpopedal spasms, twitching (possibly progressing to tetany), and muscle weakness. Severe respiratory alkalosis may cause arrhythmias that fail to respond to conventional treatment, seizures, or both.

DIAGNOSTIC TESTS
Arterial blood gas (ABG) analysis confirms respiratory alkalosis and rules out respiratory compensation for metabolic acidosis. Findings include a $PaCO_2$ level below 35 mm Hg, a pH value that's elevated in proportion to the fall in $PaCO_2$ during the acute stage but drops toward normal in the chronic stage, and a bicarbonate level that's normal in the acute stage but below normal in the chronic stage.

TREATMENT
The treatment goal is to eradicate the underlying condition — for example, by removing ingested toxins, correcting fever or sepsis, or treating CNS disease. In severe respiratory alkalosis, the patient may be instructed to breathe into a paper bag to relieve acute anxiety and increase carbon dioxide levels.

SPECIAL CONSIDERATIONS
• ABG and serum electrolyte values are monitored closely.
• Keep in mind that twitching and ar-

rhythmias may be associated with alkalemia and electrolyte imbalances.

Retinal detachment

Retinal detachment occurs when the layers of the retina become separated, creating a subretinal space. This space then fills with subretinal fluid. Retinal detachment usually involves only one eye, but may involve the other eye later.

Surgical reattachment is often successful. However, the prognosis for good vision depends on the area of the retina affected.

CAUSES

Any retinal tear or hole allows the liquid vitreous humor of the eye to seep between the retinal layers, separating the retina from its choroidal blood supply. In adults, retinal detachment usually results from degenerative changes of aging, which cause a spontaneous retinal hole.

Predisposing factors include myopia, cataract surgery, and trauma. Retinal detachment is twice as common in males.

Retinal detachment may also result from fluid seepage into the subretinal space (due to inflammation, tumors, or systemic diseases) or from traction placed on the retina by vitreous bands or membranes (from proliferative diabetic retinopathy, posterior uveitis, or a traumatic intraocular foreign body).

Retinal detachment is rare in children, but occasionally can result from retinopathy of prematurity, tumors (retinoblastomas), or trauma. It can also be inherited.

SIGNS AND SYMPTOMS

Initially, the patient may complain of seeing floating spots and recurrent flashes of light. As detachment progresses, gradual, painless vision loss may be described as a veil, curtain, or cobweb that eliminates part of the visual field.

DIAGNOSTIC TESTS

Ophthalmoscopy reveals a gray, opaque retina; in severe detachment, it reveals retinal folds and ballooning out of the area.

TREATMENT

Depending on the location and severity of the detachment, treatment may include restriction of eye movements and complete bed rest to prevent further detachment.

A hole in the peripheral retina can be treated with cryotherapy; in the posterior portion, with laser therapy. Retinal detachment usually requires scleral buckling to reattach the retina and, possibly, vitreous replacement with silicone, oil, air, or gas. (See *Scleral buckling: Two-step treatment for retinal detachment*.)

SPECIAL CONSIDERATIONS

● Provide emotional support; the patient may be upset due to vision loss.
● Postoperatively, the patient should lie on his back or unoperated side.
● Discourage activities that increase intraocular pressure, such as straining during defecation, bending down, hard coughing, sneezing, and vomiting or other activities in which the eye can be bumped or injured.

 TEACHING TIP: Instruct the patient in proper instillation of eyedrops, and emphasize compliance and follow-up care.

Rheumatic fever and rheumatic heart disease

Acute rheumatic fever is a systemic inflammatory disease of childhood that follows a streptococcal infection. Rheumatic heart disease refers to the cardiac effects of rheumatic fever, and includes pancarditis (myocarditis, pericarditis, and endocarditis) during the early acute phase and chronic valvular disease later.

Long-term antibiotic therapy can minimize recurrence of rheumatic fever, reducing the risk of permanent cardiac damage and eventual valvular deformity. However, severe pancardi-

Scleral buckling: Two-step treatment for retinal detachment

Surgical treatment for a detached retina is a two-step process. First the surgeon repairs the retinal hole or tear; then he reattaches the retina.

Repairing the retinal hole or tear
Using cryotherapy, photocoagulation, or diathermy, the surgeon creates a sterile inflammatory reaction that seals the retinal hole or tear and achieves retinal readherence.

Reattaching the retina
The surgeon then performs scleral buckling, which applies external pressure to the separated retinal lay-

ers to reunite the retina with its blood supply.

First, the surgeon severs the superior rectus muscles. This allows him to place an explant (a silicone plate or sponge) over the readherence site. A circling band keeps the explant in place. Pressure exerted on the explant indents, or "buckles," the eyeball, gently pushing the choroid and retina closer together.

This reunites the retina with its blood supply and prevents vitreous humor from seeping between the detached retinal layers. (Seepage could lead to further detachment and possible blindness.)

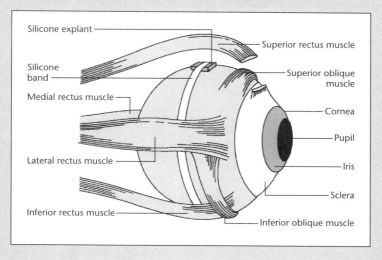

tis occasionally produces fatal heart failure during the acute phase.

CAUSES
Rheumatic fever appears to be a reaction to a streptococcal infection, in which antibodies manufactured to combat streptococci react and produce lesions at specific tissue sites — especially in the heart and joints. Altered

host resistance seems to be involved in its development or recurrence.

SIGNS AND SYMPTOMS
In 95% of cases, rheumatic fever occurs within a few days to 6 weeks of an initial streptococcal infection. Body temperature rises to at least 100.4° F (38° C), and most patients complain of pain, swelling, and red-

PATHOPHYSIOLOGY

Valvular vegetations in rheumatic fever

Rheumatic fever may lead to inflamed mitral valve leaflets, with a thin line of vegetations along the delicate leaflet edges. These vegetations form when fibrin and platelets build up on the damaged valve surface.

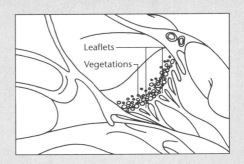

ness in the knees, ankles, elbows, or hips (polyarthritis). In about 5% of cases, rheumatic fever causes a nonirritating rash that gives rise to red lesions with blanched centers.

Later, rheumatic fever may cause transient chorea (involuntary body movements).

The most destructive effect of rheumatic fever is carditis, which develops in up to 50% of affected patients. Pericarditis may cause pain. Myocarditis leads to formation of a progressively fibrotic nodule and interstitial scars. Endocarditis causes valve leaflets to swell and erode along their edges and leads to formation of beadlike vegetations composed of platelet and fibrin deposits. (See *Valvular vegetations in rheumatic fever.*) Severe carditis may cause heart failure.

DIAGNOSTIC TESTS
Identification of one or more of the classic signs (carditis, polyarthritis, chorea, erythema marginatum, or subcutaneous nodules) and a detailed patient history allow diagnosis. Laboratory tests, including a white blood cell count, C-reactive protein, antistreptolysin O titer, and cardiac enzyme measurements, support the diagnosis. Echocardiography helps

evaluate valvular damage, chamber size, and ventricular function.

TREATMENT
Effective management eradicates the streptococcal infection, relieves symptoms, and prevents recurrence, reducing the chance of permanent heart damage.

During the acute phase, the doctor typically prescribes penicillin or (for patients with penicillin hypersensitivity) erythromycin. Salicylates, such as aspirin, relieve fever and minimize joint swelling and pain. If carditis is present or salicylates fail to relieve pain and inflammation, corticosteroids may be used.

Supportive treatment includes strict bed rest for about 5 weeks during the acute phase with active carditis, followed by a progressive increase in physical activity.

After the acute phase subsides, the patient typically receives a monthly I.M. injection of penicillin G benzathine or daily doses of oral sulfadiazine or penicillin G to prevent recurrence. Usually, such preventive treatment continues for 5 to 10 years.

Surgery and other measures
Heart failure necessitates continued bed rest and diuretics. Severe mitral

or aortic valvular dysfunction causing persistent heart failure warrants corrective valvular surgery (commissurotomy, valvuloplasty, or valve replacement).

SPECIAL CONSIDERATIONS

 TEACHING TIP: Stress the need for bed rest during the acute phase. If the child is receiving penicillin, tell the parents to immediately report rash, fever, or chills.

• After the acute phase, encourage family and friends to spend as much time as possible with the child to minimize boredom.

• Make sure the child and family understand the importance of complying with prolonged antibiotic therapy and follow-up care and for receiving additional antibiotics during dental surgery.

Rheumatoid arthritis

A chronic, systemic, inflammatory disease, rheumatoid arthritis (RA) primarily attacks peripheral joints and surrounding muscles, tendons, ligaments, and blood vessels. Spontaneous remissions and unpredictable exacerbations mark the course of this potentially crippling disease.

In most patients, RA follows an intermittent course and allows normal activity, although 10% suffer total disability. The prognosis worsens with development of nodules, vasculitis, and high titers of rheumatoid factor (RF).

CAUSES

What causes the chronic inflammation seen in RA isn't known, but various theories point to infectious, genetic, and endocrine factors. Currently, it's believed that a genetically susceptible individual develops abnormal or altered immunoglobulin G (IgG) antibodies when exposed to an antigen. This altered IgG antibody isn't recognized as "self," and the individual forms an antibody against it — RF. By aggregating into complexes, RF generates inflammation.

SIGNS AND SYMPTOMS

RA usually develops insidiously and initially produces nonspecific symptoms — fatigue, malaise, anorexia, persistent low-grade fever, weight loss, lymphadenopathy, and vague joint symptoms.

As the disease progresses, more specific localized joint symptoms develop, frequently in the fingers at the proximal interphalangeal (PIP), metacarpophalangeal (MCP), and metatarsophalangeal joints. These symptoms may extend to the wrists, knees, elbows, and ankles. Affected joints stiffen after inactivity, especially on rising in the morning.

Fingers may assume a spindle shape. Joints become tender and painful and may feel hot to the touch. Ultimately, joint function diminishes. If active disease continues, deformities are common. The fingers may become fixed in a characteristic "swan's neck" appearance or "boutonniere" deformity. The hands appear foreshortened.

Many patients also develop extra-articular signs. (See *Extra-articular findings in rheumatoid arthritis*, page 282.)

DIAGNOSTIC TESTS

Typical clinical features suggest RA, but a firm diagnosis relies on laboratory and other test results, including blood tests (such as white blood cell count and erythrocyte sedimentation rate), synovial fluid analysis, and X-rays. The RF titer is positive in 75% to 80% of patients.

TREATMENT

Salicylates are the mainstay of RA therapy because they decrease inflammation and relieve joint pain. Other useful medications include nonsteroidal anti-inflammatory drugs (such as indomethacin, fenoprofen, and ibuprofen), antimalarials (hydroxychloroquine), gold salts, penicillamine, and corticosteroids (prednisone).

Immunosuppressants, such as cyclophosphamide, methotrexate, and azathioprine, are also therapeutic.

Extra-articular findings in rheumatoid arthritis

The effects of rheumatoid arthritis aren't limited to the joints. The most common extra-articular finding is the gradual appearance of rheumatoid nodules — subcutaneous, round or oval, nontender masses. They usually appear on the elbows and other pressure areas.

Vasculitis can lead to skin lesions, leg ulcers, and multiple systemic complications. Peripheral neuropathy may produce numbness or tingling in the feet or weakness and sensation loss in the fingers. The muscles may become stiff, weak, or painful.

Other common extra-articular effects include pericarditis, pulmonary nodules or fibrosis, pleuritis, scleritis, and episcleritis.

They're being used more commonly in early disease.

Supportive measures include 8 to 10 hours of sleep every night, frequent rest periods between activities, and splinting to rest inflamed joints. A physical therapy program, including range-of-motion exercises and carefully individualized therapeutic exercises, forestalls loss of joint function.

Heat application relaxes muscles and relieves pain. Moist heat usually works best for patients with chronic disease. Ice packs are effective during acute episodes.

Treatment in advanced disease

Advanced disease may require synovectomy, joint reconstruction, or total joint arthroplasty. Useful surgical procedures include metatarsal head and distal ulnar resectional arthroplasty, insertion of a prosthesis between MCP and PIP joints, and arthrodesis (joint fusion).

SPECIAL CONSIDERATIONS

● Tell the patient that a balanced diet is important but special diets won't cure RA. Stress the need for weight control, because obesity further stresses the joints.
● Urge the patient to perform activities of daily living, such as dressing and feeding himself. Recommend using easy-to-open cartons, lightweight cups, and unpackaged silverware.
● Encourage the patient to exercise. Exercise continued over a prolonged period can reduce pain and increase muscle strength and flexibility. Studies also show that exercise can ease depression.

 TEACHING TIP: Teach the patient how to stand, walk, and sit correctly: upright and erect. Chairs with high seats and armrests make it easier for the patient to rise. Suggest ways to conserve energy, such as pacing activities, resting for 5 to 10 minutes of each hour, and getting adequate sleep in the correct sleeping posture.

Instruct the patient to avoid putting undue stress on joints and to use the largest joint available for a given task. When performing any activity, he should support weak or painful joints as much as possible; avoid positions of flexion and promote positions of extension; hold objects parallel to the knuckles as briefly as possible; and slide — not lift — objects whenever possible.
● Inform the patient that RA is a chronic disease with no miracle cures, despite claims to the contrary.

Salmonellosis

A common infection in the United States, salmonellosis is caused by gram-negative bacilli of the genus *Salmonella,* a member of the Enterobacteriaceae family. It occurs as enterocolitis, bacteremia, localized infection, typhoid, or paratyphoid fever. Nontyphoidal forms usually produce mild to moderate illness with low mortality.

Typhoid, the most severe form of salmonellosis, usually lasts 1 to 4 weeks. Mortality is about 3% in persons who are treated and 10% in those untreated.

A typhoid attack confers lifelong immunity, although the patient may become a carrier.

Enterocolitis and bacteremia are common among infants, elderly people, and people already weakened by other infections. Salmonellosis occurs 20 times more commonly in patients with acquired immunodeficiency syndrome.

CAUSES

Of an estimated 1,700 serotypes of *Salmonella,* 10 cause the diseases most common in the United States; all 10 can survive for weeks in water, ice, sewage, or food. Nontyphoidal salmonellosis generally follows ingestion of contaminated or inadequately processed foods; proper cooking reduces the risk.

Other causes include contact with infected people or animals and ingestion of contaminated dry milk, chocolate bars, or drugs of animal origin. Salmonellosis may occur in children under age 5 from fecal-oral spread.

Typhoid results most commonly from drinking water contaminated by excretions of a carrier.

SIGNS AND SYMPTOMS

Clinical features vary but usually include fever, abdominal pain, and severe diarrhea with enterocolitis. Headache, increasing fever, and constipation are more common with typhoidal infection.

DIAGNOSTIC TESTS

Generally, diagnosis depends on isolating the organism in a culture, particularly blood (in typhoid, paratyphoid, and bacteremia) or feces (in enterocolitis, paratyphoid, and typhoid).

TREATMENT

Antimicrobial therapy for typhoid, paratyphoid, and bacteremia depends on the organism's sensitivity. It may include amoxicillin, chloramphenicol and, in severely toxemic patients, co-trimoxazole, ciprofloxacin, or ceftriaxone. Localized abscesses may call for surgical drainage.

Enterocolitis requires a short course of antibiotics only if it causes septicemia or prolonged fever. Other treatments include bed rest and replacement of fluids and electrolytes. Camphorated opium tincture, kaolin with pectin, diphenoxylate, codeine, or small morphine doses may relieve diarrhea and control cramps in patients who must remain active.

SPECIAL CONSIDERATIONS

• Follow enteric precautions. Wash your hands thoroughly before and after contact with the patient. Teach the patient to use proper hand-washing technique, especially after defecating and before eating or handling food. Wear gloves and a gown when disposing of feces or fecally contaminated objects.
• During acute infection, use safety measures because the patient may become delirious.

• Provide comfort measures, such as good skin and mouth care, frequent turning, mild passive exercises, and application of mild heat to the abdomen to relieve cramps.

 TEACHING TIP: If the patient has positive stool cultures on discharge, instruct him to use a different bathroom than other family members, if possible (during antibiotic therapy); to wash his hands thoroughly; and to avoid preparing uncooked foods for family members.

 PREVENTION: To help prevent salmonellosis, recommend prompt refrigeration of meat and cooked foods and teach the importance of proper hand washing. Advise those at high risk of contracting typhoid (laboratory workers, travelers) to seek vaccination.

Sarcoidosis

Sarcoidosis is a multisystemic, granulomatous disorder that causes lymphadenopathy, pulmonary infiltration, and skeletal, liver, eye, or skin lesions. It occurs mostly in young adults.

Acute sarcoidosis usually resolves within 2 years. Chronic, progressive sarcoidosis (rare) is associated with pulmonary fibrosis and progressive pulmonary disability.

CAUSES

Although the cause of sarcoidosis is unknown, the following possible causes have been considered:
• hypersensitivity response to such agents as atypical mycobacteria, fungi, and pine pollen
• genetic predisposition (suggested by a slightly higher incidence of sarcoidosis within the same family)
• chemicals, such as zirconium or beryllium, which can lead to illnesses resembling sarcoidosis, suggesting an extrinsic cause for this disease.

SIGNS AND SYMPTOMS

Initial signs include arthralgia, fatigue, malaise, and weight loss. Other clinical features vary with the extent and location of fibrosis. (See *Other signs and symptoms of sarcoidosis.*)

DIAGNOSTIC TESTS

Typical clinical features with appropriate laboratory data and X-ray findings suggest sarcoidosis. An abnormal Kveim-Siltzbach skin test result supports the diagnosis.

Other relevant diagnostic tests include chest X-ray, pulmonary function tests, blood tests (such as serum calcium), arterial blood gas studies, and lymph node, skin, or lung biopsy. A negative tuberculin skin test reaction, fungal serologies, sputum cultures for mycobacteria and fungi, and negative biopsy cultures help rule out infection.

TREATMENT

Asymptomatic sarcoidosis requires no treatment. Sarcoidosis that causes ocular, respiratory, central nervous system, cardiac, or systemic symptoms (such as fever and weight loss) requires treatment with systemic or topical steroids, as does sarcoidosis that produces hypercalcemia or destructive skin lesions. Such therapy usually continues for 1 to 2 years, but some patients may need lifelong therapy.

Other treatment includes a low-calcium diet and avoidance of direct exposure to sunlight in patients with hypercalcemia.

SPECIAL CONSIDERATIONS

• The patient requires a nutritious, high-calorie diet and plenty of fluids. If he has hypercalcemia, suggest a low-calcium diet.
• Remind the patient on long-term or high-dose steroid therapy that he is vulnerable to infection.

 TEACHING TIP: Stress the need for compliance with prescribed steroid therapy and regular, careful follow-up examinations and treatment.

• Refer the patient with failing vision to community support and resource groups and the American Foundation for the Blind, if necessary.

Other signs and symptoms of sarcoidosis

Besides joint aches and systemic features, such as fatigue and malaise, a patient with sarcoidosis may have these additional signs and symptoms.

Respiratory features
- Breathlessness
- Cough (usually nonproductive)
- Substernal pain
- Complications such as pulmonary hypertension and cor pulmonale (in advanced pulmonary disease)

Skin features
- Erythema nodosum
- Subcutaneous skin nodules with maculopapular eruptions
- Extensive nasal mucosal lesions

Ophthalmic features
- Anterior uveitis (common)
- Glaucoma or blindness (rare)

Musculoskeletal features
- Muscle weakness

- Polyarthralgia
- Pain
- Punched-out lesions on phalanges

Cardiovascular features
- Arrhythmias (premature beats, bundle-branch heart block, or complete heart block)
- Cardiomyopathy (rare)

Central nervous system features
- Cranial or peripheral nerve palsies
- Basilar meningitis
- Seizures
- Pituitary and hypothalamic lesions, producing diabetes insipidus

Other features
- Granulomatous hepatitis
- Hypercalciuria
- Bilateral hilar and right paratracheal lymphadenopathy and splenomegaly

Scabies

An age-old skin infection, scabies results from infestation with *Sarcoptes scabiei* var. *hominis* (itch mite), which provokes a sensitivity reaction. The infection occurs worldwide, is predisposed by overcrowding and poor hygiene, and can be endemic.

CAUSES

Mites can live their entire life cycles in the skin of humans, causing chronic infection. The female mite burrows into the skin to lay her eggs, from which larvae emerge to copulate and then reburrow under the skin.

Transmission of scabies occurs through skin or sexual contact. The adult mite can survive without a human host for only 2 or 3 days.

SIGNS AND SYMPTOMS

Typically, scabies causes itching that intensifies at night. Characteristic lesions are usually excoriated and may appear as erythematous nodules.

These threadlike lesions are approximately ⅜" long and generally occur between fingers, on flexor surfaces of the wrists, on elbows, in axillary folds, at the waistline, on nipples in females, and on genitalia in males. In infants, the burrows (lesions) may appear on the head and neck.

Intense scratching can lead to severe excoriation and secondary bacterial infection. Itching may become generalized secondary to sensitization.

DIAGNOSTIC TESTS

Visual examination of the contents of the scabietic burrow may reveal the itch mite. If not, a drop of miner-

Teaching patients about scabies treatment

If the doctor prescribes permethrin or lindane treatment for your patient, provide the following instructions:

• Apply permethrin or lindane cream from the neck down, making sure it covers the entire body. Wait 15 minutes before dressing, and avoid bathing for 8 to 12 hours.

• Wash contaminated clothing and linens in hot water, or have them dry-cleaned.

• Don't apply lindane cream if the skin is raw or inflamed. Immediately report any skin irritation or hypersensitivity reaction; then discontinue using the drug, and wash it off thoroughly.

al oil placed over the burrow, followed by superficial scraping and examination of expressed material under a low-power microscope, may reveal ova or mite feces. However, excoriation or inflammation of the burrow often makes such identification difficult.

If diagnostic tests offer no positive identification of the mite and if scabies is still suspected (for example, close contacts of the patient also report itching), skin clearing after a therapeutic trial of a pediculicide confirms the diagnosis.

TREATMENT

Generally, treatment of scabies consists of application of a pediculicide — permethrin or lindane cream — in a thin layer over the entire skin surface. The pediculicide is left on for 8 to 12 hours. (See *Teaching patients about scabies treatment*.) To make sure that all areas have been treated, this application should be repeated in approximately 1 week. Another pediculicide,

crotamiton cream, may be applied on 4 consecutive nights.

Approximately 10% of a pediculicide is absorbed systemically; therefore, a 6% to 10% solution of sulfur, which is less toxic, applied for 3 consecutive days is an alternative therapy for infants and pregnant women. Widespread bacterial infections call for systemic antibiotics.

Persistent pruritus (from mite sensitization or contact dermatitis) may develop from repeated use of pediculicides rather than from continued infection. An antipruritic emollient or topical steroid can reduce itching; intralesional steroids may resolve erythematous nodules.

SPECIAL CONSIDERATIONS

• Family members and other close contacts of the patient should be checked for possible symptoms.

 PREVENTION: If a hospitalized patient has scabies, measures must be taken to prevent transmission to other patients. For instance, staff must practice good hand-washing technique or wear gloves when touching the patient, observe wound and skin precautions for 24 hours after treatment with a pediculicide, gas autoclave blood pressure cuffs before using them on other patients, isolate linens until the patient is noninfectious, and thoroughly disinfect the patient's room after discharge.

Scoliosis

Scoliosis, a lateral curvature of the spine, may be found in the thoracic, lumbar, or thoracolumbar spinal segment. The curve may be convex to the right (more common in thoracic curves) or to the left (more common in lumbar curves). Rotation of the vertebral column around its axis occurs and may cause rib cage deformity. Scoliosis is often associated with kyphosis (humpback) and lordosis (swayback).

CAUSES

Scoliosis may be functional or structural. Functional (postural) scoliosis usually results from poor posture or a discrepancy in leg lengths, not fixed deformity of the spinal column. In structural scoliosis, curvature results from a deformity of the vertebral bodies.

Structural scoliosis may occur in one of four types. (See *Types of structural scoliosis*.)

SIGNS AND SYMPTOMS
The most common curve in functional or structural scoliosis arises in the thoracic segment, with convexity to the right, and compensatory curves (S curves) in the cervical segment above and the lumbar segment below — both with convexity to the left. As the spine curves laterally, compensatory curves develop to maintain body balance and mark the deformity.

Scoliosis rarely produces subjective symptoms until it's well established. When symptoms do occur, they include backache, fatigue, and dyspnea. Because many teenagers are shy about their bodies, their parents may suspect something is wrong only after they notice uneven hemlines, pantlegs that appear unequal in length, or subtle physical signs, such as one hip appearing higher than the other.

Untreated scoliosis may result in pulmonary insufficiency (the curvature may decrease lung capacity), back pain, degenerative arthritis of the spine, disk disease, and sciatica.

DIAGNOSTIC TESTS
Anterior, posterior, and lateral spinal X-rays, taken with the patient standing upright and bending, confirm scoliosis and determine the degree of curvature (Cobb method) and flexibility of the spine. A scoliometer can also be used to measure the angle of trunk rotation.

A physical examination reveals unequal shoulder heights, elbow levels, and heights of the iliac crests. Muscles on the convex side of the curve may be rounded; those on the concave side, flattened, producing asymmetry of paraspinal muscles.

Types of structural scoliosis

Structural scoliosis occurs as congenital scoliosis, paralytic or musculoskeletal scoliosis, and idiopathic scoliosis.

Congenital scoliosis
Congenital scoliosis is usually related to a congenital defect, such as wedge vertebrae, fused ribs or vertebrae, or hemivertebrae.

Paralytic or musculoskeletal scoliosis
Paralytic or musculoskeletal scoliosis develops several months after asymmetric paralysis of the trunk muscles from polio, cerebral palsy, or muscular dystrophy.

Idiopathic scoliosis
The most common form of scoliosis, idiopathic scoliosis may be transmitted as an autosomal dominant or multifactorial trait. It appears in a previously straight spine during the growing years.

Idiopathic scoliosis can be classified as:
• *infantile,* which affects mostly male infants between birth and age 3 and causes left thoracic and right lumbar curves
• *juvenile,* which affects both sexes between ages 4 and 10 and causes varying types of curvature
• *adolescent,* which generally affects girls between age 10 and achievement of skeletal maturity and causes varying types of curvature.

TREATMENT
The severity of the deformity and potential spine growth determine appropriate treatment, which may include such noninvasive measures as close observation, exercise, or a brace. For a more serious deformity,

surgery or a combination of methods may be needed. To be most effective, treatment should begin early, when spinal deformity is still subtle.

Noninvasive measures

A curve of less than 25 degrees is mild and can be monitored by X-rays and an examination every 3 months. An exercise program that includes sit-ups, pelvic tilts, spine hyperextension, pushups, and breathing exercises may strengthen torso muscles and prevent curve progression. A heel lift may also help.

A curve of 30 to 50 degrees requires management with spinal exercises and a brace. (Transcutaneous electrical nerve stimulation may be used as an alternative.)

A brace halts progression in most patients but doesn't reverse the established curvature. Such devices passively strengthen the patient's spine by applying asymmetric pressure to the skin, muscles, and ribs. Braces can be adjusted as the patient grows and can be worn until bone growth is complete.

Surgery

A curve of 40 degrees or more requires surgery (spinal fusion with instrumentation), because a lateral curve continues to progress at the rate of 1 degree a year even after skeletal maturity.

Some surgeons prescribe Cotrel dynamic traction for 7 to 10 days for preoperative preparation. This traction consists of a belt-pulley-weight system. While in traction, the patient should exercise for 10 minutes every hour, increasing muscle strength while keeping the vertebral column immobile.

Surgery corrects lateral curvature by posterior spinal fusion and internal stabilization with a Harrington rod. A distraction rod on the concave side of the curve "jacks" the spine into a straight position and provides an internal splint. A Cotrel-Dubousset rod system may also be used.

An alternative procedure, anterior spinal fusion with Dwyer or Zielke instrumentation, corrects curvature with vertebral staples and an anterior stabilizing cable. Some spinal fusions may require postoperative immobilization in a brace.

Postoperatively, periodic checkups are required for several months to monitor stability of the correction.

SPECIAL CONSIDERATIONS

• Keep in mind that scoliosis often affects adolescent girls, who are likely to find activity limitations and treatment with orthopedic appliances distressing. Be sure to provide emotional support, along with meticulous skin and cast care and patient teaching.
• A patient who needs a brace requires thorough teaching. (See *What to tell the patient about a brace*.)

If the patient needs traction or a cast before surgery:
• These procedures should be explained to the patient and family. Remember that application of a body cast can be traumatic, because it's done on a special frame and the patient's head and face are covered throughout the procedure.
• The cast must be kept clean and dry and its edges must be "petaled" (padded). The skin around the cast edge should be checked daily.
• Warn the patient not to insert anything under the cast or let anything get under it and to immediately report cracks in the cast, pain, burning, skin breakdown, numbness, or odor.

After corrective surgery:
• Encourage deep-breathing exercises to avoid pulmonary complications.
• Promote active range-of-motion (ROM) arm exercises to help maintain muscle strength. Inform the patient that any exercise, even brushing the hair or teeth, is helpful. Encourage her to perform quadriceps-setting, calf-pumping and active ROM exercises of the ankles and feet.
• Offer emotional support to help prevent depression, which may result from altered body image and immo-

What to tell the patient about a brace

A patient who must wear a brace to treat scoliosis requires the help of a physical therapist, a social worker, and an orthopedic appliance specialist (orthotist). Before she goes home, the staff must make sure she and her family understand what the brace does and how to care for it. Follow the patient-teaching guidelines below.

• Show the patient how to check the screws for tightness and pad the uprights to prevent excessive wear on clothing.

• Suggest that the patient wear loose-fitting, oversized clothes for greater comfort.

• Tell her to wear the brace 23 hours a day and to remove it only for bathing and exercise. While she's still adjusting to the brace, tell her to lie down and rest several times a day.

• Advise the patient to use a soft mattress if a firm one is uncomfortable.

• To prevent skin breakdown, caution the patient not to use lotions, ointments, or powders on areas where the brace contacts the skin. Instead, suggest that she use rubbing alcohol or tincture of benzoin to toughen the skin. Tell her to keep the skin dry and clean and to wear a snug T-shirt under the brace.

• Instruct the patient to increase activities gradually and to avoid strenuous sports. Emphasize the importance of conscientiously performing prescribed exercises. Recommend swimming during the 1 hour out of the brace — but strongly warn against diving.

• Tell the patient to turn her whole body, instead of just her head, when looking to the side. To make reading easier, instruct her to hold the book so she can look straight ahead at it instead of down. If she finds this difficult, help her to obtain prism glasses.

bility. Encourage the patient to wear her own clothes, wash her hair, and use makeup.

• If the patient is being discharged with a Harrington rod and cast and must have bed rest, staff should arrange for a social worker and a visiting nurse to provide home care.

Severe combined immunodeficiency disease

In severe combined immunodeficiency disease (SCID), both cell-mediated (T-cell) and humoral (B-cell) immunity are deficient or absent. This causes susceptibility to infection from all classes of microorganisms during infancy.

SCID occurs in at least three types — reticular dysgenesis (most severe), Swiss type agammaglobulinemia, and enzyme deficiency (such as adenosine deaminase (ADA) deficiency).

The estimated incidence of SCID is 1 in every 100,000 to 500,000 births. Most untreated patients die from infection within 1 year of birth.

CAUSES

SCID is usually transmitted as an autosomal recessive trait, although it may be X-linked. Less commonly, it results from an enzyme deficiency.

SIGNS AND SYMPTOMS

An extreme susceptibility to infection becomes obvious in the first months of the infant's life. The infant fails to thrive and develops chronic ear infection, sepsis, watery diarrhea, recurrent pulmonary infections, persistent oral candidiasis and, possibly, fatal viral infections such as chickenpox. (See Pneumocystis carinii: *Threat to the SCID infant,* page 290.)

Pneumocystis carinii: Threat to the SCID infant

Pneumocystis carinii pneumonia usually strikes an infant with severe combined immunodeficiency disease (SCID) within the first 3 to 5 weeks of life. Onset is typically insidious, with gradually worsening cough, low-grade fever, tachypnea, and respiratory distress. Typically, a chest X-ray shows pulmonary infiltrates in both lungs.

DIAGNOSTIC TESTS
Diagnosis is generally made clinically because most affected infants suffer recurrent overwhelming infections within 1 year of birth. Some infants are diagnosed after a severe reaction to vaccination.

Defective humoral immunity is hard to detect before an infant is 5 months old. However, a severe decrease in the number and function of T-cells and lymph node biopsy showing lymphocyte absence can confirm the diagnosis.

TREATMENT
Restoring immune response and preventing infection are the first treatment goals. Histocompatible bone marrow transplantation is the only satisfactory treatment available.

Because bone marrow cells must be matched according to human leukocyte antigen and mixed leukocyte culture, the most common donors are histocompatible siblings. But a bone marrow transplant can produce a potentially fatal graft-versus-host (GVH) reaction, so newer methods of bone marrow transplant that eliminate GVH reaction are being evaluated.

Fetal thymus and liver transplants have achieved limited success. Immune globulin can also play a role in treatment. Some SCID infants have received long-term protection by being isolated in a completely sterile environment. However, this approach isn't effective if the infant already has had recurring infections.

Gene therapy is being used for ADA deficiency.

SPECIAL CONSIDERATIONS
• The infant must be monitored constantly for early signs of infection. Vaccinations should be avoided.
• Although SCID infants must remain in strict protective isolation, a stimulating atmosphere promotes growth and development. Explain the condition to the parents and encourage them to visit their child often, to hold him, and to bring toys that can be easily sterilized. If the parents can't visit, frequent reports on their infant's condition can ease their anxiety.
• Refer parents for genetic counseling. Refer parents and siblings for psychological and spiritual counseling to help them cope with the child's inevitable long-term illness and early death.
• For assistance in coping with the financial burden of the child's long-term hospitalization, refer the parents to social services.

Sickle cell anemia

Sickle cell anemia is a congenital hemolytic anemia that occurs primarily in blacks. The disease results from a defective hemoglobin molecule (hemoglobin S) that causes red blood cells (RBCs) to roughen and become sickle shaped. Such cells impair circulation, resulting in chronic ill health, periodic crises, long-term complications, and premature death. One-half of all patients with sickle cell anemia die by their early twenties; few live to middle age.

Sickle cell anemia is most common in tropical Africans and in people of African descent; about 1 in 10 blacks carries the abnormal gene. If two such carriers have offspring, each child has a 1 in 4 chance of having the disease.

The disease also occurs in Puerto Rico, Turkey, India, the Middle East, and the Mediterranean. The defective hemoglobin S gene may have persisted in areas where malaria is endemic because the heterozygous sickle cell trait provides resistance to malaria.

CAUSES

Sickle cell anemia results from homozygous inheritance of the hemoglobin S gene. Heterozygous inheritance of this gene results in sickle cell trait, usually an asymptomatic condition.

Altered cells

Whenever hypoxia occurs, hemoglobin S becomes insoluble. As a result, RBCs grow rigid, rough, and elongated, forming a crescent, or sickle, shape. Such sickling can cause hemolysis (cell destruction).

These altered cells also tend to pile up in capillaries and smaller blood vessels, making the blood more viscous. Normal circulation is impaired, causing pain, tissue infarctions, and swelling. Such blockage causes anoxic changes that lead to further sickling and obstruction.

SIGNS AND SYMPTOMS

Sickle cell anemia typically causes tachycardia, cardiomegaly, systolic and diastolic murmurs, pulmonary infarctions, chronic fatigue, unexplained dyspnea or dyspnea on exertion, hepatomegaly, jaundice, pallor, joint swelling, aching bones, chest pains, ischemic leg ulcers, and increased susceptibility to infection.

Infection, stress, dehydration, and conditions that provoke hypoxia — strenuous exercise, high altitude, unpressurized aircraft, cold, and vasoconstrictive drugs — may all provoke periodic crises. Four types of crises can occur.

Painful crisis

Also called a vaso-occlusive crisis or infarctive crisis, painful crisis is the hallmark of this disease. It usually appears periodically after age 5. (See *What happens in painful crisis*, page 292.)

Aplastic crisis

Also called megaloblastic crisis, aplastic crisis results from bone marrow depression and is associated with infection. This crisis causes pallor, lethargy, sleepiness, dyspnea, possible coma, markedly decreased bone marrow activity, and RBC hemolysis.

Acute sequestration crisis

In infants between 8 months and 2 years old, an acute sequestration crisis may cause sudden, massive entrapment of RBCs in the spleen and liver. If untreated, this rare crisis commonly progresses to hypovolemic shock and death.

Hemolytic crisis

Hemolytic crisis (rare) usually occurs in patients who also have glucose-6-phosphate dehydrogenase deficiency. It probably results from complications of sickle cell anemia such as infection, rather than from the disorder itself. Hemolytic crisis causes liver congestion and hepatomegaly and worsens chronic jaundice.

Long-term complications

Sickle cell anemia also causes long-term complications. Typically, the affected child is small for his age, and puberty is delayed. If he reaches adulthood, he tends to have narrow shoulders and hips, long arms and legs, curved spine, barrel chest, and an elongated skull.

Adults usually have such complications as retinopathy and nephropathy. Premature death commonly results from infection or repeated blockage of small blood vessels and consequent infarction or necrosis of major organs.

DIAGNOSTIC TESTS

A positive family history and typical clinical features suggest sickle cell anemia. Hemoglobin electrophoresis showing hemoglobin S or other hemoglobinopathies can confirm it.

Additional laboratory studies show a low RBC count, elevated white blood cell and platelet counts, decreased erythrocyte sedimentation rate, in-

PATHOPHYSIOLOGY

What happens in painful crisis

Painful (vaso-occlusive) crisis occurs when red blood cells (RBCs) release oxygen to the tissues. In response, abnormal hemoglobin S associates to form fibers that cause RBCs to take on a sickle shape. The sickled cells clump together and reduce or block blood flow to the area fed by the vessel. If this persists, microscopic obstructions eventually produce widespread ischemia.

Meanwhile, increased oxygen demand causes further sickling, compounding the problem. This, in turn, produces severe pain from tissue infarction and possible organ damage.

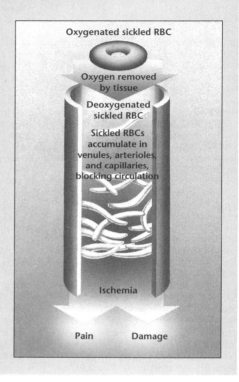

Oxygenated sickled RBC

Oxygen removed by tissue

Deoxygenated sickled RBC

Sickled RBCs accumulate in venules, arterioles, and capillaries, blocking circulation

Ischemia

Pain   Damage

creased serum iron level, decreased RBC survival, and reticulocytosis.

TREATMENT
Prophylactic penicillin is given before age 4 months. If the patient's hemoglobin drops suddenly or if his condition deteriorates rapidly, a transfusion of packed RBCs is needed.

In a sequestration crisis, treatment may include sedation, analgesics, blood transfusion, oxygen administration, and oral or I.V. fluids.

SPECIAL CONSIDERATIONS
• During a painful crisis, promote comfort by applying warm compress-

es to painful areas and covering the child with a blanket. (Never use cold compresses; this aggravates the condition.)

During remission
• Advise the patient to avoid tight clothing that restricts circulation.
• Warn against strenuous exercise, vasoconstricting medications, cold temperatures (even from swimming or drinking large amounts of ice water), unpressurized aircraft, high altitudes, and other conditions that provoke hypoxia.
• Stress the importance of normal childhood immunizations, meticu-

lous wound care, good oral hygiene, regular dental checkups, and a balanced diet as safeguards against infection.

• Tell the parents to encourage the child to drink more fluids, especially in the summer.

• Refer parents of children with sickle cell anemia for genetic counseling about the risk to future offspring. Recommend screening of other family members to determine if they're heterozygote carriers. In addition, suggest they join an appropriate community support group.

Sideroblastic anemias

Sideroblastic anemias are a group of disorders marked by a common defect — failure to use iron in hemoglobin synthesis, despite the availability of adequate iron stores. This failure causes iron deposition in the mitochondria of normoblasts, which are then termed *ringed sideroblasts*.

These anemias may be hereditary or acquired; the acquired form can be primary or secondary.

CAUSES

Hereditary sideroblastic anemia appears to be transmitted by X-linked inheritance, occurring mostly in young males.

The acquired form may arise secondary to ingestion of, or exposure to, toxins (such as alcohol and lead) or to drugs (such as isoniazid and chloramphenicol). It can also occur as a complication of other diseases, such as rheumatoid arthritis, lupus erythematosus, multiple myeloma, tuberculosis, and severe infections.

The primary acquired form is most common in elderly people and in those with a myelodysplastic syndrome.

SIGNS AND SYMPTOMS

Sideroblastic anemias usually produce nonspecific clinical effects, such as anorexia, fatigue, weakness, dizziness, pale skin and mucous membranes and, occasionally, enlarged lymph nodes.

Heart and liver failure may develop from excessive iron accumulation in these organs, causing dyspnea, exertional angina, slight jaundice, and hepatosplenomegaly. Additional features of secondary sideroblastic anemia depend on the underlying cause.

DIAGNOSTIC TESTS

Ringed sideroblasts, revealed in microscopic examination of bone marrow aspirate stained with Prussian blue or alizarin red dye, confirm the diagnosis.

Microscopic examination of blood shows red blood cells (RBCs) that are hypochromic or normochromic, and slightly macrocytic. RBC precursors may be megaloblastic, with abnormal variation in RBC size and shape.

TREATMENT

The underlying cause determines the type of treatment.

Hereditary form

Hereditary sideroblastic anemia usually responds to several weeks of treatment with high doses of pyridoxine (vitamin B_6).

Primary acquired form

Elderly patients with sideroblastic anemia are less likely to improve quickly and are more likely to develop serious complications. Selected patients with chronic iron overload may receive deferoxamine.

Carefully crossmatched transfusions or high doses of androgens are effective palliative measures for some patients. However, the primary acquired form resists treatment and usually leads to death from acute leukemia or from respiratory or cardiac complication.

Some patients may benefit from phlebotomy to prevent hemochromatosis. Phlebotomy speeds erythropoiesis and uses up excess iron stores; thus, it reduces serum and total-body iron levels.

Secondary acquired form

The secondary acquired form generally subsides after the causative drug or

Silica in the workplace

Industrial sources of silica in its pure form include the manufacture of ceramics (flint) and building materials (sandstone). Silica occurs in mixed form in the production of construction materials (cement); it's found in powder form (silica flour) in paints, porcelain, scouring soaps, and wood fillers and in the mining of gold, coal, lead, zinc, and iron. Foundry workers, boiler scalers, and stonecutters are all at high risk for developing silicosis from exposure to silica dust.

toxin is removed or the underlying condition is adequately treated. Folic acid supplements may prove beneficial when megaloblastic nuclear changes in RBC precursors are present.

SPECIAL CONSIDERATIONS
• Urge the patient to continue prescribed therapy, even after he begins to feel better. Advise frequent rest periods if he becomes easily fatigued.
• If the patient must undergo frequent phlebotomy, recommend a high-protein diet to help replace lost protein.

Silicosis

Silicosis is a progressive disease marked by nodular lesions. Frequently progressing to fibrosis, it's the most common form of pneumoconiosis.

Silicosis can be classified according to the severity of pulmonary disease and the speed of onset and progression; it usually occurs as a simple asymptomatic illness.

Acute silicosis develops after 1 to 3 years in workers exposed to high concentrations of respirable silica. Workers at risk include sandblasters and

tunnel workers. *Accelerated silicosis* appears after an average of 10 years of exposure to lower concentrations of free silica. *Chronic silicosis* develops after 20 or more years of exposure to lower concentrations of free silica.

CAUSES
Silicosis results from inhalation and pulmonary deposition of respirable crystalline silica dust, mostly from quartz. The danger to the worker depends on the concentration of dust in the atmosphere, the percentage of respirable free silica particles in the dust, and the duration of exposure. Respirable particles are less than 10 microns in diameter, but disease-causing particles deposited in the alveolar space are usually 1 to 3 microns in diameter.

Silica exposure occurs in numerous industries. (See *Silica in the workplace.*)

SIGNS AND SYMPTOMS
Initially, silicosis may be asymptomatic or it may produce dyspnea on exertion.

If the disease progresses to the chronic and complicated stage, dyspnea on exertion worsens, and the patient develops other signs — usually tachypnea and an insidious, dry cough that's most pronounced in the morning. Progression to the advanced stage causes dyspnea on minimal exertion, worsening cough, and pulmonary hypertension, which in turn leads to right-sided heart failure and cor pulmonale.

Patients with silicosis have a high incidence of active tuberculosis. With advanced silicosis, central nervous system changes — confusion, lethargy, and a decrease in respiratory rate and depth — may occur.

DIAGNOSTIC TESTS
The patient's history reveals occupational exposure to silica dust. A physical examination is normal in simple silicosis; in chronic silicosis with conglomerate lesions, it may reveal signs of lung damage. Diagnostic tests include pulmonary function studies,

chest X-rays, and arterial blood gas studies.

TREATMENT
The goal of treatment is to relieve respiratory symptoms, to manage hypoxia and cor pulmonale, and to prevent respiratory tract irritation and infections. Treatment also includes careful observation for development of tuberculosis.

Respiratory problems may be relieved through daily use of bronchodilating aerosols and increased fluid intake. Steam inhalation and chest physiotherapy techniques, such as controlled coughing and segmental bronchial drainage with chest percussion and vibration, help clear secretions.

In severe cases, oxygen may be given by cannula or mask for the patient with chronic hypoxia or by mechanical ventilation if warranted. Respiratory infections call for prompt antibiotic administration.

SPECIAL CONSIDERATIONS

TEACHING TIP: Encourage regular activity to raise the patient's exercise tolerance. Instruct him to plan daily activities to decrease the work of breathing. Advise him to pace himself, rest often, and move slowly through the daily routine.
● Stress the importance of preventing infections by avoiding crowds and people with respiratory infections and by getting influenza and pneumococcal vaccines.

Sinusitis
Sinusitis refers to inflammation of the paranasal sinuses. The condition may be acute, subacute, chronic, allergic, or hyperplastic.

Acute sinusitis usually results from the common cold and lingers in subacute form in only about 10% of patients. *Chronic sinusitis* follows persistent bacterial infection, *allergic sinusitis* accompanies allergic rhinitis, and *hyperplastic sinusitis* is a combination

of purulent acute sinusitis and allergic sinusitis or rhinitis.

CAUSES
Sinusitis usually results from viral or bacterial infection. Bacteria responsible for acute sinusitis include pneumococci, other streptococci, *Haemophilus influenzae,* and *Moraxella catarrhalis.*

Predisposing factors include any condition that interferes with sinus drainage and ventilation, such as chronic nasal edema, deviated septum, viscous mucus, nasal polyps, allergic rhinitis, nasal intubation, or debilitation related to chemotherapy, malnutrition, diabetes, blood dyscrasias, chronic steroid use, or immunodeficiency.

Bacterial invasion commonly occurs from the conditions listed above or after viral infection. It may also result from swimming in contaminated water.

SIGNS AND SYMPTOMS
Features vary with sinusitis type. (See *Comparing the five sinusitis types,* page 296.)

DIAGNOSTIC TESTS
Diagnosis requires nasal examination for inflammation and pus. Other studies may include X-rays, sinus puncture to obtain a specimen for culture and sensitivity testing (rarely done), ultrasonography, and computed tomography scans to identify suspected complications.

TREATMENT
Effective treatment depends on the type of sinusitis.

Acute sinusitis
Local decongestants usually are tried before systemic decongestants; steam inhalation may also be helpful. Local heat application may relieve pain and congestion.

Antibiotics are necessary to combat purulent or persistent infection. Amoxicillin, ampicillin, and amoxicillin–clavulanate potassium are usu-

Comparing the five sinusitis types

Signs and symptoms vary with the type of sinusitis present.

Acute sinusitis

The primary symptom is nasal congestion, followed by gradual build-up of pressure in the affected sinus. For 24 to 48 hours after onset, nasal discharge may be present and later may become purulent. Associated effects include malaise, sore throat, headache, and low-grade fever (temperature of 99° to 99.5° F [37.2° to 37.5° C]).

The nature of the pain depends on the affected sinus: maxillary sinusitis causes pain over the cheeks and upper teeth; ethmoid sinusitis, pain over the eyes; frontal sinusitis, pain over the eyebrows; and sphenoid sinusitis (rare), pain behind the eyes.

Subacute sinusitis

Purulent nasal drainage that continues for longer than 3 weeks after an acute infection subsides suggests subacute sinusitis. The patient also may have a stuffy nose, vague facial discomfort, fatigue, and a nonproductive cough.

Chronic sinusitis

The effects of chronic sinusitis resemble those of acute sinusitis, but the chronic form causes continuous mucopurulent discharge.

Allergic sinusitis

Signs and symptoms of allergic sinusitis include sneezing, frontal headache, watery nasal discharge, and a stuffy, burning, itchy nose.

Hyperplastic sinusitis

Bacterial growth on diseased tissue causes pronounced tissue edema in hyperplastic sinusitis. Mucosal thickening and mucosal polyps combine to produce chronic nasal stuffiness and headaches.

---

ally the antibiotics of choice. Sinusitis is a deep-seated infection, so antibiotic therapy should continue for 2 to 3 weeks.

Subacute sinusitis

In subacute sinusitis, antibiotics and decongestants may be helpful.

Other types

Treatment of allergic sinusitis must include treatment of allergic rhinitis — administration of antihistamines, identification of allergens by skin testing, and desensitization by immunotherapy. Severe allergic symptoms may call for corticosteroids and epinephrine.

In both chronic sinusitis and hyperplastic sinusitis, antihistamines, antibiotics, and a steroid nasal spray may relieve pain and congestion. If irrigation fails to relieve symptoms, one or more sinuses may require surgery.

SPECIAL CONSIDERATIONS

● Advise the patient to rest in bed, with the head of the bed elevated no more than 30 degrees. Encourage high fluid intake to promote sinus drainage.
● Instruct the patient to apply warm compresses continuously or four times daily for 2-hour intervals to ease pain and promote drainage.

Sjögren's syndrome

Sjögren's syndrome (SS) is the second most common autoimmune rheumatic disorder after rheumatoid arthritis. It is marked by diminished lacrimal and salivary gland secretion (sicca complex). SS occurs mainly in women (90% of patients).

SS may be a primary disorder or may be associated with a connective tissue disorder, such as rheumatoid arthritis, scleroderma, or systemic lupus erythe-

Ocular and oral effects of Sjögren's syndrome

Patients with Sjögren's syndrome may experience discomfort related to severe dryness of the eyes and mouth.

Ocular effects

Ocular dryness (xerophthalmia) leads to foreign body sensation, redness, burning, photosensitivity, eye fatigue, itching, and mucoid discharge. The patient may also complain of a film across his field of vision.

Oral effects

Oral dryness leads to difficulty swallowing and talking; abnormal taste or smell sensation, or both; thirst; ulcers of the tongue, buccal mucosa, and lips (especially at the corners of the mouth); and severe dental caries.

Dryness of the respiratory tract leads to epistaxis, hoarseness, chronic nonproductive cough, recurrent otitis media, and increased incidence of respiratory infections.

---

matosus. In some patients, the disorder is limited to the exocrine glands; in others, it also involves other organs, such as the lungs and kidneys.

CAUSES

The cause of SS is unknown. Most likely, genetic and environmental factors contribute to its development. Viral or bacterial infection or perhaps exposure to pollen may trigger SS in a genetically susceptible individual.

SIGNS AND SYMPTOMS

About 50% of patients with SS have confirmed rheumatoid arthritis and a history of slowly developing sicca complex. However, some seek medical help for rapidly progressive and severe oral and ocular dryness, commonly accompanied by periodic parotid gland enlargement. (See *Ocular and oral effects of Sjögren's syndrome.*)

Other features

Other effects may include dyspareunia and pruritus (associated with vaginal dryness), generalized itching, fatigue, recurrent low-grade fever, and arthralgia or myalgia. Lymph node enlargement may be the first sign of malignant lymphoma or pseudolymphoma.

About 50% of patients show evidence of hypothyroidism related to

autoimmune thyroid disease. A few patients develop systemic necrotizing vasculitis.

DIAGNOSTIC TESTS

A patient with SS has at least two of the following three conditions: xerophthalmia, xerostomia (oral dryness, with a salivary gland biopsy showing lymphocytic infiltration), and an associated autoimmune or lymphoproliferative disorder. Diagnosis must rule out other causes of oral and ocular dryness. Cancer must be ruled out in patients with salivary gland enlargement and severe lymphoid infiltration.

TREATMENT

Usually symptomatic, treatment includes conservative measures to relieve ocular or oral dryness.

Mouth dryness can be relieved by using a methylcellulose swab or spray and by drinking plenty of fluids, especially at meals. Meticulous oral hygiene is essential.

Instillation of artificial tears as often as every half hour prevents eye damage from insufficient tears. Some patients also benefit from using an eye ointment at bedtime or from twice-a-day sustained-release cellulose capsules.

Other measures

Other treatment measures vary with associated extraglandular findings. Parotid gland enlargement requires local heat and analgesics; pulmonary and renal interstitial disease, corticosteroids; accompanying lymphoma, a combination of chemotherapy, surgery, and radiation.

SPECIAL CONSIDERATIONS

 TEACHING TIP: Advise the patient to avoid drugs that decrease saliva production, such as atropine derivatives, antihistamines, anticholinergics, and antidepressants.

If mouth lesions make eating painful, recommend high-protein, high-calorie liquid supplements to maintain adequate nutrition. Instruct the patient to avoid sugar (which contributes to dental caries), tobacco, alcohol, and spicy, salty, or highly acidic foods, which cause mouth irritation.
• Sunglasses can protect the patient's eyes from dust, wind, and strong light. Moisture chamber spectacles may also be helpful.
• Humidifying the home and work environments can help relieve respiratory dryness.

Spinal neoplasms

A spinal neoplasm is any one of many tumor types that are similar to intracranial tumors and involve the spinal cord or its roots. If untreated, such a tumor can eventually cause paralysis.

Primary spinal neoplasms originate in the meningeal coverings, the parenchyma of the cord or its roots, the intraspinal vasculature, or the vertebrae. They can also occur as metastases from primary tumors.

CAUSES

Primary spinal cord tumors may be extramedullary (occurring outside the spinal cord) or intramedullary (occurring within the cord itself). Extramedullary tumors may be intradural (meningiomas and schwannomas) or extradural (metastatic tumors from the breasts, lungs, or prostate; leukemia; or lymphomas).

Intramedullary tumors, or gliomas, are comparatively rare, accounting for only about 10% of tumors.

SIGNS AND SYMPTOMS

Pain is most severe directly over the tumor, radiates around the trunk or down the limb on the affected side, and is unrelieved by bed rest.

Motor symptoms include spastic muscle weakness, decreased muscle tone, exaggerated reflexes, and a positive Babinski's sign. A tumor at the level of the cauda equina causes muscle flaccidity, muscle wasting, weakness, and a progressive decrease in tendon reflexes.

Sensory deficits include contralateral loss of pain, temperature, and touch sensation.

Bladder symptoms vary with the tumor stage. Early signs include incomplete emptying or difficulty with the urinary stream. Urine retention is an inevitable late sign with cord compression. Cauda equina tumors cause bladder and bowel incontinence from flaccid paralysis.

DIAGNOSTIC TESTS

Tests to confirm the diagnosis include lumbar puncture to investigate spinal fluid flow and spinal X-rays to assess cord distortions and vertebral changes. Myelography determines the anatomic relationship of the tumor to the cord and the dura. Computed tomography scans reveal cord compression and tumor location. Radioisotope bone scan is used to confirm cancer spread to the vertebrae. Frozen section biopsy helps identify the tumor type.

TREATMENT

Spinal cord tumors usually require decompression or radiation. Laminectomy is indicated for primary tumors that cause spinal cord or cauda equina compression.

If the tumor is slowly progressive or treated before the cord degenerates from compression, symptoms are likely to disappear and complete restoration of function is possible.

If the patient has incomplete paraplegia of rapid onset, emergency surgical decompression may save cord function. Steroid therapy minimizes cord edema until surgery can be performed. Partial removal of intramedullary gliomas, followed by radiation, may relieve symptoms for a short time.

Metastatic extradural tumors can be controlled with radiation, analgesics and, in the case of hormone-mediated tumors (breast and prostate), appropriate hormone therapy.

Transcutaneous electrical nerve stimulation (TENS) may control radicular pain from spinal cord tumors and may serve as an alternative to narcotic analgesics. In TENS, an electrical charge is applied to the skin to stimulate large-diameter nerve fibers and thereby inhibit transmission of pain impulses through small-diameter nerve fibers.

SPECIAL CONSIDERATIONS

• Advise the patient with impaired sensation and motor deficits to wear flat shoes and remove scatter rugs and clutter to prevent falls.
• Encourage the patient to perform activities of daily living as independently as possible. Avoid aggravating pain by moving the patient slowly and by making sure his body is well aligned.

Sporotrichosis

A chronic disease, sporotrichosis is caused by the fungus *Sporothrix schenckii.* It occurs in three forms:
• *cutaneous-lymphatic,* which produces nodular erythematous primary lesions and secondary lesions along lymphatic channels
• *pulmonary,* a rare form that causes a productive cough and pulmonary lesions
• *disseminated,* another rare form, which may cause arthritis or osteomyelitis.

The course of sporotrichosis is slow, the prognosis is good, and fatalities are rare. However, untreated skin lesions may cause secondary bacterial infection.

CAUSES

S. schenckii is found in soil, wood, sphagnum moss, and decaying vegetation throughout the world. Because this fungus usually enters through broken skin (the pulmonary form through inhalation), sporotrichosis is more common in horticulturists, agricultural workers, and home gardeners.

Perhaps because of occupational exposure, it is more prevalent in adult men than in women and children. The typical incubation period lasts from 1 week to 3 months.

SIGNS AND SYMPTOMS

Cutaneous-lymphatic sporotrichosis produces characteristic skin lesions, usually on the hands or fingers. Each lesion begins as a small, painless, movable subcutaneous nodule but grows progressively larger, discolors, and eventually ulcerates. Later, additional lesions form along the adjacent lymph node chain.

Pulmonary sporotrichosis causes a productive cough, lung cavities and nodules, hilar adenopathy, pleural effusion, fibrosis, and the formation of a fungus ball. It's often associated with sarcoidosis and tuberculosis.

Disseminated sporotrichosis produces multifocal lesions that spread from the primary lesion in the skin or lungs. Onset is insidious. Typically, it causes weight loss, anorexia, synovial or bony lesions and, possibly, arthritis or osteomyelitis.

DIAGNOSTIC TESTS

Typically, clinical findings and culture of *S. schenckii* in sputum, pus, or bone drainage confirm this diagnosis. Histologic identification is difficult. The diagnosis must rule out tuberculosis, sarcoidosis and, in patients with the disseminated form, bacterial osteomyelitis and neoplasm.

TREATMENT

Sporotrichosis doesn't require isolation. The cutaneous-lymphatic form

PATHOPHYSIOLOGY

From premalignant skin lesion to squamous cell carcinoma

Transformation from a premalignant lesion to squamous cell carcinoma may start with induration and inflammation of the preexisting lesion. When squamous cell carcinoma arises from normal skin, the nodule grows slowly on a firm, indurated base.

If untreated, the nodule eventually ulcerates and invades underlying tissues. Metastasis can occur to the regional lymph nodes, producing systemic symptoms of pain, malaise, fatigue, weakness, and anorexia.

usually responds to application of a saturated solution of potassium iodide, generally continued for 1 to 2 months after lesions heal. Occasionally, cutaneous lesions must be excised or drained.

The disseminated form responds to I.V. amphotericin B but may require several weeks of treatment. Local heat application relieves pain. Cavitary pulmonary lesions may warrant surgery.

SPECIAL CONSIDERATIONS
• The lesions must be kept clean. Contaminated dressings must be disposed of carefully.
• Advise the patient about the possible adverse effects of drugs. Because amphotericin B may cause fever, chills, nausea, and vomiting, the doctor may order antipyretics and antiemetics.

 PREVENTION: To help prevent sporotrichosis, advise horticulturists and home gardeners to wear gloves while working.

Squamous cell carcinoma

Squamous cell carcinoma of the skin is an invasive tumor with the potential to spread. Arising from the keratinizing epidermal cells, it occurs most often in fair-skinned white men over age 60. Outdoor employment

and residence in a sunny, warm climate greatly increase the risk of developing this cancer.

CAUSES
Predisposing factors include overexposure to the sun's ultraviolet rays and the presence of premalignant lesions (such as actinic keratosis). (See *From premalignant skin lesion to squamous cell carcinoma.*)

Other predisposing factors include X-ray therapy, ingestion of herbicides containing arsenic, chronic skin irritation and inflammation, exposure to local carcinogens, and hereditary diseases (such as xeroderma pigmentosum and albinism).

SIGNS AND SYMPTOMS
Squamous cell carcinoma commonly develops on the face, ears, backs of the hands and forearms, and other sun-damaged areas.

Lesions on sun-damaged skin tend to be less invasive and less likely to metastasize than lesions on unexposed skin. Notable exceptions are squamous cell lesions on the lower lip and the ears. These are almost invariably markedly invasive metastatic lesions with a generally poor prognosis.

DIAGNOSTIC TESTS
An excisional biopsy provides a definitive diagnosis. Other laboratory tests depend on systemic signs and symptoms.

TREATMENT

The size, shape, location, and invasiveness of a squamous cell tumor and the condition of the underlying tissue determine the treatment method used.

Premalignant lesions respond well to fluorouracil cream or solution. A deeply invasive tumor may require a combination of techniques.

All major treatment methods have excellent cure rates; the prognosis is usually better with a well-differentiated lesion than with a poorly differentiated one in an unusual location.

Depending on the lesion, treatment may consist of:
• wide surgical excision
• micrographic surgery (Mohs' surgery)
• electrodesiccation and curettage
• radiation therapy (generally for elderly or debilitated patients)
• chemosurgery (for resistant or recurrent lesions).

SPECIAL CONSIDERATIONS

 TEACHING TIP: Instruct the patient to keep the wound dry and clean. Describe ways to control odor such as using balsam of Peru, yogurt flakes, oil of cloves, or other odor-masking substances.
• Disfiguring lesions are distressing to both the patient and others. To increase his self-esteem, show that you accept him as he is.
• Instruct the patient to have periodic skin examinations for precancerous lesions and to have any removed promptly.

 PREVENTION: Advise all patients to avoid excessive sun exposure, to wear protective clothing outdoors, and to apply a sunblock 30 to 60 minutes before sun exposure.

Staphylococcal scalded skin syndrome

A severe skin disorder, staphylococcal scalded skin syndrome (SSSS) is marked by redness, peeling, and necrosis of the skin, giving the skin a scalded appearance.

SSSS is most prevalent in infants ages 1 to 3 months but may develop in children; it's uncommon in adults. The disease follows a consistent pattern of progression and most patients recover fully.

CAUSES

The causative organism in SSSS is group 2 *Staphylococcus aureus*. Predisposing factors may include impaired immunity and renal insufficiency — present to some extent in the normal neonate because of immature development of these systems.

SIGNS AND SYMPTOMS

SSSS can commonly be traced to a prodromal upper respiratory tract infection. Cutaneous changes progress through three stages. (See *Three stages of staphylococcal scalded skin syndrome.* page 302.)

DIAGNOSTIC TESTS

Careful observation of the three-stage progression of SSSS allows diagnosis. Results of exfoliative cytology and a biopsy help rule out erythema multiforme and drug-induced toxic epidermal necrolysis, both of which resemble SSSS. Isolation of group 2 *S. aureus* on cultures of skin lesions confirms the diagnosis.

TREATMENT

Systemic antibiotics — usually penicillinase-resistant penicillin — are used to treat the underlying infection. Replacement measures maintain fluid and electrolyte balance.

SPECIAL CONSIDERATIONS

 ACTION STAT: Notify the doctor or nurse right away if the patient's body temperature rises suddenly. This signals sepsis and calls for prompt, aggressive treatment.
• Maintain the patient's skin integrity. Use strict aseptic technique to help prevent secondary infection.

Three stages of staphylococcal scalded skin syndrome

The skin changes that occur in staphylococcal scalded skin syndrome (SSSS) pass through three stages before resolving.

Erythema

In the first stage, erythema becomes visible, usually around the mouth and other orifices, and may spread in widening circles over the entire body surface. The skin becomes tender; Nikolsky's sign (sloughing of the skin when friction is applied) may appear.

Exfoliation

About 24 to 48 hours later, exfoliation occurs. In the more common,

localized form of SSSS, superficial erosions and minimal crusting develop, generally around body orifices, and may spread to exposed areas of the skin.

In the more severe disease forms, large, flaccid bullae erupt and may spread to cover extensive areas of the body. These bullae eventually rupture, revealing sections of denuded skin.

Desquamation

In this final stage, affected areas dry up and powdery scales form. Normal skin replaces these scales in 5 to 7 days.

• To prevent friction and skin sloughing, leave affected areas uncovered or loosely covered. To prevent webbing, place cotton between fingers and toes that are severely affected.
• Warm baths and soaks may promote comfort during recovery.
• Reassure parents that complications are rare and residual scars are unlikely.

Stomatitis and other oral infections

Stomatitis is an inflammation of the oral mucosa that may extend to the buccal mucosa, lips, and palate. A common infection, it may occur alone or as part of a systemic disease.

Stomatitis occurs in two main types: acute herpetic stomatitis and aphthous stomatitis. Acute herpetic stomatitis is common in children ages 1 to 3; aphthous stomatitis, in girls and female adolescents.

Acute herpetic stomatitis is usually self-limiting; however, it may be severe and, in neonates, generalized and potentially fatal. Aphthous stomatitis usually heals spontaneously without a scar in 10 to 14 days.

Other oral infections include gingivitis, periodontitis, Vincent's angina, and glossitis.

CAUSES

Acute herpetic stomatitis results from herpes simplex virus. Predisposing factors include stress, fatigue, anxiety, febrile states, trauma, and sun overexposure.

SIGNS AND SYMPTOMS

Acute herpetic stomatitis begins suddenly with mouth pain, malaise, lethargy, anorexia, irritability, and fever, which may persist for 1 to 2 weeks. Gums are swollen and bleed easily, and the mucous membranes are extremely tender. Papulovesicular ulcers appear in the mouth and throat and eventually become punched-out lesions with reddened centers. Another common finding is submaxillary lymphadenitis.

Pain usually disappears 2 to 4 days before healing of ulcers is complete. If the child with stomatitis sucks his thumb, these lesions spread to the hand.

A patient with aphthous stomatitis typically reports burning, tingling, and slight swelling of the mucous membrane. Single or multiple shallow ulcers with whitish centers and red borders appear and heal at one site but then appear at another.

DIAGNOSTIC TESTS
Physical examination allows diagnosis. In Vincent's angina, a smear of ulcer exudate allows identification of the causative organism.

TREATMENT
For acute herpetic stomatitis, treatment is conservative. For local symptoms, management includes warmwater mouth rinses (antiseptic mouthwashes are contraindicated because they are irritating) and a topical anesthetic to relieve mouth ulcer pain. Supplementary treatment includes a bland or liquid diet and, in severe cases, I.V. fluids and bed rest.

For aphthous stomatitis, primary treatment involves application of a topical anesthetic.

SPECIAL CONSIDERATIONS
 TEACHING TIP: For effective long-term treatment, advise the patient to avoid conditions that trigger stomatitis, such as stress, fatigue, anxiety, and sun overexposure.

Syndrome of inappropriate antidiuretic hormone secretion

Excessive release of antidiuretic hormone (ADH) disturbs fluid and electrolyte balance in the syndrome of inappropriate antidiuretic hormone secretion (SIADH). Such disturbances result from an inability to excrete dilute urine, retention of free water, expansion of extracellular fluid volume, and hyponatremia.

SIADH occurs secondary to diseases that affect the osmoreceptors (supraoptic nucleus) of the hypothalamus. The prognosis depends on the underlying disorder and response to treatment.

CAUSES
The most common cause of SIADH (80% of patients) is oat cell carcinoma of the lung, which secretes excessive levels of ADH or vasopressin-like substances. Other neoplastic diseases — such as pancreatic and prostatic cancer, Hodgkin's disease, and thymoma — may also trigger SIADH, as may various other conditions. (See *Less common causes of SIADH,* page 304.)

SIGNS AND SYMPTOMS
SIADH may produce weight gain despite anorexia, nausea, and vomiting; muscle weakness; restlessness; and, possibly, seizures and coma. Edema is rare unless water overload exceeds 4 L, because much of the free-water excess is within cellular boundaries.

DIAGNOSTIC TESTS
A complete medical history revealing positive water balance may suggest SIADH. Serum osmolality less than 280 mOsm/kg of water and serum sodium less than 123 mEq/L confirm it. (Normal urine osmolality is 1½ times serum values.)

Supportive laboratory values include high urine sodium secretion (more than 20 mEq/L) without diuretics. In addition, diagnostic studies show normal renal function and no evidence of dehydration.

TREATMENT
Symptomatic treatment begins with restricted water intake (500 to 1,000 ml/day). With severe water intoxication, administration of 200 to 300 ml of 5% saline solution may be necessary to raise the serum sodium level.

When possible, treatment should include correction of the underlying cause of SIADH. If SIADH results from cancer, success in alleviating water retention may be obtained by surgical resection, radiation, or chemotherapy.

If fluid restriction is ineffective, demeclocycline or lithium may be helpful by blocking the renal response to ADH.

PATHOPHYSIOLOGY

Less common causes of SIADH

Although the syndrome of inappropriate antidiuretic hormone secretion (SIADH) most commonly results from lung cancer, it can also be caused by the conditions below.

Central nervous system disorders
• Brain tumor or abscess
• Cerebrovascular accident
• Guillain-Barré syndrome
• Head injury

Pulmonary disorders
• Lung abscess
• Positive-pressure ventilation
• Pneumonia
• Tuberculosis

Drugs
• Carbamazepine
• Chlorpropamide
• Clofibrate
• Cyclophosphamide
• Morphine
• Vincristine

Miscellaneous conditions
• Myxedema
• Psychosis

SPECIAL CONSIDERATIONS
• The patient is observed for restlessness, irritability, seizures, heart failure, and unresponsiveness resulting from hyponatremia and water intoxication.

PREVENTION: To help prevent water intoxication, explain to the patient and his family why he *must* restrict his intake.

Syphilis

Syphilis is a chronic, infectious, sexually transmitted disease. It begins in the mucous membranes and quickly becomes systemic, spreading to nearby lymph nodes and the bloodstream. Untreated, the disease progresses through four stages: primary, secondary, latent, and late (formerly called tertiary).

About 34,000 cases of syphilis, in primary and secondary stages, are reported annually in the United States. Incidence is highest among urban populations, especially in persons between ages 15 and 39, drug users, and those infected with the human immunodeficiency virus (HIV).

Untreated syphilis leads to crippling or death, but the prognosis is excellent with early treatment.

CAUSES
Infection from the spirochete *Treponema pallidum* causes syphilis. Transmission occurs primarily through sexual contact during the primary, secondary, and early latent stages of infection. Prenatal transmission from an infected mother to her fetus is also possible.

SIGNS AND SYMPTOMS
Each stage produces distinctive signs and symptoms. (See *Assessing syphilis stage by stage.*)

DIAGNOSTIC TESTS
Microscopic identification of *T. pallidum* from a lesion confirms the diagnosis. Other tests may identify this organism in tissue, eye fluid, cerebrospinal fluid, tracheobronchial secretions, and discharges from lesions.

Additional procedures may include the Venereal Disease Research Laboratory (VDRL) slide test, rapid plasma reagin test, and cerebrospinal fluid analysis.

Assessing syphilis stage by stage

Signs and symptoms of syphilis vary with the disease stage.

Primary syphilis

After an incubation period of about 3 weeks, features of primary syphilis develop. Initially, one or more chancres (small, fluid-filled lesions) erupt on the genitalia. Others may erupt on the anus, fingers, lips, tongue, nipples, tonsils, or eyelids. Usually painless, these chancres start as papules and then erode. They have indurated, raised edges and clear bases.

Chancres typically disappear after 3 to 6 weeks, even when untreated. In women, many chancres are commonly overlooked because they often develop on internal structures — the cervix or vaginal wall.

Secondary syphilis

Symmetrical mucocutaneous lesions and general lymphadenopathy signal the onset of secondary syphilis, which may develop within a few days or up to 8 weeks after onset of the initial chancres.

The rash of secondary syphilis can be macular, papular, pustular, or nodular. Lesions are uniform in size, well defined, and generalized. Macules commonly erupt between rolls of fat on the trunk and on the arms, palms, soles, face, and scalp. In warm, moist areas, the lesions enlarge and erode, producing highly contagious, pink, or grayish white lesions (condylomata lata).

In the second stage, mild constitutional symptoms of syphilis appear — headache, malaise, anorexia, weight loss, nausea, vomiting, sore throat and, possibly, slight fever. Nails become brittle and pitted.

Latent syphilis

During latent syphilis, no clinical effects appear, but the patient has a reactive serologic test for syphilis. Because infectious mucocutaneous lesions may reappear with infection of less than 4 years' duration, early latent syphilis is considered contagious.

Approximately two-thirds of patients remain asymptomatic in the late latent stage until death. The rest develop late-stage signs and symptoms.

Late syphilis

The final, destructive, but noninfectious stage of the disease, late syphilis has three subtypes, any or all of which may affect the patient: late benign syphilis, cardiovascular syphilis, and neurosyphilis.

Late benign syphilis

The lesions of late benign syphilis develop 1 to 10 years after infection. They may appear on the skin, bones, mucous membranes, upper respiratory tract, liver, or stomach.

The typical lesion is a gumma — a chronic, superficial nodule or deep, granulomatous lesion that is solitary, asymmetric, painless, and indurated. Gummas can be found on any bone and in any organ.

If late syphilis involves the liver, it can cause epigastric pain, tenderness, enlarged spleen, and anemia; if it involves the upper respiratory tract, it may cause perforation of the nasal septum or palate. In severe cases, late benign syphilis results in destruction of bones or organs, eventually causing death.

Cardiovascular syphilis

This subtype develops about 10 years after the initial infection in approximately 10% of patients with late, untreated syphilis. It leads to fibrosis of elastic tissue of the aorta and results in aortitis, most com-

(continued)

Assessing syphilis stage by stage *(continued)*

monly in the ascending and transverse sections of the aortic arch. Cardiovascular syphilis may be asymptomatic or may cause aortic regurgitation or aneurysm.

Neurosyphilis
About 8% of patients with late, untreated syphilis develop signs and symptoms of neurosyphilis 5 to 35 years after infection. These consist of meningitis and widespread central nervous system damage that may include general paresis, personality changes, and arm and leg weakness.

TREATMENT
Penicillin I.M. is the treatment of choice. For early syphilis, treatment may consist of a single injection of penicillin G benzathine I.M. Syphilis of more than 1 year's duration should be treated with penicillin G benzathine I.M. (2.4 million U/week for 3 weeks).

Nonpregnant patients who are allergic to penicillin may be treated with oral tetracycline or doxycycline for 15 days for early syphilis; 30 days for late infections. Tetracycline is contraindicated in pregnant women.

SPECIAL CONSIDERATIONS
• Emphasize the importance of completing the entire course of therapy, even after symptoms subside.
• Tell the patient to inform sexual partners of his disease, and urge him to get tested for HIV.
• Urge the patient to seek VDRL testing after 3, 6, 12, and 24 months to detect possible relapse. Instruct a patient treated for latent or late syphilis to have blood tests at 6-month intervals for 2 years.

Taeniasis

Also called tapeworm disease or ces-
todiasis, taeniasis is a parasitic infestation by *Taenia saginata* (beef tapeworm), *Taenia solium* (pork tapeworm), *Diphyllobothrium latum* (fish
tapeworm), or *Hymenolepis nana*
(dwarf tapeworm).

Taeniasis is usually a chronic, benign intestinal disease; however, infestation with *T. solium* may cause
dangerous systemic and central nervous system symptoms if larvae invade the brain and striated muscle of
vital organs.

CAUSES

T. saginata, T. solium, and *D. latum*
are transmitted to humans by ingestion of beef, pork, or fish containing
tapeworm cysts. Gastric acids break
down these cysts in the stomach, lib-
erating them to mature. Mature tape-
worms fasten to the intestinal wall
and produce ova that are passed in
the feces.

Transmission of *H. nana* is direct
from person to person and requires
no intermediate host; it completes
its life cycle in the intestine.

SIGNS AND SYMPTOMS

H. nana may cause diarrhea and abdominal discomfort in children with
massive infection. *T. saginata* and *T.
solium* are usually asymptomatic;
some patients have abdominal distress. *D. latum* may lead to mild GI
distress.

DIAGNOSTIC TESTS

Tapeworm infestations are diagnosed
by laboratory observation of tapeworm ova or body segments in feces.
Because ova aren't secreted continuously, confirmation may require
multiple specimens. A supporting dietary or travel history aids confirmation.

TREATMENT

Niclosamide offers a cure in up to
95% of patients. In beef, pork, and
fish tapeworm infestation, the drug
is given once; in severe dwarf tapeworm infestations, twice (5 to 7 days
each time, spaced 2 weeks apart).
Another anthelmintic agent, prazi-
quantel, may also be effective.

After drug therapy, all types of
tapeworm infestations require a follow-up laboratory examination of
stool specimens during the next 3 to
5 weeks to check for any remaining
ova or worm segments. Of course,
persistent infestation typically requires a second course of medication.

SPECIAL CONSIDERATIONS

● Be sure to wear gloves when giving
personal care and handling the patient's fecal excretions, bedpans, and
bed linens. Wash your hands thoroughly and instruct the patient to do
the same. Dispose of the patient's excretions carefully.
● The patient should not consume
anything after midnight on the day
niclosamide therapy is to start, because the drug must be given on an
empty stomach.
● Pork tapeworm infestation calls for
enteric and secretion precautions.
Children and incontinent patients
require a private room.

 TEACHING TIP: To prevent reinfestation, teach proper
handwashing technique and
the need to cook meat and fish thoroughly. Stress the importance of follow-up evaluations to monitor the
success of therapy and to detect possible reinfestation.

Tendinitis and bursitis

Tendinitis is a painful inflammation of the tendons and of tendon-muscle attachments to bone. It usually occurs in the shoulder rotator cuff, hip, Achilles tendon, or hamstring.

Bursitis is a painful inflammation of one or more of the bursae — closed sacs lubricated with synovial fluid that aid the motion of muscles and tendons over bony prominences.

CAUSES

Tendinitis commonly results from trauma (such as strain during sports activity), another musculoskeletal disorder (rheumatic disease, congenital defects), postural misalignment, abnormal body development, or hypermobility.

Bursitis usually occurs in middle age from recurring trauma that stresses or pressures a joint or from an inflammatory joint disease (rheumatoid arthritis, gout). Chronic bursitis follows attacks of acute bursitis or repeated trauma and infection. Septic bursitis may result from wound infection or from bacterial invasion of skin over the bursa.

SIGNS AND SYMPTOMS

Tendinitis of the shoulder causes of restricted shoulder movement, especially abduction, and localized pain, which is most severe at night. The pain extends from the acromion (the shoulder's highest point) to the deltoid muscle insertion, especially when the patient abducts his arm 50 to 130 degrees. Fluid accumulation causes swelling.

In calcific tendinitis, calcium deposits in the tendon cause proximal weakness and, if calcium erodes into adjacent bursae, acute calcific bursitis.

Bursitis causes irritation, inflammation, sudden or gradual pain, and limited movement. Other signs and symptoms depend on the affected site. Subdeltoid bursitis impairs arm abduction; prepatellar bursitis produces pain when the patient climbs stairs.

DIAGNOSTIC TESTS

In tendinitis, X-rays may be normal at first but later show bony fragments, bone changes, or calcium deposits. Diagnosis must rule out other causes of shoulder pain. Typically, heat application worsens the shoulder pain of tendinitis, in contrast to other painful joint disorders, in which heat relieves pain.

With bursitis, localized pain and inflammation occur; the patient typically has a history of unusual strain or injury 2 to 3 days before pain begins. During early stages, X-rays may appear normal (except in calcific bursitis).

TREATMENT

Therapy to relieve pain includes resting the joint (by immobilization with a sling, splint, or cast), systemic analgesics, cold or heat application, ultrasound, or local injection of an anesthetic and corticosteroids to reduce inflammation.

A mixture of a corticosteroid and an anesthetic such as lidocaine commonly provides immediate pain relief. Extended-release injections of a corticosteroid such as prednisolone offer longer pain relief. Until the patient is free from pain and can perform range-of-motion exercises easily, treatment also includes oral anti-inflammatory agents, such as sulindac and indomethacin. Short-term analgesics include codeine and acetaminophen with codeine.

Supplementary treatment

Other treatment measures include fluid removal by aspiration, physical therapy to preserve motion and prevent frozen joints, and heat therapy; for calcific tendinitis, ice packs.

Long-term control of chronic bursitis and tendinitis may require lifestyle changes.

SPECIAL CONSIDERATIONS

● After an intra-articular injection, advise the patient to apply ice intermittently for about 4 hours to reduce pain. Tell him to avoid applying heat to the area for 2 days.

 TEACHING TIP: Instruct the patient to perform strengthening exercises and to avoid activities that aggravate the joint. To maintain joint mobility and prevent muscle atrophy, advise him to perform exercises or physical therapy when free from pain.

Testicular cancer

Cancerous testicular tumors primarily affect young to middle-aged men and are the most common solid tumor in this group. Most testicular tumors originate in gonadal cells. About 40% are seminomas — uniform, undifferentiated cells. The remainder are nonseminomas — tumor cells showing various degrees of differentiation.

Testicular cancer spreads through the lymphatic system and may metastasize to the lungs, liver, viscera, and bone.

The prognosis varies with the cell type and disease stage. For almost all patients with localized disease, surgery and radiation provide survival beyond 5 years.

CAUSES

The cause of testicular cancer isn't known, but incidence is higher in men with cryptorchidism and in men whose mothers used diethylstilbestrol during pregnancy.

SIGNS AND SYMPTOMS

The first sign is usually a firm, painless, smooth testicular mass, varying in size and sometimes producing a sensation of testicular heaviness. Some patients have gynecomastia and nipple tenderness.

In advanced stages, signs and symptoms include ureteral obstruction, abdominal mass, cough, hemoptysis, shortness of breath, weight loss, fatigue, pallor, and lethargy.

DIAGNOSTIC TESTS

Regular self-examinations and testicular palpation during a routine physical examination can detect a testicular tumor. Transillumination can distinguish between a tumor and a hydrocele or spermatocele.

Serum alpha-fetoprotein and beta-human chorionic gonadotropin levels indicate testicular tumor activity. These tests provide a baseline for measuring response to therapy and determining the prognosis.

Surgical excision and biopsy of the tumor and testicle permit verification of the tumor cell type — essential for effective treatment. Groin examination determines the extent of lymph node involvement.

TREATMENT

The extent of surgery, radiation, and chemotherapy vary with tumor cell type and stage.

Surgery

Surgical procedures include orchiectomy and retroperitoneal node dissection. Most surgeons remove the testis, not the scrotum. Hormone replacement therapy may be needed after bilateral orchiectomy.

Radiation

Retroperitoneal and homolateral iliac nodes may receive radiation after seminoma removal. All positive nodes receive radiation after nonseminoma removal. Patients with retroperitoneal extension receive prophylactic radiation to the mediastinal and supraclavicular nodes.

Chemotherapy

Essential for tumors beyond the earliest stage, chemotherapy combinations include bleomycin, etoposide, and cisplatin; cisplatin, vindesine, and bleomycin; cisplatin, vinblastine, and bleomycin; and cisplatin, vincristine, methotrexate, bleomycin, and leucovorin.

Chemotherapy and radiation followed by autologous bone marrow transplantation may help unresponsive patients.

SPECIAL CONSIDERATIONS

• Before orchiectomy, reassure the pa-

Tetanus: Lethal threat to newborns

Tetanus is one of the most common causes of neonatal death in developing countries, where infants of unimmunized mothers are delivered in unsterile conditions. In such newborns, the unhealed umbilical cord is the portal of entry.

Neonatal tetanus is always generalized. The first sign is difficulty in sucking, which usually appears 3 to 10 days after birth. It progresses to total inability to suck, with excessive crying, irritability, and nuchal rigidity.

tient that sterility and impotence need not follow unilateral orchiectomy, that synthetic hormones can restore hormonal balance, and that most surgeons don't remove the scrotum.

• During chemotherapy, antiemetics may be needed for nausea and vomiting. Advise the patient to eat small, frequent meals to maintain oral intake despite anorexia.

• To prevent renal damage, encourage increased fluid intake.

Tetanus

Tetanus, or lockjaw, is an acute exotoxin-mediated infection caused by the anaerobic, spore-forming, gram-positive bacillus *Clostridium tetani*. Usually, such infection is systemic. Tetanus is fatal in up to 60% of unimmunized persons, usually within 10 days of onset.

Tetanus is more prevalent in developing countries that lack mass immunization programs. It takes a special toll on newborns in developing countries. (See *Tetanus: Lethal threat to newborns*.)

CAUSES

Normally, transmission is through a puncture wound contaminated by soil, dust, or animal excreta containing *C. tetani*, or by way of burns and minor wounds. After *C. tetani* enters the body, it causes local infection and tissue necrosis. It also produces toxins that enter the bloodstream and lymphatics and eventually spread to the central nervous system.

SIGNS AND SYMPTOMS

The incubation period varies from 3 to 4 weeks in mild tetanus to under 2 days in severe tetanus. When symptoms occur within 3 days after injury, death is more likely. If tetanus remains localized, signs of onset are spasm and increased muscle tone near the wound.

Generalized (systemic) tetanus produces marked muscle hypertonicity, hyperactive deep tendon reflexes, tachycardia, profuse sweating, low-grade fever, and painful, involuntary muscle contractions. For example, contractions of neck and facial muscles cause a locked jaw and a grotesque, grinning expression. Contractions of somatic muscles lead to arched-back rigidity (opisthotonos). Intermittent tonic convulsions may result in cyanosis and sudden death by asphyxiation.

Complications include atelectasis, pneumonia, pulmonary emboli, acute gastric ulcers, flexion contractures, and arrhythmias.

DIAGNOSTIC TESTS

Frequently, the diagnosis must rest on clinical features and a history of injury and no previous tetanus immunization. Blood cultures and tetanus antibody test reactions are commonly negative; only one-third of infected people have a positive wound culture. The doctor must rule out meningitis, rabies, phenothiazine or strychnine poisoning, and other conditions that mimic lockjaw.

TREATMENT

Within 72 hours after a puncture wound, a patient with no previous history of tetanus immunization first requires tetanus immune globulin (TIG) or tetanus antitoxin to confer temporary protection. Next, he needs active immunization with tetanus toxoid. A patient who has not received tetanus immunization within 5 years needs a tetanus toxoid booster.

If tetanus develops despite immediate postinjury treatment, the patient requires airway maintenance and a muscle relaxant such as diazepam to decrease muscle rigidity and spasm. If muscle relaxants don't relieve muscle contractions, a neuromuscular blocker may be needed. High-dose antibiotic therapy is given (penicillin I.V. if the patient isn't allergic to it).

SPECIAL CONSIDERATIONS
● All puncture wounds should be thoroughly debrided and cleaned with 3% hydrogen peroxide. The patient's immunization history should be checked. If the cause of injury was a dog bite, the case must be reported to local public health authorities.

 PREVENTION: Stress the importance of maintaining active immunization with a tetanus toxoid booster every 10 years.

Thalassemia

A hereditary group of hemolytic anemias, thalassemia is characterized by defective synthesis in the polypeptide chains necessary for hemoglobin production. Consequently, red blood cell (RBC) synthesis is also impaired. Thalassemia is most common in persons of Mediterranean ancestry (especially Italian and Greek), but also occurs in blacks and persons from southern China, southeast Asia, and India.

ß-Thalassemia is the most common form of this disorder, resulting from defective beta polypeptide chain synthesis. It occurs in three clinical forms: thalassemia major, intermedia, and minor. The severity of the resulting anemia depends on whether the patient is homozygous or heterozygous for the thalassemic trait.

Prognosis for ß-thalassemia varies. Patients with thalassemia major seldom survive to adulthood; children with thalassemia intermedia develop normally into adulthood, although puberty is usually delayed. Persons with thalassemia minor can expect a normal life span.

CAUSES
Thalassemia major and thalassemia intermedia result from homozygous inheritance of the partially dominant autosomal gene responsible for this trait. Thalassemia minor results from heterozygous inheritance of the same gene.

In all these disorders, total or partial deficiency of beta polypeptide chain production impairs hemoglobin (Hb) synthesis and results in continual production of fetal hemoglobin (Hb F), lasting even past the neonatal period.

SIGNS AND SYMPTOMS
The three clinical forms of ß-thalassemia have different signs and symptoms. (See *Comparing clinical features of three thalassemia types,* page 312.)

DIAGNOSTIC TESTS
In *thalassemia major,* laboratory results show a lowered RBC count and Hb level, microcytosis, and elevations in the reticulocyte, bilirubin, and urinary and fecal urobilinogen levels. A low serum folate level indicates increased folate utilization by the hypertrophied bone marrow. A peripheral blood smear reveals target cells, microcytes, pale nucleated RBCs, and marked anisocytosis.

X-rays of the skull and long bones show thinning and widening of the marrow space because of overactive bone marrow. The bones of the skull and vertebrae may appear granular; long bones may show areas of osteoporosis. The phalanges may also be deformed.

Quantitative Hb studies show a significant rise in Hb F and a slight increase in Hb A_2. Diagnosis must rule out iron deficiency anemia, which also produces hypochromia (slightly lowered Hb) and microcytic (notably small) RBCs.

In *thalassemia intermedia,* laboratory results show hypochromia and microcytic RBCs, but the anemia is less

Comparing clinical features of three thalassemia types

Signs and symptoms of ß-thalassemia vary with the form of the disease.

Thalassemia major

In thalassemia major (also known as Cooley's anemia, Mediterranean disease, and erythroblastic anemia), the infant is well at birth but develops severe anemia, bone abnormalities, failure to thrive, and life-threatening complications. Commonly, the first signs are pallor and yellow skin and sclerae in infants aged 3 to 6 months.

Later clinical features, in addition to severe anemia, include splenomegaly or hepatomegaly, with abdominal enlargement; frequent infections; bleeding tendencies (especially toward epistaxis); and anorexia.

Children with thalassemia major typically have small bodies and large heads and may be mentally retarded. Infants may have mongoloid features because bone marrow hyperactivity has thickened the bone at the base of the nose. As these children grow older, they become susceptible to pathologic fractures as a result of expansion of the marrow cavities with thinning of the long bones.

They are also subject to cardiac arrhythmias, heart failure, and other complications that result from iron deposits in the heart and in other tissues from repeated blood transfusions.

Thalassemia intermedia

Thalassemia intermedia comprises moderate thalassemic disorders in homozygotes. Patients show some degree of anemia, jaundice, splenomegaly and, possibly, signs of hemosiderosis from increased intestinal absorption of iron.

Thalassemia minor

Thalassemia minor may cause mild anemia but usually produces no symptoms and is often overlooked.

---

severe than that in thalassemia major.

In *thalassemia minor,* laboratory results show hypochromia and microcytic RBCs. Quantitative Hb studies show a significant increase in Hb A_2 levels and a moderate rise in Hb F levels.

TREATMENT

Therapy for thalassemia major is essentially supportive. For example, infections require prompt treatment with appropriate antibiotics. Folic acid supplements help maintain folic acid levels in the face of increased requirements.

Transfusions of packed RBCs raise Hb levels but must be used judiciously to minimize iron overload. Splenectomy and bone marrow transplantation have been tried, but their effectiveness has not been confirmed.

Thalassemia intermedia and thalassemia minor generally don't require treatment. Iron supplements are contraindicated in all forms of thalassemia.

SPECIAL CONSIDERATIONS

● During and after RBC transfusions for thalassemia major, the patient must be observed for adverse reactions — shaking chills, fever, rash, itching, and hives.

 PREVENTION: To help prevent infection, stress the importance of good nutrition, meticulous wound care, and periodic dental checkups.

• Discuss with the parents of a young patient various options for healthy physical and creative outlets. Such a child must avoid strenuous athletic activity because of increased oxygen demand and the tendency toward pathologic fractures, but he may participate in less stressful activities.

TEACHING TIP: Instruct parents to watch for signs of hepatitis and iron overload — always possible with frequent transfusions.

• Because parents may have questions about the vulnerability of future offspring, they should be referred for genetic counseling. Adult patients with thalassemia minor and thalassemia intermedia should also be referred for such counseling; they need to recognize the risk of transmitting thalassemia major to their children if they marry another person with thalassemia. If such persons choose to marry and have children, all of their children should be evaluated for thalassemia by age 1.

Thoracic aortic aneurysm

Thoracic aortic aneurysm is an abnormal widening of the ascending, transverse, or descending part of the aorta. Aneurysm of the ascending aorta is most common and usually fatal.

The aneurysm may be *dissecting,* a hemorrhagic separation in the aortic wall, usually within the medial layer; *saccular,* an outpouching of the arterial wall, with a narrow neck; or *fusiform,* a spindle-shaped enlargement encompassing the entire aortic circumference.

Some aneurysms progress to serious and eventually lethal complications such as rupture of an untreated thoracic dissecting aneurysm into the pericardium, with resulting tamponade.

CAUSES

Commonly, a thoracic aortic aneurysm results from atherosclerosis, which weakens the aortic wall and distends the lumen. An intimal tear in the ascending aorta triggers a dissecting aneurysm in about 60% of cases.

An ascending aortic aneurysm, the most common type, usually affects hypertensive men under age 60. A descending aortic aneurysm is most common in elderly hypertensive men. Transverse aortic aneurysm is the rarest.

Other causes of aneurysm include:
• fungal infection of the aortic arch and descending segments
• congenital disorders such as coarctation of the aorta
• trauma that shears the aorta transversely
• syphilis, usually of the ascending aorta
• hypertension (in dissecting aneurysm).

SIGNS AND SYMPTOMS

Pain most commonly accompanies a thoracic aortic aneurysm. (See *Clinical features of thoracic dissection,* page 314.)

DIAGNOSTIC TESTS

Diagnosis relies on patient history, clinical findings, and results of appropriate tests. In many asymptomatic patients, diagnosis comes accidentally when chest X-rays show widening of the aorta. Other tests, such as aortography and echocardiography, help confirm the aneurysm.

TREATMENT

A dissecting aortic aneurysm is an emergency that requires prompt surgery and stabilizing measures: antihypertensives such as nitroprusside, negative inotropic agents that decrease contractility force such as propranolol, oxygen for respiratory distress, narcotics for pain, I.V. fluids and, possibly, whole blood transfusions.

Surgery consists of resecting the aneurysm, restoring normal blood flow through a Dacron or Teflon graft replacement and, with aortic valve insufficiency, replacing the aortic valve.

Clinical features of thoracic dissection

ASCENDING AORTA	DESCENDING AORTA	TRANSVERSE AORTA
Character of pain		
Severe, boring, ripping; extending to neck, shoulders, lower back, or abdomen (rarely to jaw and arms); more severe on right side	Sudden onset, sharp, tearing, usually between shoulder blades; may radiate to chest	Sudden onset, sharp, boring, tearing; radiates to shoulders
Other effects		
If dissection involves carotid arteries, abrupt onset of neurologic deficits; pericardial friction rub; unequal intensity of right and left carotid pulses and radial pulses; difference in blood pressure between right and left arms	Aortic insufficiency without murmur, hemopericardium, or pleural friction rub; carotid and radial pulses and blood pressure in both arms typically equal	Hoarseness, dyspnea, pain, difficulty swallowing, and dry cough (from compression of surrounding structures)

SPECIAL CONSIDERATIONS

 TEACHING TIP: Encourage compliance with antihypertensive therapy by explaining the need for such drugs. Teach the patient how to monitor blood pressure.

Thrombocytopenia

The most common cause of bleeding disorders, thrombocytopenia is a deficiency of circulating platelets. Because platelets play a vital role in coagulation, this disease poses a serious threat to blood clotting.

Prognosis is excellent in drug-induced thrombocytopenia if the offending drug is withdrawn. Otherwise, prognosis depends on response to treatment for the underlying cause.

CAUSES

Thrombocytopenia may be congenital or acquired; the acquired form is more common. In either case, it usually results from one of the following:
• decreased or defective production of platelets in the marrow (such as occurs in leukemia, aplastic anemia, or toxicity with certain drugs)
• increased destruction outside the marrow caused by an underlying disorder (such as cirrhosis, disseminated intravascular coagulation, or severe infection)
• less commonly, sequestration (hypersplenism, hypothermia) or platelet loss.

Acquired thrombocytopenia may result from such drugs as nonsteroidal anti-inflammatory agents, sulfonamides, histamine blockers, alkylating agents, and antibiotic chemotherapeutic agents.

Precautions in thrombocytopenia

Because thrombocytopenia puts the patient at risk for serious consequences of bleeding, special precautions such as the following are required:

● Warn the patient to avoid aspirin in any form as well as other drugs that impair coagulation. Teach him how to recognize aspirin or ibuprofen compounds on labels of over-the-counter remedies.

● Advise the patient to avoid straining at stool or coughing because both can lead to increased intracranial pressure, possibly causing cerebral hemorrhage. A stool softener can be used to prevent constipation.

● If thrombocytopenia is drug-induced, stress the importance of avoiding the offending drug.

● If the patient must receive long-term steroid therapy, instruct him to watch for and report cushingoid symptoms (acne, moon face, hirsutism, buffalo hump, hypertension, girdle obesity, thinning arms and legs, glycosuria, and edema). Emphasize that he must never stop taking steroids abruptly; instead, he must discontinue them gradually under the doctor's guidance.

An idiopathic form of thrombocytopenia commonly occurs in children. A transient form may follow viral infection (Epstein-Barr or infectious mononucleosis).

SIGNS AND SYMPTOMS

Thrombocytopenia typically causes sudden onset of petechiae or bruises or bleeding into any mucous membrane. Nearly all patients are otherwise asymptomatic, although some complain of malaise, fatigue, and general weakness.

In adults, large blood-filled bullae commonly appear in the mouth. In severe thrombocytopenia, hemorrhage may lead to tachycardia, shortness of breath, loss of consciousness, and death.

DIAGNOSTIC TESTS

Diagnosis requires patient history (including a drug history), physical examination, and coagulation studies. If increased platelet destruction is causing the low platelet count, bone marrow studies are ordered.

TREATMENT

Treatment varies with the underlying cause and may include corticosteroids or immune globulin to increase platelet production. When possible, the underlying cause is corrected; in drug-induced thrombocytopenia, the offending agents are removed. Platelet transfusions are helpful only in treating complications of severe hemorrhage.

SPECIAL CONSIDERATIONS

● Take every possible precaution against bleeding. (See *Precautions in thrombocytopenia.*) Stay alert for signs of bleeding, such as petechiae, bruises, and abnormally heavy menstrual periods.

● During periods of active bleeding, the patient may require strict bed rest.

● To guard against trauma, advise the patient to use an electric razor and a soft toothbrush. Invasive procedures such as venipuncture should be avoided if possible. When venipuncture is unavoidable, pressure must be exerted on the puncture site for at least 20 minutes or until bleeding stops.

Thrombophlebitis

Thrombophlebitis, or a blood clot in a vein, is an acute condition marked by inflammation and thrombus formation. It may occur in deep or superficial veins.

Deep vein thrombophlebitis can affect small or large veins. In many cases, the disorder is progressive, leading to pulmonary embolism, a potentially lethal complication.

Superficial thrombophlebitis is usually self-limiting and rarely leads to pulmonary embolism. Thrombophlebitis commonly begins with localized inflammation alone (phlebitis), but such inflammation rapidly provokes thrombus formation.

CAUSES

A thrombus occurs when an alteration in the epithelial lining causes platelet aggregation and consequent fibrin entrapment of blood cells and additional platelets. The enlarging clot may block the vessel lumen partially or totally, or it may detach and embolize, to lodge elsewhere in the systemic circulation.

Deep vein thrombophlebitis

Deep vein thrombophlebitis may be idiopathic but usually results from endothelial damage, accelerated blood clotting, and reduced blood flow. Predisposing factors include prolonged bed rest, trauma, surgery, childbirth, and oral contraceptive use.

Superficial thrombophlebitis

Causes include trauma, infection, I.V. drug abuse, and chemical irritation from extensive use of the I.V. route for medications and diagnostic tests.

SIGNS AND SYMPTOMS

Clinical features vary with the site and length of the affected vein. Although deep vein thrombophlebitis is sometimes asymptomatic, it may produce severe pain, fever, chills, malaise and, possibly, swelling and cyanosis of the affected limb.

Superficial thrombophlebitis causes visible and palpable signs and symptoms, such as heat, pain, swelling, redness, tenderness, and hardening along the affected vein.

DIAGNOSTIC TESTS

Some patients have signs of inflammation and, possibly, a positive Homans' sign (pain on dorsiflexion of the foot); others lack symptoms. Laboratory tests include Doppler ultrasonography, plethysmography, and phlebography.

Diagnosis of superficial thrombophlebitis rests on physical findings — redness and warmth over the affected area, a palpable vein, and pain during palpation or compression.

TREATMENT

Treatment aims to control thrombus development, prevent complications, relieve pain, and prevent recurrences. Symptomatic measures include bed rest with elevation of the affected limb; warm, moist soaks to the affected area; and analgesics.

Deep vein thrombophlebitis

After the acute episode subsides, the patient may resume activity while wearing antiembolism stockings. Treatment may include anticoagulants to prolong clotting time. For lysis of acute, extensive deep vein thrombosis, treatment should include streptokinase.

Rarely, deep vein thrombophlebitis may warrant venous interruption through simple ligation to vein plication, or clipping. Embolectomy and insertion of a vena caval umbrella or filter may also be done.

Superficial thrombophlebitis

Therapy may include an anti-inflammatory drug such as indomethacin, antiembolism stockings, warm soaks, and limb elevation.

SPECIAL CONSIDERATIONS

ACTION STAT: Call for immediate help if the patient shows signs of pulmonary embolism — dyspnea, hemoptysis, sudden changes in mental status, restlessness, or hypotension.

• Enforced bed rest and elevation of the affected limb reduce the risk of thrombus formation. Warm soaks applied to the affected area increase circulation and relieve pain and inflammation.

TEACHING TIP: Emphasize the importance of follow-up blood studies to monitor anticoagulant therapy. Advise the patient to avoid prolonged sitting or standing to help prevent recurrences. Make sure he knows how to apply antiembolism stockings properly.

Thyroid cancer

Cancer of the thyroid occurs in all age-groups, especially in persons who have had radiation treatment to the neck. Papillary and follicular carcinomas, the most common thyroid tumors, are usually associated with prolonged survival. (See *Types of thyroid cancer*.)

CAUSES

Predisposing factors include radiation exposure, prolonged thyrotropin stimulation (through radiation or heredity), familial predisposition, and chronic goiter.

SIGNS AND SYMPTOMS

The primary signs of thyroid cancer are a painless nodule, a hard nodule in an enlarged thyroid gland, or palpable lymph nodes with thyroid enlargement. Eventually, the pressure of such a nodule or enlargement causes hoarseness, dysphagia, dyspnea, and pain on palpation.

If the tumor is large enough to destroy the gland, hypothyroidism follows, with typical symptoms of low metabolism (mental apathy and cold intolerance). However, if the tumor stimulates excess thyroid hormone production, it induces symptoms of hyperthyroidism (sensitivity to heat, restlessness, and hyperactivity).

Other clinical features include diarrhea, anorexia, irritability, vocal cord paralysis, and effects of distant metastasis.

DIAGNOSTIC TESTS

The first clue to thyroid cancer is usually an enlarged node palpable in the thyroid gland, neck, lymph nodes of the neck, or vocal cords. Patient his-

PATHOPHYSIOLOGY

Types of thyroid cancer

Thyroid cancers include papillary, follicular, and medullary carcinomas.

● *Papillary carcinoma* accounts for one-half of all thyroid cancers in adults. It is most common in young adult females and metastasizes slowly.

● *Follicular carcinoma* is less common than papillary carcinoma but more likely to recur and metastasize.

● *Medullary carcinoma* arises in the parafollicular cells derived from the last branchial pouch. It can produce calcitonin, histaminase, corticotropin (causing Cushing's syndrome), and prostaglandins (causing diarrhea). This rare form of thyroid cancer is familial, associated with pheochromocytoma, and completely curable when detected before it causes symptoms. Untreated, it progresses rapidly.

● *Giant and spindle cell cancer (anaplastic tumor)* is seldom curable by resection. It resists radiation and metastasizes rapidly.

tory may reveal radiation therapy or a family history of thyroid cancer.

Before confirming thyroid cancer, the doctor must rule out noncancerous thyroid enlargements. A thyroid scan can determine if nodes are functional (rarely malignant) or hypofunctional (commonly malignant).

Other tests include needle biopsy, computed tomography scan, ultrasonography, chest X-ray, and laboratory tests, such as serum alkaline phosphatase and serum calcitonin assay.

TREATMENT

Treatment may involve total or partial removal of the thyroid and removal of some lymph nodes. In some cases, the surgeon must also remove some neck tissue. Radioiodine (^{131}I) with external radiation may be used for inoperable cancer and sometimes after surgery.

To increase tolerance of surgery and radiation, the patient may receive drugs that suppress the thyroid, along with an adrenergic blocking agent such as propranolol. Chemotherapy is given to some patients whose symptoms suggest widespread metastases.

SPECIAL CONSIDERATIONS
• Explain that the patient can expect temporary voice loss or hoarseness for several days after surgery.

Thyroiditis

Thyroiditis is an inflammation of the thyroid gland. It occurs as autoimmune thyroiditis (long-term inflammatory disease), subacute granulomatous thyroiditis (self-limiting inflammation), Riedel's thyroiditis (rare, invasive fibrotic process), and miscellaneous thyroiditis (acute suppurative, chronic infective, and chronic noninfective).

CAUSES
Autoimmune thyroiditis results from antibodies to thyroid antigens in the blood. It may cause inflammation and lymphocytic infiltration (Hashimoto's thyroiditis). Glandular atrophy (myxedema) and Graves' disease are linked to autoimmune thyroiditis.

Postpartum thyroiditis is an autoimmune disorder associated with transient thyroiditis in women within 1 year after delivery.

Subacute granulomatous thyroiditis usually follows mumps, influenza, coxsackievirus, or adenovirus infection. *Riedel's thyroiditis* is a rare condition of unknown cause.

Miscellaneous thyroiditis results from bacterial invasion of the gland in acute suppurative thyroiditis; tuberculosis, syphilis, actinomycosis, or other infectious agents in the chronic infective form; and sarcoidosis and amyloidosis in chronic noninfective thyroiditis.

SIGNS AND SYMPTOMS
Autoimmune thyroiditis is usually asymptomatic and commonly occurs in women. It's the most prevalent cause of spontaneous hypothyroidism.

In subacute granulomatous thyroiditis, moderate thyroid enlargement may follow an upper respiratory tract infection or a sore throat. The thyroid may be painful and tender, and the patient may have difficulty swallowing.

In Riedel's thyroiditis, the gland enlarges slowly as it is replaced by hard, fibrous tissues, which may compress the trachea or esophagus. The thyroid feels firm.

Clinical effects of miscellaneous thyroiditis include fever, pain, tenderness, and reddened skin over the gland.

DIAGNOSTIC TESTS
Laboratory tests are the key to accurate diagnosis. Test results vary with the type of thyroiditis.

TREATMENT
Treatment varies with the type of thyroiditis. Drug therapy includes levothyroxine for accompanying hypothyroidism, analgesics and anti-inflammatory drugs for mild subacute granulomatous thyroiditis, propranolol for transient hyperthyroidism, and steroids for severe episodes of acute inflammation. Suppurative thyroiditis requires antibiotic therapy.

In Riedel's thyroiditis, a partial thyroidectomy may be necessary to relieve tracheal or esophageal compression.

SPECIAL CONSIDERATIONS
• If hypothyroidism occurs, inform the patient that he will need lifelong thyroid hormone replacement therapy. Tell him to watch for symptoms of overdose, such as nervousness and palpitations.

TEACHING TIP: Instruct the patient to stay alert for signs and symptoms of hypothyroidism (lethargy, restlessness, cold intolerance, forgetfulness, dry skin) and hyperthyroidism (nervousness, tremor, weakness).

Tonsillitis

Tonsillitis, an inflammation of the tonsils, can be acute or chronic. The uncomplicated acute form usually lasts 4 to 6 days and commonly affects children from ages 5 to 10.

CAUSES

Tonsillitis typically results from infection with group A beta-hemolytic streptococci, but it can result from other bacteria or viruses or from oral anaerobes.

SIGNS AND SYMPTOMS

Acute tonsillitis commonly begins with a mild to severe sore throat. A very young child, unable to complain about a sore throat, may stop eating. Acute tonsillitis may also produce difficulty swallowing, fever, swelling and tenderness of submandibular lymph nodes, muscle and joint pain, chills, malaise, headache, and pain.

Chronic tonsillitis causes a recurrent sore throat and purulent drainage in the tonsillar crypts. Frequent attacks of acute tonsillitis may occur. Complications include obstruction from tonsillar hypertrophy and peritonsillar abscess.

DIAGNOSTIC TESTS

Diagnostic confirmation requires a thorough throat examination, which reveals generalized inflammation of the pharyngeal wall, swollen tonsils, and drainage with pus. Cultures may determine the infecting organism and guide antibiotic therapy.

TREATMENT

Acute tonsillitis calls for rest, adequate fluid intake, aspirin or acetaminophen and, for bacterial infection, antibiotics.

When the causative organism is group A beta-hemolytic streptococcus, penicillin is the drug of choice (another broad-spectrum antibiotic may be substituted). To prevent complications, antibiotic therapy continues for 10 to 14 days.

Proven chronic tonsillitis justifies tonsillectomy, the only effective treatment.

SPECIAL CONSIDERATIONS

• Urge the patient to drink plenty of fluids, especially if he has a fever. A child may respond better to offers of ice cream and flavored drinks and ices. Suggest gargling to soothe the throat, unless it makes the pain worse.
• Make sure the patient or his parents understand the importance of completing the entire course of antibiotic therapy. Tell them to expect a white scab to form in the patient's throat 5 to 10 days after surgery. Instruct them to report bleeding, ear discomfort, or a fever that lasts longer than 3 days.

Toxic shock syndrome

Toxic shock syndrome (TSS) is an acute bacterial infection caused by toxin-producing, penicillin-resistant strains of *Staphylococcus aureus,* such as TSS toxin-1 and staphylococcal enterotoxins B and C. The disease primarily affects menstruating women under age 30 and is associated with continuous use of tampons during menstruation.

TSS incidence peaked in the mid-1980s and has since declined, probably because high-absorbency tampons were withdrawn from the market.

CAUSES

Although tampons are clearly implicated in TSS, their role is uncertain. Theoretically, tampons may contribute to TSS development by introducing *S. aureus* into the vagina or by traumatizing the vaginal mucosa during insertion (thus leading to infec-

Identifying toxoplasmosis in newborns

Toxoplasmosis acquired during the first trimester of pregnancy commonly results in stillbirth. About one-third of infants who survive have congenital toxoplasmosis. The later in pregnancy maternal infection occurs, the greater the risk of congenital infection.

Obvious signs of congenital toxoplasmosis include retinochoroiditis, hydrocephalus or microcephalus, cerebral calcification, seizures, lymphadenopathy, fever, enlargement of the spleen and liver, jaundice, and rash. Other complications which may become apparent months or years later, include strabismus, blindness, epilepsy, and mental retardation.

tion), by absorbing toxin from the vagina, or by providing a favorable environment for *S. aureus* growth.

When TSS isn't related to menstruation, it seems to be linked to *S. aureus* infections, such as abscesses, osteomyelitis, and postsurgical infections.

SIGNS AND SYMPTOMS

Typically, TSS produces intense myalgias, fever over 104° F (40° C), vomiting, diarrhea, headache, decreased level of consciousness, rigors, conjunctival redness, and vaginal redness and discharge. Severe hypotension occurs with hypovolemic shock. Within a few hours of onset, a deep red rash develops — especially on the palms and soles — and later exfoliates.

Major complications include neuropsychological abnormalities, renal failure, rash, and cyanotic arms and legs.

DIAGNOSTIC TESTS

Diagnosis depends on clinical findings and the presence of at least three of the following:

- GI effects, including vomiting and profuse diarrhea
- muscular effects, with severe muscle ache or a fivefold or greater increase in creatine kinase, an enzyme in the muscles and brain
- mucous membrane effects such as swelling
- kidney involvement with blood urea nitrogen or creatinine at least twice their normal levels
- liver involvement with elevated levels of bilirubin and other substances
- blood involvement with a platelet count below 100,000 per microliter
- central nervous system effects such as disorientation.

Isolation of *S. aureus* from vaginal discharge or lesions supports the diagnosis.

TREATMENT

TSS is treated with I.V. antistaphylococcal antibiotics that are beta-lactamase-resistant, such as oxacillin and nafcillin. To reverse shock, fluids are replaced with saline solution and colloids.

SPECIAL CONSIDERATIONS

- Instruct the patient to avoid using tampons.

Toxoplasmosis

One of the most common infectious diseases, toxoplasmosis results from the protozoa *Toxoplasma gondii*. Distributed worldwide, it's less common in cold or hot arid climates and at high elevations. It usually causes localized infection but may produce significant generalized infection, especially in immunodeficient patients or neonates.

Congenital toxoplasmosis, characterized by central nervous system lesions, may result in stillbirth or serious birth defects.

CAUSES

T. gondii exists in trophozoite forms in acute stages of infection and in cystic forms in latent stages. Ingestion of tissue cysts in raw or undercooked meat or fecal-oral contamination from infected cats transmits toxoplasmosis.

However, toxoplasmosis also occurs in vegetarians who aren't exposed to cats, so other transmission modes may exist.

Congenital toxoplasmosis follows transplacental transmission from a chronically infected mother or one who acquired toxoplasmosis shortly before or during pregnancy.

SIGNS AND SYMPTOMS

Acquired toxoplasmosis may cause localized (mild lymphatic) or generalized (fulminating, disseminated) infection. Localized infection produces fever and a mononucleosis-like syndrome (malaise, myalgia, headache, fatigue, sore throat) and lymphadenopathy.

Generalized infection produces encephalitis, fever, headache, vomiting, delirium, seizures, and a diffuse maculopapular rash. Generalized infection may lead to myocarditis, pneumonitis, hepatitis, and polymyositis. (For findings in congenital toxoplasmosis, see *Identifying toxoplasmosis in newborns*.)

DIAGNOSTIC TESTS

Identification of *T. gondii* in an appropriate tissue specimen confirms toxoplasmosis. Serologic tests may be useful. In patients with toxoplasmosis encephalitis, computed tomography and magnetic resonance imaging scans disclose lesions.

TREATMENT

Acute disease is treated with sulfonamides and pyrimethamine for about 4 weeks and, possibly, folinic acid to control adverse effects. In patients who also have acquired immunodeficiency syndrome, treatment continues indefinitely. No safe, effective treatment exists for chronic toxoplasmosis or toxoplasmosis occurring in the first trimester of pregnancy.

SPECIAL CONSIDERATIONS

 TEACHING TIP: Instruct the patient about using measures to prevent complications and to control spread of the disease.

• All cases of toxoplasmosis must be reported to the local public health department.

Trichinosis

An infection caused by larvae of intestinal roundworm *Trichinella spiralis,* trichinosis (trichiniasis, trichinellosis) occurs worldwide, especially in populations that eat pork or bear meat. Trichinosis may produce multiple symptoms; respiratory, central nervous system (CNS), and cardiovascular complications; and, rarely, death.

CAUSES

Transmission is through ingestion of uncooked or undercooked meat that contains *T. spiralis* cysts. Such cysts are found primarily in swine, less often in dogs, cats, bears, foxes, wolves, and marine animals. These cysts result from the animals' ingestion of similarly contaminated flesh. In swine, such infection results from eating table scraps or raw garbage.

After gastric juices free the worm from the cyst capsule, it reaches sexual maturity in a few days. The female roundworm burrows into the intestinal mucosa and reproduces. Larvae are then transported through the lymphatic system and the bloodstream. They become embedded as cysts in striated muscle, especially in the diaphragm, chest, arms, and legs. Human-to-human transmission does not take place.

SIGNS AND SYMPTOMS

In the United States, trichinosis is usually mild and seldom produces symptoms. When symptoms do occur, they vary with the stage and degree of infection. (See *Stages of trichinosis infection,* page 322.)

Stages of trichinosis infection

The clinical features of trichinosis depend on the stage and degree of the patient's infection.

Stage 1: Invasion

The first stage occurs 1 week after ingestion. Release of larvae and reproduction of adult *T. spiralis* cause anorexia, nausea, vomiting, diarrhea, abdominal pain, and cramps.

Stage 2: Dissemination

The second stage takes place 7 to 10 days after ingestion. *T. spiralis* penetrates the intestinal mucosa and begins to migrate to striated muscle.

Signs and symptoms include:
• edema, especially of the eyelids or face
• muscle pain, particularly in extremities
• occasionally, itching and burning skin, sweating, skin lesions, a temperature of 102° F (38.9° C), and delirium
• palpitations and lethargy in severe respiratory, cardiovascular, or central nervous system infections.

Stage 3: Encystment

The third stage occurs during convalescence, generally 1 week later. *T. spiralis* larvae invade muscle fiber and become encysted.

DIAGNOSTIC TESTS

A history of ingestion of raw or improperly cooked pork or pork products, with typical clinical features, suggests trichinosis, but infection may be difficult to prove. Stools may contain mature worms and larvae during the invasion stage.

Skeletal muscle biopsies can show encysted larvae 10 days after inges-

tion; if available, analyses of contaminated meat also show larvae.

Skin testing may show a positive histamine-like reactivity 15 minutes after intradermal injection of the antigen (within 17 to 20 days after ingestion). However, such a result may remain positive for up to 5 years after exposure.

Other abnormal results include elevated alanine aminotransferase, aspartate aminotransferase, creatine kinase, and lactate dehydrogenase levels during the acute stages and an elevated eosinophil count. A normal or increased cerebrospinal fluid lymphocyte level and increased protein levels indicate CNS involvement.

TREATMENT

Thiabendazole effectively combats this parasite during the intestinal stage. Severe infection (especially CNS invasion) may warrant glucocorticoids to fight possible inflammation.

SPECIAL CONSIDERATIONS

• The patient may require reduction of fever through alcohol rubs, tepid baths, cooling blankets, and antipyretics.
• To relieve muscular pain, the doctor may prescribe analgesics, enforced bed rest, and proper body alignment.
• Frequent patient repositioning and massage of bony prominences can help ward off pressure sores.

 PREVENTION: To help prevent trichinosis, educate the public about proper cooking and storing methods — not only for pork and pork products, but also for meat from carnivores. To kill trichinae, internal meat temperatures should reach 150° F (66° C) and its color should change from pink to gray (unless the meat has been cured or frozen for at least 10 days at lower temperatures).

Also, warn travelers to foreign countries or to very poor areas in the Untied States to avoid eating pork; swine in these areas are often fed raw garbage.

Trichomoniasis

Trichomoniasis is a protozoal infection of the lower genitourinary tract. It affects about 15% of sexually active females and 10% of sexually active males. In females, the condition may be acute or chronic. Treating sexual partners concurrently minimizes recurrence.

CAUSES

Trichomonas vaginalis — a flagellated, motile protozoan — causes trichomoniasis in females by infecting the vagina, the urethra and, possibly, the endocervix, Bartholin's glands, Skene's glands, or the bladder. In males, it infects the lower urethra and, possibly, the prostate gland, seminal vesicles, or epididymis.

T. vaginalis grows best when the vaginal mucosa is more alkaline than normal (pH about 5.5 to 5.8). Therefore, factors that raise the vaginal pH — use of oral contraceptives, pregnancy, bacterial overgrowth, exudative cervical or vaginal lesions, or frequent douching — may predispose a woman to trichomoniasis.

Trichomoniasis is usually transmitted by intercourse; less commonly, by contaminated douche equipment or moist washcloths. Occasionally, the neonate of an infected mother develops the condition during vaginal delivery.

SIGNS AND SYMPTOMS

Approximately 70% of females, including those with chronic infections, and most males with trichomoniasis are asymptomatic. In females, acute infection may produce variable signs, such as a gray or greenish yellow, malodorous and, possibly, profuse and frothy vaginal discharge.

Other effects include severe itching, redness, swelling, tenderness, dyspareunia, dysuria, urinary frequency and, occasionally, postcoital spotting, menorrhagia, or dysmenorrhea.

Such signs and symptoms may persist for a week to several months and may be more pronounced just after menstruation or during pregnancy. If trichomoniasis is untreated, symptoms may subside, although *T. vaginalis* infection persists and may be associated with an abnormal cytologic smear of the cervix.

In males, trichomoniasis may cause mild to severe transient urethritis, possibly with dysuria and urinary frequency.

DIAGNOSTIC TESTS

Direct microscopic examination of vaginal or seminal discharge and examination of clear urine specimens may reveal the infecting organism. Physical examination of the vagina and cervix may reveal signs of illness.

TREATMENT

The treatment of choice is a single 2-g dose of oral metronidazole given to both sexual partners. Alternative treatment is 500 mg of oral metronidazole twice daily for 7 days. Oral metronidazole has not been proven safe during the first trimester of pregnancy.

Effective alternatives aren't available for patients who are allergic to metronidazole. Sitz baths may relieve symptoms.

After treatment, both sexual partners require a follow-up examination to check for residual signs of infection.

SPECIAL CONSIDERATIONS

• Urge abstinence from intercourse until the patient is cured. Instruct the patient to have sexual partners receive treatment.

 TEACHING TIP: Tell the female patient to avoid using tampons. Warn patients to abstain from alcoholic beverages while taking metronidazole because alcohol consumption may provoke a disulfiram-type reaction (confusion, headache, cramps, vomiting, seizures). Tell the patient that this drug may turn urine dark brown.

 PREVENTION: Caution patients to avoid over-the-counter douches and vaginal sprays, because chronic use can alter vaginal pH. Tell the patient she can

What to teach the patient after surgery

After resection of the *first division* of the trigeminal nerve, caution the patient to avoid rubbing his eyes and using aerosol spray. Also advise him to wear glasses or goggles outdoors and to blink often.

After surgery to severe the *second division* or *third division* of the trigeminal nerve, tell the patient to avoid hot foods and drinks, which could burn his mouth, and to chew carefully to avoid biting his mouth.

reduce the risk of genitourinary bacterial growth by wearing loose-fitting, cotton underwear that allows ventilation.

Trigeminal neuralgia

Also called tic douloureux, trigeminal neuralgia is a painful disorder of one or more branches of the fifth cranial (trigeminal) nerve. It produces paroxysmal attacks of excruciating facial pain precipitated by stimulation of a trigger zone.

Trigeminal neuralgia occurs mostly in people over age 40, in women more often than men, and on the right side of the face more often than the left. It may subside spontaneously, with remissions lasting from several months to years.

CAUSES

Although the cause of trigeminal neuralgia remains undetermined, some researchers suspect that the condition reflects an afferent reflex phenomenon located centrally in the brain stem or more peripherally in the sensory root of the trigeminal nerve. Another theory links trigeminal neuralgia to compression of the nerve root by posterior fossa tumors, middle fossa tumors, or vascular lesions (subclinical aneurysm), although such lesions usually produce simultaneous loss of sensation.

SIGNS AND SYMPTOMS

Typically, the patient reports a searing or burning pain that occurs in lightning-like jabs and lasts 1 to 15 minutes (usually 1 to 2 minutes) in an area innervated by one of the divisions of the trigeminal nerve, primarily the superior mandibular or maxillary division.

The pain rarely affects more than one division, and seldom the first division (ophthalmic) or both sides of the face. It affects the second (maxillary) and third (mandibular) divisions of the trigeminal nerve equally.

These attacks typically follow stimulation of a trigger zone, usually by a light touch to a hypersensitive area, such as the tip of the nose, the cheeks, or the gums. Although attacks can occur at any time, they may follow a draft of air, exposure to heat or cold, eating, smiling, talking, or drinking hot or cold beverages.

The frequency of attacks varies greatly, from many times a day to several times a month or year. Between attacks, most patients are free from pain, although some have a constant, dull ache. No patient is ever free of the fear of the next attack.

DIAGNOSTIC TESTS

The patient's pain history is the basis for diagnosis, because trigeminal neuralgia produces no objective clinical or pathologic changes. Physical examination shows no impairment of sensory or motor function; indeed, sensory impairment implies a space-occupying lesion as the cause of pain.

Observation during the examination shows the patient favoring (splinting) the affected area. To ward off a painful attack, the patient often holds his face immobile when talking. He may also leave the affected side of his face unwashed or unshaven, or protect it with a coat or shawl.

When asked where the pain occurs, he points to — but doesn't touch —

the affected area. Witnessing a typical attacks helps to confirm the diagnosis. Rarely, a tumor in the posterior fossa can produce pain that is clinically indistinguishable from trigeminal neuralgia. Skull X-rays, tomography, and computed tomography scan rule out sinus or tooth infections as well as tumors.

TREATMENT
Oral administration of carbamazepine or phenytoin may temporarily relieve or prevent pain. Narcotics may be helpful during the pain episode.

When these medical measures fail or attacks become increasingly frequent or severe, neurosurgical procedures may provide permanent relief. The preferred procedure is percutaneous electrocoagulation of nerve rootlets under local anesthesia.

New treatments include a percutaneous radio frequency procedure, which causes partial root destruction and relieves pain, and microsurgery for vascular decompression of the trigeminal nerve.

SPECIAL CONSIDERATIONS
• The patient who is receiving carbamazepine must be observed for cutaneous and hematologic reactions (erythematous and pruritic rashes, urticaria, photosensitivity, exfoliative dermatitis, leukopenia, agranulocytosis, eosinophilia, aplastic anemia, thrombocytopenia) and, possibly, urine retention and transient drowsiness.
• Provide appropriate teaching for the patient who has undergone surgery to treat trigeminal neuralgia. (See *What to teach the patient after surgery.*)
• Advise the patient to place food in the unaffected side of his mouth when chewing, to brush his teeth and rinse his mouth often, and to see a dentist twice a year to detect cavities. (Cavities in the area of the severed nerve won't cause pain.)
• Provide emotional support, and encourage the patient to express his fear and anxiety. Promote independence

through self-care and maximum physical activity. Reinforce natural avoidance of stimulation (air, heat, cold) of trigger zones (lips, cheeks, gums).

Tuberculosis
Tuberculosis (TB) is an acute or chronic infection caused by *Mycobacterium tuberculosis,* marked by pulmonary infiltrates, granulomas with caseation, fibrosis, and cavitation. People living in crowded, poorly ventilated conditions are most likely to become infected.

In patients with strains that are sensitive to the usual antitubercular agents, the prognosis is excellent with correct treatment. In those with resistant strains, mortality is 50%.

CAUSES
After exposure to *M. tuberculosis,* roughly 5% of infected people develop active TB within 1 year; in the remainder, microorganisms cause a latent infection. The host's immune system usually controls the tubercle bacillus by killing it or walling it up in a tiny nodule (tubercle). However, the bacillus may lie dormant within the tubercle for years and later reactivate and spread. (See *How tuberculosis develops,* page 326.)

Reactivation risk factors
Although the primary infection site is the lungs, mycobacteria commonly exist in other parts of the body. Conditions that increase the risk of infection and reactivation include gastrectomy, uncontrolled diabetes mellitus, Hodgkin's disease, leukemia, silicosis, acquired immunodeficiency syndrome, and steroid or immunosuppressive therapy.

SIGNS AND SYMPTOMS
In primary infection, after an incubation period of 4 to 8 weeks, TB is usually asymptomatic but may produce nonspecific signs and symptoms, such as fatigue, weakness, anorexia, weight loss, night sweats, and low-grade fever.

PATHOPHYSIOLOGY

How tuberculosis develops

Tuberculosis (TB) is transmitted by droplet nuclei produced when infected persons cough or sneeze. After inhalation, if a tubercle bacillus settles in an alveolus, infection occurs. Cell-mediated immunity to the mycobacteria, which develops about 3 to 6 weeks later, usually contains the infection and arrests the disease.

Response to reactivation

If the infection reactivates, the body's response typically leads to caseation — conversion of necrotic tissue to a cheeselike material. The caseum may localize, undergo fibrosis, or excavate and form cavities whose walls are studded with multiplying tubercle bacilli. If this happens, infected caseous debris may spread throughout the lungs.

Sites of extrapulmonary TB include pleurae, meninges, joints, lymph nodes, peritoneum, genitourinary tract, and bowel.

In reactivation, signs and symptoms may include a productive cough, occasional hemoptysis, and chest pain.

DIAGNOSTIC TESTS

A chest X-ray shows nodules, patchy infiltrates, cavity formation, scar tissue, and calcium deposits. However, it may not be able to distinguish active from inactive TB.

A tuberculin skin test detects TB infection. Purified protein derivative or 5 tuberculin units are injected into the skin of the forearm. Test results are read in 48 to 72 hours; a positive reaction develops 2 to 10 weeks after infection. (However, people with severe immunosuppression may never develop a positive reaction.)

TREATMENT

Antitubercular therapy with daily oral doses of isoniazid, rifampin, and pyrazinamide for at least 6 months usually cures TB. After 2 to 4 weeks, the disease generally is no longer infectious. The patient can resume a normal lifestyle while taking medication.

Patients with atypical mycobacterial disease or drug-resistant TB may require treatment with second-line drugs, such as capreomycin, streptomycin, para-aminosalicylic acid, cycloserine, amikacin, and quinoline drugs.

SPECIAL CONSIDERATIONS

• The infectious patient must be isolated in a well-ventilated room until no longer contagious. He must cough and sneeze into tissues and dispose of all secretions properly.
• The patient must wear a mask when outside his room. Visitors and hospital personnel should wear masks in the patient's room.
• Adequate rest and a balanced diet promote recovery. If the patient is anorectic, urge him to eat small meals throughout the day.
• Emphasize the importance of regular follow-up examinations, and make sure the patient and family know how to recognize signs and symptoms of recurring TB.

 PREVENTION: Advise persons who have been exposed to infected TB patients to receive tuberculin tests and, if necessary, chest X-rays and prophylactic isoniazid.

Ulcerative colitis

An inflammatory, often chronic disease, ulcerative colitis affects the mucosa of the colon. Beginning in the rectum and sigmoid colon, it commonly extends upward into the entire colon. It rarely affects the small intestine, except for the terminal ileum. Patients with ulcerative colitis are at increased risk of developing colorectal cancer.

Ulcerative colitis produces edema and ulcerations. Severity ranges from a mild, localized disorder to a severe disease that may cause a perforated colon, progressing to potentially fatal peritonitis and toxemia.

CAUSES

The cause of ulcerative colitis is unknown, but seems to be related to an abnormal immune response in the GI tract. Stress may increase the severity of attacks.

Ulcerative colitis occurs primarily in young adults. Prevalence is greater among Jews and higher socioeconomic groups.

SIGNS AND SYMPTOMS

The hallmark of ulcerative colitis is recurrent bloody diarrhea, often containing pus and mucus, interspersed with asymptomatic remissions. The intensity of these attacks varies with the extent of inflammation. Other signs and symptoms include spastic rectum and anus, abdominal pain, irritability, weight loss, weakness, anorexia, nausea, and vomiting.

Ulcerative colitis may lead to complications in other organs. (See *Complications of ulcerative colitis,* page 328.)

DIAGNOSTIC TESTS

Sigmoidoscopy reveals changes in the mucous lining of the lower intestine and detects thick pus. Biopsy can help confirm the condition. Colonoscopy may be used to determine the extent of the disease. A barium enema X-ray shows the extent of the disease and detects certain complications. Laboratory values and blood tests reveal the severity of the attack.

TREATMENT

The treatment goals are to control inflammation, replace nutritional losses and blood volume, and prevent complications.

Supportive treatment includes bed rest, I.V. fluid replacement, and a clear-liquid diet. For patients who are awaiting surgery or who are dehydrated and debilitated from excessive diarrhea, total parenteral nutrition rests the GI tract, decreases stool volume, and restores positive nitrogen balance.

Drug therapy

Medications to control inflammation include corticotropin and adrenal corticosteroids such as prednisone. Sulfasalazine, which has anti-inflammatory and antimicrobial properties, may be used.

Antispasmodics such as tincture of belladonna and antidiarrheals such as diphenoxylate compound are used only for patients with frequent, troublesome diarrheal stools whose ulcerative colitis is under control. (These drugs may trigger toxic megacolon and are generally contraindicated.)

Surgery

If the patient has toxic megacolon, fails to respond to drugs and supportive measures, or finds symptoms unbearable, surgery is the treatment of last resort. The common surgical technique simply removes the diseased section of intestine. Another

Complications of ulcerative colitis

Ulcerative colitis may cause such intestinal complications as strictures, pseudopolyps, stenosis, and perforated colon, leading to peritonitis and toxemia.

However, effects of the disease may extend beyond the intestines.

- *Blood:* anemia from iron deficiency, coagulation defects from vitamin K deficiency
- *Eye:* uveitis
- *Liver:* pericholangitis, sclerosing cholangitis, cirrhosis, possible cholangiocarcinoma
- *Musculoskeletal:* arthritis, ankylosing spondylitis, loss of muscle mass
- *Skin:* erythema nodosum on the face and arms, pyoderma gangrenosum on the legs and ankles

type of surgery, called pouch ileostomy (Kock pouch or continent ileostomy), creates a reservoir (Kock pouch) from a loop of small intestine that empties through a tube opening just above the pubic hairline.

A colectomy may be performed after 10 years of active ulcerative colitis because of the increased incidence of colon cancer in these patients. Performing a partial colectomy to prevent colon cancer is controversial.

SPECIAL CONSIDERATIONS

 Teaching tip: After a proctocolectomy and ileostomy, teach the patient about stoma care. Instruct him to wash the skin around the stoma with soapy water and dry it thoroughly. Tell him to apply karaya gum around the stoma's base to avoid irritation, and make a watertight seal. After attaching the pouch over the karaya ring, instruct him to cut an opening in the ring to fit over the stoma and then secure the pouch to the skin. Advise him to empty the pouch when it's one-third full.

Urinary tract infection, lower

Lower urinary tract infections (UTIs) are bacterial infections that are nearly 10 times more common in women than in men. Cystitis and urethritis, the two forms of lower UTIs, affect approximately 10% to 20% of all women at least once. Lower UTI is also common in children.

Many UTIs respond readily to treatment, but recurrence and resistant bacterial flare-up during therapy are possible.

CAUSES

Most lower UTIs result from ascending infection by a single gram-negative enteric bacteria, such as *Escherichia coli, Klebsiella, Proteus, Enterobacter, Pseudomonas,* or *Serratia.*

Recent studies suggest that infection results from a breakdown in local defense mechanisms in the bladder that allows bacteria to invade the bladder mucosa and multiply. These bacteria cannot be washed out by normal urination. Recurrent lower UTI almost always results from reinfection by the same organism or from some new pathogen.

The high incidence of lower UTI among women probably results from the short female urethra and the ease with which bacteria can travel from the vagina, rectum, pudendal and perineal skin, or a sexual partner. Men are less vulnerable because their urethras are longer and their prostatic fluid has antibacterial properties.

SIGNS AND SYMPTOMS

Lower UTI usually produces urinary urgency, frequency, and dysuria along with bladder cramps or spasms, itching, a feeling of warmth during urination, nocturia, and possibly urethral discharge in males.

Other common features include low back pain, malaise, nausea, vomiting, abdominal pain or tenderness over the bladder area, chills, and flank pain.

DIAGNOSTIC TESTS
Typical clinical features and a microscopic urinalysis showing red blood cells and white blood cells greater than 5/high-power field suggest lower UTI.

TREATMENT
Antimicrobials are the treatment of choice for most initial lower UTIs. A 7- to 10-day course of antibiotic therapy is standard, but recent studies suggest that a single antibiotic dose or a 3- to 5-day regimen may render the urine sterile. After 3 days of antibiotic therapy, urine culture should show no organisms.

If the urine isn't sterile, bacterial resistance has probably occurred, necessitating a change in antimicrobials.

SPECIAL CONSIDERATIONS
• Suggest warm sitz baths or application of a warm heating pad to the abdomen and sides to soothe pain and burning.

 TEACHING TIP: Advise the patient to drink 2½ to 3½ qt (2½ to 3½ L) of fluid a day. Recommend foods and fluids with a high acid content, such as meats, nuts, plums, prunes, whole grain breads and cereals, and fruit juices. Tell the patient to limit intake of milk and other products with a high calcium content and to avoid caffeine, carbonated beverages, and alcohol because these substances irritate the bladder.

 PREVENTION: To help prevent lower UTIs, instruct the patient to wipe from front to back after using the toilet, to wear cotton undergarments and change them daily, to take showers instead of baths, and to avoid bubble baths, bath oils, perfumed vaginal sprays,

and strong bleaches and cleaning powders in the laundry. Also instruct her to urinate frequently to completely empty the bladder and to urinate as soon as she feels the urge and right after sexual intercourse.

Urticaria and angioedema

Also called hives, *urticaria* is an episodic, usually self-limited skin reaction characterized by local dermal wheals surrounded by erythematous flare.

Angioedema is a subcutaneous and dermal eruption that produces deeper, large wheals (usually on the hands, feet, lips, genitalia, and eyelids) and a more diffuse swelling of loose subcutaneous tissue.

Urticaria and angioedema can occur simultaneously but angioedema may last longer.

CAUSES
Urticaria and angioedema may arise from allergic reactions or may have nonallergic causes. (See *Triggers for urticaria and angioedema,* page 330.)

Mechanisms of action
Several different mechanisms and underlying disorders may provoke urticaria and angioedema. These include immunoglobulin E (IgE)-induced release of mediators from cutaneous mast cells and binding of IgG or IgM to antigen, resulting in complement activation.

Disorders include localized or secondary infection (respiratory infection), neoplastic disease (Hodgkin's lymphoma), connective tissue diseases (systemic lupus erythematosus), collagen vascular disease, and psychogenic diseases.

SIGNS AND SYMPTOMS
Characteristic features of urticaria are distinct, raised, evanescent dermal wheals surrounded by an erythematous flare. These lesions may vary in

PATHOPHYSIOLOGY

Triggers for urticaria and angioedema

Urticaria and angioedema may result from a wide range of allergic reactions or from such nonallergic causes as external stimuli.

Allergic reactions

Urticaria and angioedema from allergies may occur in roughly 20% of the general population at some time or other. The causes of these reactions include allergy to drugs, foods, insect stings and, occasionally, inhalant allergens (animal danders, cosmetics) that provoke an immunoglobulin E (IgE)-mediated response to protein allergens. However, certain drugs may cause urticaria without an IgE response.

When urticaria and angioedema are part of an anaphylactic reaction, they almost always persist long after the systemic response has subsided.

This occurs because circulation to the skin is the last to be restored after an allergic reaction, which results in slow histamine reabsorption at the reaction site.

Nonallergic causes

Urticaria and angioedema from nonallergic causes are probably also related to histamine release by some still-unknown mechanism. External physical stimuli, such as cold (usually in young adults), heat, water, or sunlight, may also provoke urticaria and angioedema.

Dermatographic urticaria, which develops after stroking or scratching the skin, occurs in up to 20% of the population. Such urticaria develops with varying pressure, most often under tight clothing, and is aggravated by scratching.

---

size. In cholinergic urticaria, the wheals may be tiny and blanched, surrounded by erythematous flares.

Angioedema characteristically produces nonpitted swelling of deep subcutaneous tissue, usually on the eyelids, lips, genitalia, and mucous membranes. These swellings usually don't itch but may burn and tingle.

DIAGNOSTIC TESTS

An accurate patient history can help determine the cause of hives. Diagnosis also requires physical assessment to rule out similar conditions, and a complete blood count, urinalysis, erythrocyte sedimentation rate, and chest X-ray to rule out inflammatory infections.

Skin testing, an elimination diet, and a food diary (recording the time and amount of food eaten, and the circumstances) can pinpoint provoking allergens. The food diary may also

suggest other allergies. For instance, a patient who is allergic to fish may also be allergic to iodine contrast materials.

Recurrent angioedema without urticaria, along with a family history, point to hereditary angioedema. Decreased serum levels of C4 and C1 esterase inhibitor confirm this diagnosis.

TREATMENT

The aim of treatment is to prevent or limit contact with triggering factors or, if this is impossible, to desensitize the patient to them and to relieve symptoms. Once the triggering stimulus has been removed, urticaria usually subsides in a few days — except for drug reactions, which may persist as long as the drug is in the bloodstream.

During desensitization, progressively larger doses of specific antigens (determined by skin testing) are injected intradermally.

SPECIAL CONSIDERATIONS
● Corticosteroid therapy may be necessary for some patients.
● Advise the patient with urticaria that hydroxyzine or another antihistamine can ease itching and swelling.
● Inform the patient receiving antihistamines of the possibility of drowsiness.

Uterine cancer

Uterine cancer (cancer of the endometrium) is the most common gynecologic cancer. Usually, it affects postmenopausal women between ages 50 and 60; it's extremely rare before age 30.

Generally, uterine cancer is an adenocarcinoma that metastasizes late, usually from the endometrium to the cervix, ovaries, fallopian tubes, and other peritoneal structures. It may spread to distant organs, such as the lungs and the brain, through the blood or lymphatic system. Lymph node involvement can also occur.

CAUSES
Uterine cancer seems to be linked to several predisposing factors:
● low fertility index and anovulation
● abnormal uterine bleeding
● obesity, hypertension, or diabetes
● familial tendency
● history of uterine polyps or endometrial hyperplasia
● estrogen therapy (controversial).

SIGNS AND SYMPTOMS
Uterine enlargement and persistent and unusual premenopausal bleeding, or any postmenopausal bleeding, are the most common signs of uterine cancer. Discharge may be watery and blood-streaked at first, but gradually becomes bloodier. Other signs and symptoms, such as pain and weight loss, don't appear until the cancer is well advanced.

DIAGNOSTIC TESTS
Unfortunately, a Papanicolaou smear, so useful for detecting cervical cancer, doesn't dependably predict early-stage uterine cancer. Diagnosis of uterine cancer requires endometrial, cervical, and endocervical biopsies. Negative biopsies call for a fractional dilatation and curettage to determine diagnosis. Positive diagnosis requires additional tests for baseline data and disease staging.

TREATMENT
Uterine cancer treatment varies with the extent of the disease.

Surgery
Rarely curative, surgery generally involves total abdominal hysterectomy, bilateral salpingo-oophorectomy, or possibly omentectomy with or without pelvic or para-aortic lymphadenectomy. Total exenteration — removal of all pelvic organs, including the vagina — is done only when the disease is sufficiently contained to allow surgical removal of diseased parts.

Radiation therapy
When the tumor isn't well differentiated, intracavitary or external radiation (or both), given 6 weeks before surgery, may inhibit recurrence and lengthen survival time.

Hormonal therapy
Synthetic progesterones, such as medroxyprogesterone or megestrol, may be given for systemic disease. Tamoxifen (which produces a 20% to 40% response rate) may be used as an auxiliary treatment.

Chemotherapy
Varying combinations of cisplatin, doxorubicin, etoposide, and dactinomycin are usually tried when other treatments have failed.

SPECIAL CONSIDERATIONS
● If the patient will receive internal radiation, explain the procedure and an-

Understanding radiation therapy

A patient with uterine cancer may receive internal or external radiation.

Internal radiation

An internal radiation implant usually requires a 2- to 3-day hospital stay. The implant may be placed in the vagina by the doctor, or it may be implanted by a member of the radiation team in the patient's room. Internal radiation therapy lasts 48 to 72 hours, depending on the dosage.

Patient restrictions

The patient must limit her movements while the implant is in place because certain body movements could dislodge it. To compensate for immobility, she should be encouraged to do active range-of-motion exercises with both arms — but must avoid leg exercises and other body movements. To help her relax and remain still, she may receive a tranquilizer.

An indwelling urinary catheter will be inserted, and the patient's linens shouldn't be changed unless they're soiled. She should receive only partial bed baths, and the call bell, phone, water, or anything else she needs should be kept within easy reach. The doctor will order a clear liquid or low-residue diet and an antidiarrheal drug to prevent bowel movements.

Ensuring safety

Safety precautions, including time, distance, and shielding, will be imposed immediately after the radioactive source has been implanted. The patient will require a private room, and all visitors must be informed about safety precautions when visiting her. A sign should be posted on the patient's door listing safety precautions.

Because radiation effects are cumulative, caregivers should wear a radiosensitive badge and a lead shield (if available) when entering the patient's room. They should check with the radiation therapist to find out the maximum recommended time they can safely spend with the patient when giving direct care.

External radiation

External radiation is usually given 5 days a week for 6 weeks. The patient's body will be marked at certain places to ensure that treatment is directed at exactly the same area each time. Tell her not to wash off the marks.

To minimize skin breakdown and reduce the risk of skin infection, the patient must keep the treatment area dry, avoid wearing clothes that rub against the area, and avoid using heating pads, alcohol rubs, and skin creams.

---

swer her questions. (See *Understanding radiation therapy*.)

● If the patient will receive external radiation, urge her to maintain a high-protein, high-carbohydrate, low-residue diet to reduce bulk while maintaining calories.

 TEACHING TIP: Teach the patient how to use a vaginal dilator to prevent vaginal

stenosis and promote vaginal examinations and sexual intercourse.

Uterine leiomyomas

Also called fibroids, myomas, and fibromyomas, uterine leiomyomas are the most common benign tumors in women. These smooth-muscle tumors usually occur in multiples in the uterine body.

Uterine leiomyomas occur in 20% to 25% of women of reproductive age and affect three times as many blacks as whites. The tumors become malignant in only 0.1% of patients.

CAUSES

The cause of uterine leiomyomas is unknown, but steroid hormones, including estrogen and progesterone, and several growth factors, including epidermal growth factor, have been implicated as regulators of leiomyoma growth.

Leiomyomas typically arise after menarche and regress after menopause, implicating estrogen in their growth.

SIGNS AND SYMPTOMS

Leiomyomas may be located within the uterine wall or may protrude into the endometrial cavity or from the serosal surface of the uterus. Most leiomyomas produce no signs or symptoms. The most common sign is abnormal bleeding, which typically presents as abnormally heavy or long menstrual periods. Pelvic pressure and impingement on adjacent viscera are common indications for treatment.

DIAGNOSTIC TESTS

Clinical findings and patient history suggest uterine fibroids. Bimanual examination may reveal an enlarged, firm, nontender, and irregularly contoured uterus. Ultrasonography allows accurate assessment of the dimensions, number, and location of tumors. Other diagnostic procedures may include hysterosalpingography, dilatation and curettage, endometrial biopsy, and laparoscopy.

TREATMENT

Treatment depends on symptom severity, the size and location of the tumors, and the patient's age, parity, pregnancy status, desire to have children, and general health. Treatment may involve conservative measures or surgery. (See *Nonsurgical treatment for uterine leiomyomas*.)

Nonsurgical treatment for uterine leiomyomas

Many women with uterine leiomyomas require only conservative treatment. Such treatment includes taking serial histories, performing physical assessments at clinically indicated intervals, and administering gonadotropin-releasing hormone (GnRH) analogues.

GnRH analogues rapidly suppress pituitary gonadotropin release, leading to profound hypoestrogenemia and a 50% reduction in uterine volume. These agents may be given to reduce tumor size before surgery and to decrease intraoperative blood loss.

Surgery includes abdominal, laparoscopic, or hysteroscopic myomectomy — for patients who want to preserve fertility — and hysterectomy, the definitive treatment for symptomatic women who have completed childbearing.

If the patient is pregnant, but her uterus is no longer than a 6-month normal uterus by the 16th week of pregnancy, the outcome for the pregnancy is favorable, and surgery is usually unnecessary. However, if a pregnant woman has a leiomyomatous uterus the size of a 5- to 6-month normal uterus by the 9th week of pregnancy, spontaneous abortion will probably occur, especially with a cervical leiomyoma. If surgery is necessary, a hysterectomy is usually performed 5 to 6 months after delivery (when involution is complete), with preservation of the ovaries, if possible.

SPECIAL CONSIDERATIONS

• Tell the patient to report abnormal bleeding or pelvic pain immediately.

● If a hysterectomy or oophorectomy is indicated, inform the patient about the effects of surgery on menstruation, menopause, and sexual activity. Reassure her that she won't experience premature menopause if her ovaries are left intact, and explain that even if she will have a multiple myomectomy, pregnancy is still possible. However, if the uterine cavity is entered during surgery, explain that cesarean delivery may be necessary.

Vaginal cancer

Cancer of the vagina accounts for approximately 2% of all gynecologic malignancies. It usually appears as squamous cell carcinoma, but occasionally as melanoma, sarcoma, or adenocarcinoma.

The disease varies in severity according to its location and effect on lymphatic drainage. (The vagina is a thin-walled structure with a rich lymphatic drainage.) Vaginal cancer is similar to cervical cancer in that it may progress from an intraepithelial tumor to an invasive cancer. However, it spreads more slowly than cervical cancer. (See *Metastasis patterns in vaginal cancer,* page 336.)

Vaginal cancer generally occurs in women in their early to mid-50s, but some of the rare types occur in younger women, and rhabdomyosarcoma appears in children.

CAUSES
Clear cell adenocarcinoma has an increased incidence in young women whose mothers took diethylstilbestrol. Otherwise, the cause is unknown.

SIGNS AND SYMPTOMS
Commonly, the patient with vaginal cancer experiences abnormal bleeding and discharge. Also, she may have a small or large, commonly firm, ulcerated lesion in any part of the vagina. As the cancer progresses, it typically spreads to the bladder (producing frequent voiding and bladder pain, the rectum (causing bleeding), vulva (causing lesions), pubic bone (producing pain), or other surrounding tissues.

DIAGNOSTIC TESTS
The diagnosis of vaginal cancer is based on the presence of abnormal cells on a vaginal Pap smear. Careful examination and biopsy rule out the cervix and vulva as the primary sites of the lesion. In many cases, however, the cervix contains the primary lesion that has metastasized to the vagina. Then any visible lesion is biopsied and evaluated histologically.

The entire vagina may be difficult to visualize because the speculum blades may hide a lesion, or the patient may be uncooperative due to discomfort.

When lesions are not visible, colposcopy is used to search out abnormalities. Painting the suspected vaginal area with Lugol's solution also helps identify malignant areas by staining glycogen-containing normal tissue while leaving abnormal tissue unstained.

TREATMENT
Vaginal cancer may be treated with chemotherapy, surgery, or radiation, depending on its stage.

Early-stage cancer
In the early stages, treatment aims to preserve the normal parts of the vagina. (Preservation of a functional vagina is generally possible only in the early stages).

Topical chemotherapy with fluorouracil and laser surgery can be used for carcinoma in situ and carcinoma limited to the vaginal wall (the earliest stages of vaginal cancer). Radiation or surgery varies with the size, depth, and location of the lesion and the patient's desire to maintain a functional vagina. Survival rates are the same for patients treated with radiation as for those with laser surgery.

Late-stage cancer
Surgery is usually recommended only when the tumor is so extensive

Metastasis patterns in vaginal cancer

A cancerous lesion in the upper third of the vagina (the most common site) usually metastasizes to lymph nodes in the groin. A lesion in the lower third (the second most common site) usually metastasizes to the hypogastric and iliac nodes. A lesion in the middle third of the vagina metastasizes erratically.

A posterior lesion displaces and distends the vaginal posterior wall before spreading to deep layers. By contrast, an anterior lesion spreads more rapidly into other structures and deep layers because, unlike the posterior wall, the anterior wall of the vagina is not flexible.

that exenteration is needed, because close proximity to the bladder and rectum permits only minimal tissue margins around resected vaginal tissue.

Radiation therapy is the preferred treatment for advanced vaginal cancer. Most patients need preliminary external radiation treatment to shrink the tumor before internal radiation can begin. Then, if the tumor is localized to the vault and the cervix is present, radiation (using radium or cesium) can be given with an intrauterine tandem or ovoids; if the cervix is absent, a specially designed vaginal applicator is used instead.

To minimize complications, radioactive sources and filters are carefully placed away from radiosensitive tissues, such as the bladder and rectum. Internal radiation lasts 48 to 72 hours, depending on the dosage.

SPECIAL CONSIDERATIONS
For the patient receiving internal radiation:
• answer the patient's questions, and

encourage her to express her fears and concerns.
• Because the effects of radiation are cumulative, be sure to wear a radiosensitive badge and a lead shield (if available) when you enter the patient's room.
• Check with the radiation therapist concerning the maximum recommended time that you can safely spend with the patient when giving direct care.
• While the radiation source is in place, the patient must lie flat on her back. An indwelling catheter is inserted (usually in the operating room), and the patient's bed linens changed only if they become soiled. Only partial bed baths are given. The patient's call bell, phone, water, or anything else she needs must be kept within easy reach.
• The patient will be on a clear liquid or low-residue diet and an antidiarrheal drug to prevent bowel movements.
• To compensate for immobility, encourage the patient to do active range-of-motion exercises with both arms.

 TEACHING TIP: Instruct the patient to use a stent or do prescribed exercises to prevent vaginal stenosis. Coitus is also helpful in preventing stenosis.

Valvular heart disease

In valvular heart disease, three types of mechanical disruption can occur: stenosis, or narrowing, of the valve opening; incomplete valve closure; or prolapse of the valve. These disruptions can result from such disorders as endocarditis, congenital defects, and inflammation; they can lead to heart failure.

Valvular heart disease occurs in varying forms:
• In mitral insufficiency, blood from the left ventricle flows back into the left atrium during systole, causing the atrium to enlarge to accommodate the backflow. As a result, the left ventricle dilates to allow for the increased volume of blood from the

atrium and to compensate for diminishing cardiac output.

• In *mitral stenosis,* narrowing of the valve by valvular abnormalities, fibrosis, or calcification blocks blood flow from the left atrium to the left ventricle. Consequently, left atrial volume and pressure rise and the chamber dilates. Greater resistance to blood flow causes pulmonary hypertension, right ventricular hypertrophy, and right-sided heart failure. Inadequate filling of the left ventricle produces low cardiac output.

• In *mitral valve prolapse,* one or both valve leaflets protrude into the left atrium. Mitral valve prolapse is the term used when prolapse is accompanied by signs and symptoms unrelated to the valvular abnormality.

• In *aortic insufficiency,* blood flows back into the left ventricle during diastole, causing fluid overload in the ventricle, which enlarges. Excess volume overloads the left atrium and, finally, the pulmonary system. Left-sided heart failure and pulmonary edema eventually result.

• In *aortic stenosis,* left ventricular pressure rises in an effort to overcome the resistance of the narrowed valvular opening. The added workload increases the demand for oxygen, and diminished cardiac output causes poor coronary artery perfusion, ischemia of the left ventricle, and left-sided heart failure.

• In *pulmonic insufficiency,* blood ejected into the pulmonary artery during systole flows back into the right ventricle during diastole, causing fluid overload in the ventricle, ventricular hypertrophy and, finally, right-sided heart failure.

• In *pulmonic stenosis,* obstructed right ventricular outflow causes right ventricular hypertrophy, eventually resulting in right-sided heart failure.

• In *tricuspid insufficiency,* blood flows back into the right atrium during systole, decreasing blood flow to the lungs and left side of the heart. Cardiac output also diminishes. Fluid overload in the right side of the heart can eventually lead to right-sided heart failure.

• In *tricuspid stenosis,* obstructed blood flow from the right atrium to the right ventricle causes the right atrium to enlarge. Eventually, this leads to right-sided heart failure and increased pressure in the vena cava.

CAUSES

Valvular heart disease may result from such disorders as congenital heart defects, endocarditis, rheumatic fever, myocardial infarction, ruptured chordae tendineae, hypertrophic cardiomyopathy, mitral valve prolapse, severe left ventricular failure, hypertension, syphilis, or pulmonary hypertension.

SIGNS AND SYMPTOMS

Clinical features depend on which valve is affected. For example, a patient with mitral stenosis may experience dyspnea on exertion and while sleeping, along with weakness, fatigue, arrhythmias, and a chronic, nonproductive cough. A patient with aortic insufficiency may experience dyspnea on exertion and when sleeping, along with night sweats, cough, fatigue, and anginal pain.

If valvular disease leads to heart failure, the patient will experience signs and symptoms of heart failure. (See "Heart failure," pages 132 to 135.)

DIAGNOSTIC TESTS

Tests used to diagnose valvular heart disease may include cardiac catheterization, X-rays, echocardiography, electrocardiography, and color-flow Doppler studies. Findings vary with the specific type of valvular disease.

TREATMENT

Therapy depends on the nature and severity of associated signs and symptoms. For example, heart failure warrants digoxin, diuretics, a sodium-restricted diet and, in acute cases, oxygen.

Other measures may include anticoagulant therapy to prevent thrombus formation around diseased or replaced valves, prophylactic antibiotics before and after surgery and dental care, and valvuloplasty.

If the patient has severe signs and symptoms that can't be managed medically, open-heart surgery using cardiopulmonary bypass for valve replacement is indicated.

SPECIAL CONSIDERATIONS
● Reinforce instructions on diet, medications, and follow-up care.
● If the patient will have valve replacement surgery, instruct him to report shortness of breath, chest pain, or dizziness after discharge. Assure him that he will be able to do light chores when he leaves the hospital and should be able to resume normal activities in about 6 weeks.

Vascular retinopathies

Vascular retinopathies are noninflammatory disorders of the retina resulting from interference with blood supply to the eyes. The five types of vascular retinopathy are central retinal artery occlusion (rare), central retinal vein occlusion, diabetic retinopathy, hypertensive retinopathy, and sickle cell retinopathy.

CAUSES
When one of the arteries maintaining blood circulation in the retina becomes obstructed, blood flow diminishes. This damages the eye and causes visual deficits.

Causes of *central retinal artery occlusion* include embolism, atherosclerosis, infection, or conditions that retard blood flow, such as temporal arteritis, carotid occlusion, and heart failure. Sometimes, the cause is unknown.

Central retinal vein occlusion may result from external compression of the retinal vein, trauma, diabetes, thrombosis, granulomatous diseases, generalized and localized infections, glaucoma, and atherosclerosis.

Diabetic retinopathy results from juvenile or adult diabetes. This condition is a leading cause of acquired adult blindness.

Hypertensive retinopathy results from prolonged hypertensive disease, producing retinal vasospasm, and consequent damage and arteriolar narrowing.

Sickle cell retinopathy results from impaired ability of sickled cells to pass through the microvasculature, producing vaso-occlusion. This leads to microaneurysms, chorioretinal infarction, and retinal detachment.

SIGNS AND SYMPTOMS
Central retinal artery occlusion produces sudden, painless, unilateral vision loss (partial or complete). The condition typically causes permanent blindness.

Central retinal vein occlusion leads to reduced visual acuity, allowing perception of only hand movement and light. This condition is painless, except when it results in secondary neovascular glaucoma.

Nonproliferative diabetic retinopathy produces changes leading to a decrease in or blockage of blood flow within the retina. Although the condition sometimes causes no symptoms, it can result in significant loss of central visual acuity and diminished night vision.

Proliferative diabetic retinopathy produces fragile new blood vessels on the disk and elsewhere. These vessels may grow into the vitreous and then rupture, causing sudden vision loss. Formation of scar tissue along the new blood vessels may lead to macular distortion and even retinal detachment.

Signs and symptoms of hypertensive retinopathy depend on the location of retinopathy. For example, mild visual disturbances such as blurred vision result from retinopathy located near the macula. Without treatment, 50% of patients become blind within 5 years. With treatment, prognosis varies with the severity of the disorder; severe, prolonged disease eventually produces blindness.

DIAGNOSTIC TESTS
Diagnostic studies depend on the type of vascular retinopathy. Diagno-

PATHOPHYSIOLOGY

Viewing vascular retinopathies

Ophthalmoscopic examination of a patient with a vascular retinopathy may reveal the changes seen here.

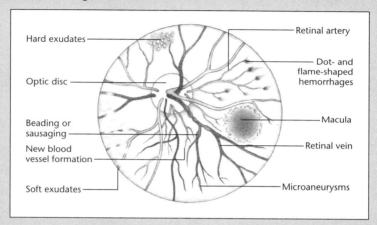

sis includes visual acuity testing and ophthalmoscopic examination. (See *Viewing vascular retinopathies.*)

TREATMENT
Treatment varies with the type of retinopathy.

Central retinal artery occlusion
No treatment has been shown to control central retinal artery occlusion. To reduce intraocular pressure, therapy includes acetazolamide, eyeball massage, anterior chamber paracentesis, and inhalation of carbogen (95% oxygen and 5% carbon dioxide).

Central retinal vein occlusion
Therapy may include aspirin, which acts as a mild anticoagulant. Laser photocoagulation can reduce the risk of neovascular glaucoma for some pa-

tients whose eyes have widespread capillary nonperfusion.

Diabetic retinopathy
Treatment for nonproliferative diabetic retinopathy is prophylactic. Careful control of blood glucose levels during the first 5 years of diabetes may reduce the severity of retinopathy or delay its onset.

The best treatment for proliferative diabetic retinopathy or severe macular edema is laser photocoagulation, which cauterizes the leaking blood vessels. Despite treatment, neovascularization doesn't always regress, and vitreous hemorrhage, with or without retinal detachment, may follow. If the blood isn't absorbed in 3 to 6 months, vitrectomy may restore partial vision.

Hypertensive retinopathy
Treatment includes control of blood

pressure with appropriate drugs, diet, and exercise.

SPECIAL CONSIDERATIONS

 ACTION STAT: A patient complaining of sudden, unilateral vision loss requires immediate ophthalmologic evaluation.
• Encourage diabetic patients to comply with the prescribed regimen to help prevent retinopathy.
• For patients with hypertensive retinopathy, stress the importance of complying with antihypertensive therapy.

Vasculitis

A broad spectrum of disorders, vasculitis is marked by inflammation and necrosis of blood vessels. Clinical effects depend on the vessels involved and reflect tissue ischemia caused by blood flow obstruction.

Prognosis varies. For example, hypersensitivity vasculitis is usually a benign disorder limited to the skin, but more extensive polyarteritis nodosa can be rapidly fatal.

Vasculitis can occur at any age, except for mucocutaneous lymph node syndrome, which affects only children. Vasculitis may be a primary disorder or may be secondary to other disorders, such as rheumatoid arthritis and systemic lupus erythematosus.

CAUSES

How vascular damage develops in vasculitis isn't well understood. It has been associated with a history of serious infectious disease, such as hepatitis B or bacterial endocarditis, and high-dose antibiotic therapy.

Excessive antigen theory

Current theory holds that vasculitis is triggered by excessive circulating antigen, which sets off a chain of events culminating in release of enzymes that cause vessel damage and necrosis, which may cause blood clot formation, occlusion, hemorrhage, and tissue ischemia.

Vascular damage may also result from the action of intracellular enzymes released by the cell-mediated (T-cell) immune response.

SIGNS AND SYMPTOMS
Clinical effects of vasculitis depend on the blood vessels involved. (See *Comparing clinical features of vasculitis types.*)

DIAGNOSTIC TESTS
Vasculitis is diagnosed from the patient history, various blood tests — especially an elevated erythrocyte sedimentation rate — and tissue biopsy showing findings characteristic of the vasculitis type present. Echocardiography is necessary to diagnose mucocutaneous lymph node syndrome.

TREATMENT
The aim of treatment is to minimize irreversible tissue damage associated with ischemia. In secondary vasculitis, treatment focuses on the underlying disorder. Primary vasculitis is treated mainly with drugs.

Treatment may involve removal of an offending antigen or use of anti-inflammatory or immunosuppressive drugs. Antigenic drugs, foods, and other environmental substances should be identified and eliminated, if possible.

Drug therapy in primary vasculitis commonly involves low-dose cyclophosphamide (2 mg/kg/day P.O.) with daily corticosteroids. In rapidly fulminant vasculitis, cyclophosphamide dosage may be increased to 4 mg/kg/day for the first 2 to 3 days, followed by the regular dose. Prednisone should be given in a dose of 1 mg/kg/day in divided doses for 7 to 10 days, with consolidation to a single morning dose by 2 to 3 weeks.

When vasculitis appears to be in remission or when prescribed cytotoxic drugs take full effect, corticosteroids are tapered to a single daily dose and then to an alternate-day schedule that may continue for 3 to 6 months before steroids are slowly discontinued.

SPECIAL CONSIDERATIONS
• Provide emotional support to help the patient and his family cope with

Comparing clinical features of vasculitis types

Signs and symptoms of vasculitis vary with the disease type.

TYPE	SIGNS AND SYMPTOMS
Polyarteritis nodosa	High blood pressure; muscle, joint, and abdominal pain; headache; weakness
Allergic angiitis and granulomatosis (Churg-Strauss syndrome)	Fever, malaise, anorexia, weight loss, severe asthmatic attacks, pulmonary infiltrates, purpura, cutaneous and subcutaneous nodules
Polyangiitis overlap syndrome	Combines symptoms of polyarteritis nodosa and allergic angiitis and granulomatosis
Wegener's granulomatosis	Fever, pulmonary congestion, cough, malaise, anorexia, weight loss, hematuria
Temporal arteritis	Fever, muscle pain, jaw muscle dysfunction, visual changes, headache (associated with polymyalgia rheumatica syndrome)
Takayasu's arteritis (aortic arch syndrome)	Malaise, pallor, nausea, night sweats, joint pain, loss of appetite, weight loss, pain or paresthesia distal to affected area, bruits, loss of distal pulses, fainting, double vision and transient blindness (if carotid artery is involved); may progress to heart failure or stroke
Hypersensitivity vasculitis	Palpable purpura, papules, nodules, vesicles, bullae, ulcers, chronic or recurrent urticaria
Mucocutaneous lymph node syndrome (Kawasaki disease)	Fever; nonsuppurative cervical adenitis; swelling; congested conjunctivae; redness of oral cavity, lips, and palms; scaly skin on fingertips; may progress to arthritis, myocarditis, pericarditis, heart attack, an enlarged heart
Behçet's disease	Recurrent oral ulcers; eye, genital, and skin lesions

an altered body image — the result of the disorder or its therapy. (For example, Wegener's granulomatosis may be associated with saddle nose, steroids may cause weight gain, and cyclophosphamide may cause alopecia.)

Ventricular aneurysm

A ventricular aneurysm is an outpouching — almost always of the left ventricle — that causes ventricular wall dysfunction. It occurs in about 20% of patients after myocardial infarction (MI), developing within weeks. Ventricular aneurysms enlarge but rarely rupture.

An untreated ventricular aneurysm can lead to arrhythmias, systemic embolization, or heart failure and may cause sudden death.

CAUSES

When MI destroys a large section of the left ventricle, necrosis reduces the ventricular wall to a thin sheath of fibrous tissue. Under pressure, this thin layer stretches and forms a separate noncontractile sac, an aneurysm.

SIGNS AND SYMPTOMS

A ventricular aneurysm may cause arrhythmias (such as premature ventricular contractions or ventricular tachycardia), palpitations, signs and symptoms of heart dysfunction (weakness on exertion, fatigue, angina) and, occasionally, a visible or palpable systolic precordial bulge.

The condition may also lead to left ventricular dysfunction, with chronic heart failure (dyspnea, fatigue, edema, neck vein distention); pulmonary edema; systemic embolization; and, with left-sided heart failure, pulsus alternans.

DIAGNOSTIC TESTS

Ventricular aneurysm is suspected in a patient with persistent ventricular arrhythmias, heart failure, or systemic embolization as well as a history of MI. Left ventriculography typically reveals ventricular enlargement, with an area of impaired movement and diminished function. Chest X-ray may show an abnormal bulge distorting the heart's contour if the aneurysm is large. Echocardiography shows abnormal left ventricular wall motion.

TREATMENT

Depending on aneurysm size and any complications, treatment may involve only routine medical examination to follow the patient's condition, or aggressive measures for intractable ventricular arrhythmias, heart failure, and emboli.

Emergency treatment for ventricular arrhythmias consists of I.V. antiarrhythmics or cardioversion. Emergency treatment for heart failure with pulmonary edema includes oxygen, digitalis glycosides I.V., furosemide I.V., morphine sulfate I.V. and, when necessary, nitroprusside I.V. and intubation. Maintenance therapy may include oral nitrates, prazosin, and hydralazine.

Systemic embolization warrants anticoagulation therapy or embolectomy. Refractory ventricular tachycardia, heart failure, recurrent arterial embolization, and persistent angina with coronary artery occlusion may call for surgery.

SPECIAL CONSIDERATIONS

 ACTION STAT: If cardiac arrest develops, cardiopulmonary resuscitation (CPR) must be initiated immediately and assistance should be obtained at once.

 TEACHING TIP: Before discharge, make sure the patient knows how to check for pulse irregularities and pulse rate changes.
● Because arrhythmias can cause sudden death, advise family members to attend a community-based CPR training program.

Vocal cord nodules and polyps

Nodules and polyps are benign growths on the vocal cords. Nodules, which result from hypertrophy of fibrous tissue, form at the point where the vocal cords come together forcibly. Polyps are swellings on the true vocal cord caused by edema in the lamina propria of the mucous membrane.

Both nodules and polyps have good prognoses, unless continued voice abuse causes recurrence with subsequent scarring and permanent hoarseness.

PATHOPHYSIOLOGY

How nodules cause hoarseness

Vocal cord nodules cause hoarseness by inhibiting proper closure of the vocal cords during phonation. The most common site of vocal cord nodules is the point of maximal vibration and impact (junction of the anterior one-third and the posterior two-thirds of the vocal cord).

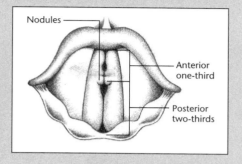

CAUSES

Vocal cord nodules and polyps usually result from voice abuse, especially in the presence of infection. Consequently, they're most common in teachers, singers, and sports fans and in energetic children who continually shout while playing. Polyps are common in adults who smoke, live in dry climates, or have allergies.

SIGNS AND SYMPTOMS

Nodules and polyps inhibit movement of the vocal cords and produce painless hoarseness. The voice may also develop a breathy or husky quality. (See *How nodules cause hoarseness.*)

DIAGNOSTIC TESTS

Persistent hoarseness suggests vocal cord nodules or polyps; visualization by indirect laryngoscopy confirms the disorder.

With nodules, laryngoscopy initially shows small red nodes and, later, white solid nodes on one or both cords. With polyps, laryngoscopy reveals sessile or pedunculated polyps of varying size, anywhere on the vocal cords.

TREATMENT

Conservative management of small vocal cord nodules and polyps includes humidification, speech therapy (voice rest, training to reduce the intensity and duration of voice production), and treatment for any underlying allergies.

When conservative treatment fails to relieve hoarseness, nodules or polyps are removed under direct laryngoscopy. For small lesions, microlaryngoscopy may be done to avoid injuring the vocal cord surface. Excision for bilateral nodules or polyps may involve two stages.

For children, treatment consists of speech therapy. If possible, surgery should be delayed until the child is old enough to benefit from voice training, or until he can understand the need to abstain from voice abuse.

SPECIAL CONSIDERATIONS

• After surgery, stress the importance of resting the voice for 10 to 14 days while the vocal cords heal. Provide an alternative means of communication, such as a Magic Slate, pad and pencil, or an alphabet board.
• A sign should be posted over the bed to remind visitors that the patient shouldn't talk.
• Minimize the need to speak by trying to anticipate the patient's needs.

TEACHING TIP: Advise the patient to use a vaporizer to increase humidity and ease throat irritation. If he smokes, encourage him to stop smoking entirely or at least to refrain from smoking during recovery.

• The patient may require speech therapy after healing because continued voice abuse causes recurrence of growths.

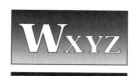

Warts

Warts (verrucae) are common, benign, viral infections of the skin and adjacent mucous membranes. Although their incidence is highest in children and young adults, warts may occur at any age.

The prognosis varies. Some warts disappear readily with treatment. Others necessitate more vigorous and prolonged treatment.

CAUSES

Warts are caused by infection with the human papillomavirus, a group of ether-resistant, DNA-containing papoviruses. The mode of transmission is probably through direct contact, but autoinoculation is possible.

SIGNS AND SYMPTOMS

Clinical manifestations depend on the type of wart and its location.

The *common* wart *(verruca vulgaris)* has a rough, elevated, rounded surface. It appears most commonly on the extremities, particularly the hands and fingers, and is most prevalent in children and young adults.

The *filiform* wart has a single, thin, threadlike projection. It commonly occurs around the face and neck.

The *periungual* wart has a rough, irregularly shaped, elevated surface. It typically appears around the edges of the fingernails and toenails. When severe, the wart may extend under the nail and lift it off the nailbed, causing pain.

The *flat* wart occurs in multiple groupings of up to several hundred slightly raised lesions with smooth, flat or slightly rounded tops. It is common on the face, neck, chest, knees, dorsa of the hands, wrists, and flexor surfaces of the forearms. Usually, flat warts occur in children but can affect adults. Distribution is commonly linear, because these warts can spread from scratching or shaving.

The *plantar* wart is slightly elevated or flat. It occurs singly or in large clusters (mosaic warts), primarily at pressure points of the feet.

The *digitate* wart is a fingerlike, horny projection arising from a pea-shaped base. It appears on the scalp or near the hairline.

Condylomata acuminatum (moist wart, also called genital wart) is usually small, pink to red, moist, and soft. For more information on this type of wart, see "Genital warts" on pages 114 and 115.

DIAGNOSTIC TESTS

Visual examination usually confirms the diagnosis. Plantar warts obliterate the natural lines of the skin, may contain red or black capillary dots that are easily discernible if the surface of the wart is shaved down with a scalpel, and are painful on application of pressure. Both plantar warts and corns have a soft, pulpy core surrounded by a thick callous ring; plantar warts and calluses are flush with the skin surface.

Recurrent anal warts require sigmoidoscopy to rule out internal involvement, which may necessitate surgery.

TREATMENT

Treatment of warts varies according to the location, size, number, pain level (present and predicted), history of therapy, the patient's age, and compliance with treatment. Treatment may include the following procedures.

• Electrodesiccation and curettage: High-frequency electric current destroys the wart, and is followed by surgical removal of dead tissue at the

base and application of an antibiotic ointment, covered with a bandage, for 48 hours. This method is effective for common, filiform and, occasionally, plantar warts.
• Cryotherapy: Liquid nitrogen kills the wart; the resulting dried blister is peeled off several days later. If initial treatment isn't successful, it can be repeated at 2- to 4-week intervals. This methods is useful for either periungual warts or for common warts on the face, extremities, penis, vagina, or anus.
• Acid therapy (primary or adjunctive): The patient applies plaster patches impregnated with acid (such as 40% salicylic acid plasters) or acid drops (such as 5% to 16.7% salicylic acid in flexible collodion) every 12 to 23 hours for 2 to 4 weeks. This method is not recommended for areas where perspiration is heavy, for those parts that are likely to get wet, or for exposed body parts where patches are cosmetically undesirable.
• 25% podophyllum in compound with tincture of benzoin (for genital warts): The podophyllum solution is applied on moist warts. The patient must lie still while it dries, leave it on for 4 hours, and then wash it off with soap and water. Treatment may be repeated every 3 to 4 days and, in some cases, must be left on a maximum of 24 hours, depending on the patient's tolerance.
  The use of antiviral drugs is under investigation. Suggestion and hypnosis are occasionally successful, especially with children. Compliance with prescribed therapy is essential.
• Carbon dioxide laser therapy: This procedure has been successful with genital warts.

SPECIAL CONSIDERATIONS

 TEACHING TIP: During acid or podophyllum therapy, instruct the patient to protect the surrounding area with petrolatum or sodium bicarbonate (baking soda).
• Podophyllum should be avoided in pregnant patients.

• Most persons eventually develop an immune response that causes warts to disappear spontaneously without treatment.

Appendices and Index

APPENDIX

1

Critical thinking self-test

Test your knowledge and skills at your own pace by answering the multiple-choice questions on pages 348 and 349. You'll find the answers along with rationales on page 349 and 350.

Mr. Jannas has diabetes mellitus and arterial occlusive disease. Yesterday, he underwent an embolectomy for a left femoral artery occlusion. Mr. Jannas is overweight and smokes heavily.

1. As you ambulate Mr. Jannas in the hall, he seems to grow short of breath. Based on what you know about him, your most appropriate action would be to:
a. run to get help.
b. ask him if he feels short of breath.
c. have him take a few deep breaths.
d. ask him to stand up straighter.

2. Mr. Jannas's blood glucose levels have been erratic since his admission to the hospital. The most likely reason is that:
a. he hasn't eaten much because he doesn't like hospital food.
b. he has just undergone surgery.
c. he's been receiving a different brand of insulin in the hospital.
d. he has lost several pounds since surgery.

3. While helping Mr. Jannas back to his bed, you notice blood on the dressing at his operative site. Your first action should be to:
a. assess the area to see if the blood is fresh or dry.
b. get help.
c. do nothing; this is a normal finding.
d. place another dressing on top of the bloody one.

When talking with your patient, Mrs. Grove, you notice that her eyes look opaque. She tells you her vision is failing, explaining, "After all, I'm old. What can I expect?"

4. Mrs. Grove says she can see better out of her left eye than her right. You suspect that's because:
a. she's left-handed, so the left side of her body is naturally stronger.
b. her symptoms suggest cataracts, which may progress at different rates bilaterally.
c. her eyeglass prescription may need to be changed or her frames adjusted.
d. she is old and somewhat confused.

5. Cataracts are most prevalent in:
a. people who have worn glasses most of their lives.
b. people over age 60.
c. people over age 70.
d. people with blue eyes.

Sally Rossi is a 56-year-old post-menopausal woman who has recently been admitted after being diagnosed with coronary artery disease (CAD). Her only previous hospitalization was during labor and delivery years ago, and she is very frightened.

6. Mrs. Rossi asks you if her heart problem is just another sign that menopause has placed her health on a downward spiral. Your best response would be to tell her:

Critical thinking self-test *(continued)*

a. "Yes, your heart and most vital organs are wearing out, but if you stay active, you should be all right."
b. "After menopause, you no longer have the natural protection against heart disease that estrogen provides. However, there may be other risk factors for CAD."
c. "I know you're upset about learning that you have heart disease, but I'm sure that everything will be OK once you start treatment."
d. "I know what you mean. My mother just started menopause, and I often wonder if she will have a heart attack."

7. Mrs. Rossi tells you she wants to learn everything she can about CAD. She mentions that she has seen some information about the disease on TV and on the Internet. Based on her statements, you should begin teaching her about CAD by:
a. asking her what she has learned so far.
b. providing a basic definition of CAD.
c. showing her a picture of the heart to help her understand the anatomy.
d. educating her about her medications.

8. After a visit by her doctor, Mrs. Rossi seems worried and upset. When you ask her what's wrong, she says, "He just told me I need a cardiac catheterization and then I might need surgery." Your best response would be to tell her:
a. not to worry, because worrying

isn't good for her heart and might cause angina.
b. that the doctor had to be truthful and that this test will tell him whether or not she needs surgery.
c. what the procedure entails, why it's necessary, what it will tell the doctor, and what the risks are.
d. that your father had a cardiac catheterization and he said it was easier to undergo than a CAT scan.

You enter the room of Mr. Vasquez, who's been admitted for pneumonia. He is coughing and appears very thin and pale.

9. He tells you that he even though he has the chills, he feels very hot. First you should:
a. check his temperature.
b. get a mask to protect yourself from his coughing.
c. give him another blanket.
d. check the thermostat in his room.

10. Mr. Vasquez has been taking his oxygen mask off frequently, complaining that it bothers him and he's fine without it. You should respond by:
a. letting him keep the mask off if this makes him more comfortable.
b. putting the mask back on him and telling him he must leave it on if he wants to get well.
c. turning down the oxygen flow rate so it won't bother him so much.
d. explaining how the humidification in the oxygen loosens his secretions and helps him breathe.

Answers and rationales

1. b. Because Mr. Jannas is overweight and a heavy smoker, he may have chronic dyspnea. Therefore, your first step is to ask him how he's feeling to determine if his shortness of breath is unusual.

2. b. Surgery is a major stressor on the body and can cause a patient's blood glucose level to fluctuate. Also, Mr. Jannas's caloric intake has been altered during his hospital stay because his oral intake has been withheld and he's been receiving I.V. fluids.

(continued)

Critical thinking self-test *(continued)*

Answers and rationales *(continued)*

3. a. You should first inspect the dressing to see if it's dry or moist. Dry blood is old and probably not a cause for concern. Moist blood is fresh and warrants closer inspection to determine the degree of bleeding. After inspection, you should report the bleeding. Because a moist dressing promotes bacterial growth, you should also place additional dressings over the original one.

4. b. Milky white pupils and visual blurring suggest cataracts. Usually occurring bilaterally, cataracts progress at different rates.

5. c. Cataracts are a normal part of aging and occur primarily in people over age 70.

6. b. Estrogen does seem to protect women against cardiovascular disease. However, a premenopausal woman who takes oral contraceptives, smokes cigarettes, and has a great deal of job stress is at increased risk for cardiovascular disease even though she's still producing estrogen.

7. a. Teaching should be geared toward the patient's current knowledge level. You should find out what the patient knows and correct any misunderstandings. Next, find out what she wants to learn — what aspects of the disease are most important to her. Then plan your teaching, making sure to include these points as well as other important topics.

8. c. You can reduce the patient's fears by providing her with accurate information about what she can expect and by explaining why this study is important in evaluating CAD. Be sure to present the information in clear, simple terms, and then give the patient a chance to ask questions.

9. a. High fever with shaking chills is common in pneumonia. Take his temperature first. The chills accompany the high fever because of evaporation of sweat and peripheral vasoconstriction.

10. d. In pneumonia, the infected area of the lungs doesn't function normally. Supplemental oxygen can support the patient's breathing effort as well as humidify the secretions by helping him cough up phlegm. Explaining the importance of oxygen therapy may motivate the patient to comply — unlike the response in option b., which provides no explanation.

APPENDIX
2

Other diseases and disorders

ADRENOGENITAL SYNDROME
Dysfunctional biosynthesis of adrenocortical steroids, leading to precocious puberty in boys and masculinization of external genitalia in girls

Causes: Inherited, or may result from another condition (usually an adrenal tumor)

Treatment: Daily cortisone or hydrocortisone therapy to normalize androgen production; in neonates with salt-losing congenital adrenal hyperplasia, immediate I.V. infusion of sodium chloride and glucose

ALCOHOLISM
Uncontrolled intake of alcoholic beverages that interferes with physical and mental health, social and familial relationships, and occupational performance

Causes: Various biological, psychological, and sociocultural factors

Treatment: Total abstinence with supportive programs offering detoxification, rehabilitation, counseling, and aftercare; disulfiram (for aversion therapy); tranquilizers; antipsychotic agents

AMYLOIDOSIS
Chronic disease in which starchlike, waxy glycoprotein (amyloid) accumulates, infiltrating organs and soft tissues and causing dysfunction of

kidneys, heart, GI tract, liver, and peripheral nerves

Causes: Inherited, or may accompany tuberculosis, chronic infection, rheumatoid arthritis, multiple myeloma, Hodgkin's disease, paraplegia, brucellosis, or Alzheimer's disease

Treatment: For associated renal failure — kidney transplantation; for cardiac amyloidosis — conservative treatment to prevent dangerous arrhythmias

APPENDICITIS
Inflammation of vermiform appendix; typically causes abdominal pain, rigidity, and tenderness accompanied by anorexia, nausea, and vomiting

Cause: Obstruction of intestinal lumen resulting from fecal mass, stricture, barium ingestion, or viral infection

Treatment: Appendectomy; if peritonitis develops — GI intubation, parenteral replacement of fluids and electrolytes, antibiotic therapy

ASCARIASIS
Infection caused by parasitic worm *Ascaris lumbricoides* (also called roundworm infection); may result in symptoms ranging from vague stomach discomfort to stomach pain, restlessness, vomiting, and intestinal obstruction

(continued)

Other diseases and disorders (continued)

Cause: Ingestion of soil contaminated with human feces that harbor *A. lumbricoides* ova

Treatment: Anthelmintic therapy (such as with pyrantel or piperazine and mebendazole)

ASPHYXIA
Life-threatening condition marked by insufficient oxygen and accumulating carbon dioxide in blood and tissues, resulting in cardiopulmonary arrest

Cause: Any condition that inhibits respiration, such as hypoventilation, intrapulmonary or extrapulmonary obstruction, or inhalation of toxic agents

Treatment: Immediate respiratory support with cardiopulmonary resuscitation, endotracheal intubation, and supplemental oxygen, along with correction of underlying cause

COCCIDIOIDOMYCOSIS
Infectious fungal disease occurring mainly as respiratory infection

Cause: Inhalation of *Coccidioides immitis* spores found in soil in endemic areas (such as southwestern United States), or inhalation of spores from dressings or plaster casts of infected persons

Treatment: For mild primary disease — bed rest and symptomatic relief; for severe primary disease with dissemination — long-term amphotericin B therapy and possibly lesion excision or drainage; for severe pulmonary lesions — lobectomy

COLD INJURIES
Injuries resulting from overexposure to cold air or water; may be localized (such as frostbite, which can lead to gangrene) or systemic (such as hypothermia, which can be fatal)

Causes: Frostbite — prolonged exposure to dry temperatures far below freezing, leading to formation and expansion of ice crystals in tissues; hypothermia — cold-water near drowning or prolonged exposure to cold temperatures, causing slowing of body functions

Treatment: For frostbite — rewarming of injured part, supportive measures, fasciotomy (if needed), or amputation (if gangrene occurs); for hypothermia — immediate resuscitation, rewarming, and careful monitoring

COLORADO TICK FEVER
Benign infection occurring in Rocky Mountain region of United States; typically causes fever, lethargy, headache with eye movement, and severe aching of back, arms, and legs

Cause: Bite from wood tick *Dermacentor andersoni* infected with Colorado tick fever virus

Treatment: Tick removal followed by supportive treatment

COMPLEMENT DEFICIENCIES
Deficiencies of proteins of complement system, which increase susceptibility to bacterial infection

Causes: Primary deficiencies — inherited; secondary deficiencies — complement-fixing immunologic reactions such as drug-induced serum sickness

Treatment: Measures to combat associated infection, collagen vascular disease, or renal disease; transfusion of fresh frozen plasma (controversial); bone-marrow transplantation

Other diseases and disorders (continued)

CRYPTOCOCCOSIS
Infectious disease resulting from fungus *Cryptococcus neoformans;* usually begins as asymptomatic pulmonary infection but may spread to other sites, such as central nervous system, kidneys, liver, skin, and bones

Cause: Inhalation of *C. neoformans* in particles of dust contaminated by pigeon feces that harbor this organism

Treatment: For pulmonary cryptococcosis — close medical observation for 1 year; for disseminated infection — amphotericin B or fluconazole

CUTANEOUS LARVA MIGRANS
Skin reaction to infestation by hookworm or roundworm that usually infects cats and dogs; usually manifests as transient rash or small vesicle followed by thin, raised, red line on skin, which may become vesicular and encrusted

Cause: Skin contact with animal feces containing hookworm or roundworm ova

Treatment: Oral or topical thiabendazole

DERMATOPHYTOSIS
Common superficial fungal infection of skin that may affect scalp (tinea capitis), body (tinea corporis), nails (tinea unguium), feet (tinea pedis), or groin (tinea cruris); results in lesions of varying appearance or duration

Causes: Direct contact with lesions infected with dermatophyte of genera *Trichophyton, Microsporum,* or *Epidermophyton* or indirect contact with contaminated articles (such as shoes, towels, or shower stalls)

Treatment: Imidazole cream, oral griseofulvin, or other antifungal agents; supportive measures (such as open wet dressings, removal of scabs and scales, and application of salicylic acid or another keratolytic)

DYSPAREUNIA
A condition in women in which sexual intercourse is accompanied by discomfort ranging from mild aches to severe pain

Causes: Physical problems (such as intact hymen, deformities or lesions of vagina or introitus, uterine retroversion, genitourinary tract infection, endometriosis, neoplasms, insufficient lubrication, or allergic reactions to condoms and other contraceptives); less commonly, psychological disorders (such as fear of pain or of injury during intercourse, recollection of painful experience, guilt feelings about sex, or fear of pregnancy, anxiety, or fatigue)

Treatment: For physical causes — creams or water-soluble gels for inadequate lubrication, appropriate medication for infection, excision of hymenal scars, gentle stretching of painful scars at vaginal opening; for psychological causes — sensate focus exercises, counseling and teaching about sexual activity and contraception

EPICONDYLITIS
Painful inflammation of forearm extensor supinator tendon fibers at their common attachment to lateral humeral epicondyle (also called tennis elbow)

Cause: Activity that requires forceful grasp, wrist extension against resistance, or frequent forearm rotation

Treatment: Pain relief through such measures as immobilization with splint, heat therapy, ultrasound,

(continued)

Other diseases and disorders *(continued)*

diathermy, physical therapy, use of "tennis elbow strap," local injection of corticosteroids and local anesthetics, and systemic anti-inflammatory therapy with aspirin or indomethacin; if necessary, surgery

ERECTILE DISORDER
Inability of a male to attain or maintain penile erection sufficient to complete intercourse (also called impotence)

Causes: Psychogenic factors (such as sexual anxiety or disturbed sexual relationship) or organic factors (such as alcohol-induced dysfunction, cardiopulmonary disease, diabetes, and multiple sclerosis)

Treatment: For psychogenic impotence — sex therapy; for organic impotence — correction of underlying cause, if possible, or psychological counseling

EXTRAOCULAR MOTOR NERVE PALSIES
Dysfunctions of third (oculomotor), fourth (trochlear), and sixth cranial (abducens) nerves

Causes: Diabetic neuropathy or pressure from aneurysm or brain tumor (most common cause); various diseases and disorders (including cerebrovascular disorders, poisoning, alcohol abuse, infections, myasthenia gravis, brain abscess, meningitis, and arterial brain occlusion); trauma to extraocular muscles; head trauma; or sinus surgery

Treatment: Treatment of underlying cause (such as neurosurgery for brain tumor or aneurysm)

GAUCHER'S DISEASE
Rare disorder of fat metabolism that results in widespread reticulum cell hyperplasia in liver, spleen, lymph nodes, and bone marrow; effects include pathologic fractures, collapsed hip joints, and severe pain in limbs and back (in type 1), motor dysfunction and spasticity (in type 2), and seizures, hypertonicity, poor coordination, and reduced mental ability (in type 3)

Cause: Inherited

Treatment: Supportive treatment as needed (such as vitamins, supplemental iron or liver extracts, blood transfusions, splenectomy, or analgesics), enzyme replacement therapy (experimental)

GOITER
Thyroid gland enlargement not caused by inflammation or a neoplasm

Causes: Endemic goiter — inadequate dietary intake of iodine; sporadic goiter — ingestion of certain drugs or foods

Treatment
Exogenous thyroid hormone replacement with levothyroxine; for endemic goiter caused by iodine deficiency — iodine therapy; for sporadic goiter — avoidance of goitrogenic drugs and foods; for either type — subtotal thyroidectomy if other treatments fail

GOODPASTURE'S SYNDROME
Chronic pulmonary hemosiderosis (deposition of antibodies against alveolar and glomerular basement membranes [GBM]) usually associated with glomerulonephritis; marked by cough with hemoptysis, dyspnea, anemia, and progressive renal failure

Cause: Unknown

Treatment: Plasmapheresis to remove GBM antibodies, immuno-

Other diseases and disorders (continued)

suppressive drugs to suppress GBM antibody production

HEAT SYNDROME
Life-threatening disorder of increased heat production or impairment of heat dissipation; may take the form of heat cramps, heat exhaustion, or heatstroke

Causes: Failure of heat loss mechanisms to offset heat production, precipitated by such conditions as high temperatures or humidity, exercise, infection, certain drugs, lack of acclimatization, excess clothing, obesity, dehydration, cardiovascular disease, or sweat gland dysfunction

Treatment: For heat cramps — salt tablets, balanced electrolyte drink, loosening of clothing, muscle massage, removal to cool place; for heat exhaustion — salt tablets, balanced electrolyte drink, loosening of clothing, placement in shock position, removal to cool place, muscle massage, and oxygen (if necessary); for heatstroke — life support, rapid cooling, replacement of fluids and electrolytes, nasogastric intubation, medications to treat severe effects of complications

HIRSCHSPRUNG'S DISEASE
Disorder of large intestine marked by absence or marked reduction of parasympathetic ganglion cells in colorectal wall; results in impaired intestinal motility and severe, intractable constipation

Cause: Congenital

Treatment: Daily colonic lavage to empty bowel until infant is old enough for corrective surgery; for total obstruction in newborn — temporary colostomy or ileostomy

HUNTINGTON'S DISEASE
Chronic progressive chorea and mental deterioration marked by degeneration in cerebral cortex and basal ganglia (also called Huntington's chorea); results in dementia

Cause: Inherited

Treatment: Supportive and symptomatic measures (such as tranquilizers or choline to control choreic movements), institutionalization (if appropriate)

HYDROCEPHALUS
Excessive accumulation of cerebrospinal fluid (CSF) in ventricles of brain, possibly resulting in brain damage; most common in neonates

Causes: Obstruction in CSF flow or faulty absorption of CSF

Treatment: Surgery (insertion of ventriculoperitoneal or ventriculoatrial shunt)

HYPERSPLENISM
Syndrome of exaggerated splenic activity and possibly spleen enlargement, resulting in peripheral blood cell deficiency

Causes: Idiopathic form — unknown; secondary form — extrasplenic disorder (such as chronic malaria, polycythemia vera, or rheumatoid arthritis)

Treatment: Splenectomy (only in transfusion-dependent patients who don't respond to medical therapy)

IMMUNOGLOBULIN A (IgA) DEFICIENCY, SELECTIVE
Deficiency of IgA leading to chronic sinopulmonary infections, GI diseases, and other disorders

Causes: Inherited, or may be associ-

(continued)

Other diseases and disorders *(continued)*

ated with autoimmune disorders (such as rheumatoid arthritis or systemic lupus erythematosus); transient IgA deficiency — use of certain drugs (such as anticonvulsants)

Treatment: Measures to control signs and symptoms of associated diseases, such as respiratory and GI infections

INCLUSION CONJUNCTIVITIS
Acute ocular inflammation resulting from infection by *Chlamydia trachomatis*

Cause: Transmission of *C. trachomatis* during sexual activity, during delivery (causing ophthalmia neonatorum in neonates), or through autoinfection (by hand-to-eye transfer of virus from genitourinary tract)

Treatment: For infants — eyedrops of 1% tetracycline in oil, erythromycin ophthalmic ointment, or sulfonamide eyedrops; for adults — oral tetracycline or erythromycin; for severe disease in adults — concomitant systemic sulfonamide therapy

INFERTILITY, FEMALE
Inability of a female to conceive after about 1 year of regular, unprotected intercourse or inability to carry pregnancy to birth

Causes: Functional factors (such as hormonal disorders), anatomic factors (such as anovulation, uterine abnormalities, tubal impairment, or cervical malfunction), or psychological factors (such as stress-induced stoppage of ovulation)

Treatment: For functional infertility — hormone therapy; for anatomic infertility — surgery, drug therapy, or such controversial methods such as surrogate mothering, frozen embryos, or in-vitro fertilization

INFERTILITY, MALE
Inability of a male to reproduce; suspected if a couple fails to achieve pregnancy after about 1 year of regular unprotected intercourse

Causes: Anatomic factors, semen disorders, sperm abnormalities, systemic diseases (such as diabetes), genital infections (such as gonorrhea and herpes), testicular disorders, genetic defects, immune disorders, endocrine imbalance, use of certain chemicals or drugs, sexual dysfunction

Treatment: For infertility caused by anatomic factors or infection — correction of underlying cause (such as through surgery, vitamin or hormonal therapy, adequate nutrition, or selective therapeutic agents); for infertility resulting from sexual dysfunction — education, counseling, or sex therapy

JUVENILE RHEUMATOID ARTHRITIS
Inflammatory disorder of connective tissues marked by joint swelling and pain or tenderness; may also involve skin, heart, lungs, liver, spleen, and eyes

Cause: Unknown

Treatment: Anti-inflammatory drugs, physical therapy, carefully planned nutrition and exercise

KERATITIS
Inflammation of cornea, which may be acute or chronic, superficial or deep; recurrent keratitis may lead to blindness if untreated

Causes: Infection by herpes simplex virus type 1, corneal exposure (due to inability to close eyelids), congenital syphilis, or bacterial or fungal infection

Other diseases and disorders (continued)

Treatment: For acute keratitis due to herpes — trifluridine eyedrops or vidarabine ointment; for chronic dendritic keratitis — vidarabine with long-term topical therapy; for fungal keratitis — natamycin; for keratitis due to exposure — moisturizing ointment applied to exposed cornea and eye shield or patch; for severe corneal scarring — corneal transplantation

LISTERIOSIS
Infectious disease caused by *Listeria monocytogenes,* a genus of gram-positive motile bacteria that infects shellfish, birds, spiders, and mammals; marked by circulatory collapse, shock, endocarditis, spleen and liver enlargement, and dark red rash over trunk and legs

Cause: Inhaling contaminated dust, drinking contaminated and unpasteurized milk, or coming in contact with infected animals, contaminated mud or sewage, or soil contaminated with feces containing *L. monocytogenes;* neonatal infection occurs in utero (through placenta) or during passage through infected birth canal

Treatment: Ampicillin or penicillin I.V.; alternatively, erythromycin, chloramphenicol, tetracycline, or trimethoprim sulfamethoxazole

MASTOIDITIS
Bacterial infection of mastoid process, usually occurring as complication of chronic middle ear infection

Causes: Infection with bacteria such as pneumococci, *Haemophilus influenzae, Moraxella catarrhalis,* beta-hemolytic streptococci, staphylococci, or gram-negative organisms

Treatment: For recurrent or persistent infection or intracranial complications — intense parenteral antibi-

otic therapy, myringotomy, simple mastoidectomy; for chronically inflamed mastoid — radical mastoidectomy

MULTIPLE ENDOCRINE NEOPLASIA
Hyperplasia, adenoma, or carcinoma of two or more endocrine glands

Cause: Inherited

Treatment: Surgical tumor removal and control of residual symptoms

MUMPS
Acute viral disease caused by a paramyxovirus; may be so mild as to go unnoticed or may cause muscle ache, headache, malaise, low-grade fever, earache, parotid gland tenderness and swelling, and pain on chewing

Cause: Airborne transmission of mumps paramyxovirus or direct contact with saliva of infected person

Treatment: Analgesics, antipyretics, adequate fluid intake

MUSCULAR DYSTROPHY
Group of congenital disorders characterized by progressive symmetric wasting of skeletal muscles without neural or sensory defects; occurs in four main types — Duchenne's, Becker's, fascioscapulohumeral, and limb-girdle

Cause: Inherited

Treatment: Orthopedic appliances, exercise, physical therapy, surgery to correct contractures

MYCOSIS FUNGOIDES
Rare, chronic, malignant T-cell lymphoma originating in reticuloendothelial system of skin and eventually affecting lymph nodes and internal organs

(continued)

Other diseases and disorders (continued)

Cause: Unknown

Treatment: Corticosteroid therapy, phototherapy, methoxsalen photochemotherapy, chlorethamine hydrochloride therapy, other systemic chemotherapy, total-body electron beam radiation

MYRINGITIS, INFECTIOUS
Inflammation of tympanic membrane; may result in gradual hearing loss (with granular myringitis)

Cause: Acute infectious myringitis — usually follows viral infection or infection with bacteria or any other organism that may cause acute otitis; chronic granular myringitis — unknown

Treatment: For acute infectious myringitis — analgesics and heat application, antibiotics to prevent or treat secondary infection, incision of blebs and evacuation of serum and blood; for chronic granular myringitis — systemic antibiotics or local anti-inflammatory antibiotic combination eardrops, surgical excision and cautery

NEUROGENIC ARTHROPATHY
Progressively degenerative disease of peripheral and axial joints resulting from impaired sensory innervation; loss of sensation in joints causes progressive deterioration from unrecognized trauma or primary disease

Causes: Diabetes mellitus (most common), tabes dorsalis, syringomyelia, myelopathy of pernicious anemia, spinal cord trauma, paraplegia, hereditary sensory neuropathy, Charcot-Marie-Tooth disease, frequent intra-articular injections of corticosteroids (theorized)

Treatment: Analgesics, restriction of weight-bearing, immobilization using crutches, splints, and braces; for severe disease — surgery or amputation (in severe diabetic neuropathy)

NEUROGENIC BLADDER
Bladder dysfunction caused by interruption of normal bladder innervation, which may lead to incontinence, residual urine retention, urinary tract infection, stone formation, and renal failure

Causes: Cerebral disorders (such as cerebrovascular accident, brain tumor, or Parkinson's disease), spinal cord disease or trauma, peripheral innervation disorders, metabolic disturbances, acute infectious diseases, heavy metal toxicity, chronic alcoholism, collagen diseases, vascular diseases, distant effects of cancer, herpes zoster, or sacral agenesis

Treatment: Bladder evacuation (such as with Credé's method or Valsalva's maneuver), drug therapy to promote bladder emptying and urine storage, or surgery to correct the structural impairment

NOCARDIOSIS
Acute, subacute, or chronic bacterial infection caused by weakly grampositive species of genus *Nocardia*; begins as pulmonary infection with cough and may spread to brain, kidneys, liver, subcutaneous tissue, and bone

Cause: Inhalation of *Nocardia* organisms suspended in dust or direct inoculation through puncture wounds or abrasions

Treatment: Long-term drug therapy with co-trimoxazole or sulfonamides (alternatively, ampicillin or erythromycin); surgical drainage of abscesses and excision of necrotic tissue

Other diseases and disorders *(continued)*

NYSTAGMUS
Recurring, involuntary eyeball movement classified as jerking or pendular; results in blurred vision and difficulty focusing

Causes: Jerking nystagmus — acute labyrinthitis, Ménière's disease, multiple sclerosis, vascular lesions, brain inflammation, drug or alcohol toxicity, congenital neurologic disorders; pendular nystagmus — corneal opacities, high astigmatism, congenital cataract, or congenital anomalies of the optic disk, bilateral macular lesions, optic atrophy, albinism

Treatment: Correction of underlying cause (if possible); eyeglasses to correct visual disturbances

OSGOOD-SCHLATTER DISEASE
Painful, incomplete separation of epiphysis of tibial tubercle from tibial shaft (also called osteochondrosis)

Causes: Trauma before complete fusion of epiphysis to main bone (between ages 10 and 15), locally deficient blood supply, genetic factors

Treatment: Leg immobilization for 6 to 8 weeks, with supportive measures such as activity restrictions, aspirin and, possibly, cortisone injections into joint; surgery if conservative measures fail

OTOSCLEROSIS
Slow formation of spongy bone in otic capsule; most common cause of conductive deafness

Cause: Inherited (presumably)

Treatment: Surgery (usually, removal of stapes and prosthesis insertion to restore partial or total hearing)

PEDICULOSIS
Infestation with parasitic lice; can occur as pediculosis capitis (head lice), pediculosis corporis (body lice), or pediculosis pubic (crab lice)

Causes: Head lice — direct contact with clothing, hats, combs, or hairbrushes infested with *Pediculus humanus* var. *capitis*; body lice — direct contact with clothing or bedsheets infested with *P. humanus*. var. *corporis*; crab lice — sexual intercourse, or contact with clothes, bedsheets, or towels harboring *Phthirus pubis*

Treatment: For head lice — permethrin creme-rinse (alternatively, pyrethrins or lindane shampoo); for body lice — bathing with soap and water, followed in severe infestation with lindane cream and removal of lice from clothes; for crab lice — lindane shampoo, repeated in 1 week

PENILE CANCER
Cancer of penis, producing ulcerative or papillary lesions that may become quite large before spreading beyond penis

Cause: Unknown

Treatment: Surgery, possibly with chemotherapy and radiation

POLIOMYELITIS
Acute communicable disease caused by poliovirus; may cause paralysis and death if it involves central nervous system

Cause: Direct contact with oropharyngeal secretions or feces contaminated with poliovirus

Treatment: For nonparalytic disease — supportive treatment (analgesics, moist heat, bed rest); for paralytic polio — bed rest, long-term rehabilitation using physical therapy, braces, corrective shoes

(continued)

Other diseases and disorders *(continued)*

and, possibly, orthopedic surgery

PSORIASIS
Chronic, recurrent disease marked by epidermal proliferations; causes plaques consisting of silver scales

Cause: Genetic tendency

Treatment: Palliative measures, such as removal of psoriatic scales, exposure to ultraviolet light (UVB or natural sunlight), drug therapy (steroid creams and ointments), Goeckerman and Ingram regimens (combinations of tar baths or anthralin with UVB treatments), PUVA therapy (psoralens and exposure to high-intensity UVA), or other drugs (such as methotrexate or etretinate)

RABIES
Acute central nervous system (CNS) infection caused by ribonucleic acid virus; almost always fatal if symptoms occur

Causes: Bite of infected animal that introduces virus through skin or mucous membrane and then spreads to CNS

Treatment: Wound treatment, tetanus-diphtheria prophylaxis (if needed), passive immunization with rabies immune globulin and active human diploid cell vaccine

RENAL INFARCTION
Formation of coagulated, necrotic area in one or both kidneys

Causes: Renal artery embolism secondary to mitral stenosis, infective endocarditis, atrial fibrillation, microthrombi in left ventricle, rheumatic valvular disease, or recent myocardial infarction; less commonly, atherosclerosis or thrombus from flank trauma, sickle-cell anemia, scleroderma, or arterionephrosclerosis

Treatment: Surgical repair of occlusion or nephrectomy, antihypertensives and low-sodium diet, intra-arterial streptokinase, lysis of blood clots, catheter embolectomy, heparin therapy

RESPIRATORY DISTRESS SYNDROME
Acute lung disease of newborn marked by airless alveoli, inelastic lungs, rapid and shallow respirations, nasal flaring, intercostal and subcostal retractions, grunting on expiration, and peripheral edema; occurs most often in premature infants and infants of diabetic mothers

Cause: Deficiency of pulmonary surfactant due to respiratory immaturity in premature newborns

Treatment: Vigorous respiratory support including warm, humidified, oxygen-enriched gases administered by oxygen hood or mechanical ventilation, thermoregulation using radiant infant warmer or an isolette, I.V. fluids, sodium bicarbonate, endotracheal administration of surfactant

RESPIRATORY SYNCYTIAL VIRUS SYNDROME
Respiratory infection that ranges in severity from mild coldlike symptoms to bronchiolitis or bronchopneumonia and, rarely, to severe, life-threatening lower respiratory tract infection; leading cause of lower respiratory tract infections in infants and young children

Cause: Infection by member of subgroup of myxoviruses that causes formation of giant cells or syncytia in tissue culture

Treatment: Respiratory support, maintenance of fluid balance, measures to relieve symptoms

Other diseases and disorders (continued)

REYE'S SYNDROME
Acute illness affecting children from infancy to adolescence that causes encephalopathy and cerebral edema

Cause: Follows an acute viral infection, such as upper respiratory infection, type B influenza, or chickenpox

Treatment: Reduction of intracranial pressure and cerebral edema, vitamin K to treat hypoprothrombinemia; if needed, endotracheal intubation, mechanical ventilation, mannitol, glycerol, barbiturate coma, decompressive craniotomy, hypothermia, or exchange transfusion

ROSACEA
Chronic skin eruption that produces flushing and dilation of small blood vessels in face; ocular involvement may result in blepharitis, conjunctivitis, uveitis, or keratitis

Cause: Unknown

Treatment: As needed, oral tetracycline, topical metronidazole gel, topical 1% hydrocortisone cream, or electrolysis to destroy dilated blood vessels

RUBELLA
Acute, mildly contagious viral disease that produces distinctive 3-day rash and lymphadenopathy (also called German measles); transplacental transmission can cause serious birth defects

Cause: Contact with blood, urine, stools, or nasopharyngeal secretions of infected persons; possibly, contact with contaminated clothing; transplacental transmission

Treatment: Aspirin to treat fever and joint pain

RUBEOLA
Acute, highly contagious paramyxovirus infection (also called measles); one of most common and most serious communicable childhood diseases

Cause: Direct contact with or inhalation of contaminated airborne respiratory droplets

Treatment: Bed rest, antipyretics, vaporizers, and warm environment; patient requires respiratory isolation throughout communicable period

SPINAL CORD DEFECTS
Congenital malformations of spine, such as spina bifida, meningocele, and myelomeningocele

Cause: Defective embryonic neural tube closure during first trimester of pregnancy

Treatment: For meningocele — surgical closure of protruding sac and continual assessment of growth and development; for myelomeningocele — repair of protruding sac and, possibly, shunt insertion to relieve associated hydrocephalus

SPRAIN
Complete or incomplete tear in supporting ligaments surrounding a joint

Cause: Overexertion or twisting of a joint beyond its normal range of motion

Treatment: For severe sprain — splinting, surgical repair (if ligaments are completely torn); for mild or moderate sprain — rest, ice application, elevation of injured limb, analgesics, minimal weight-bearing for several days

(continued)

Other diseases and disorders *(continued)*

STRAIN
Injury to a muscle or tendinous attachment

Cause: Sudden movement or overexertion

Treatment: Nonsteroidal anti-inflammatory agents, elastic bandaging, elevation of injured limb, ice application, weight-bearing restrictions (if needed)

TESTICULAR TORSION
Twisting of a testicle on its spermatic cord, impeding testicular blood supply and causing sudden, excruciating pain in or around testicle

Cause: Strenuous physical activity, other unknown factors; in newborn — abnormal development of genitourinary structures

Treatment: Manual manipulation or surgery to untwist the spermatic cord and return testicle to its normal position, followed by ice application, analgesics, scrotal support, and bed rest

TORTICOLLIS
Neck deformity in which sternocleidomastoid neck muscles are spastic or shortened, causing bending of head to affected side and chin rotation to opposite side

Causes: Congenital, or may occur secondary to muscle damage resulting from inflammatory disease, muscle spasm caused by central nervous system disorder, or psychogenic inability to control neck muscles

Treatment: For congenital torticollis passive neck stretching and proper positioning during sleep for infant, active stretching exercises for older child, surgical correction; for acquired torticollis — correction of underlying cause (such as with heat application, cervical traction, massage, stretching exercises, or neck brace)

VAGINISMUS
Involuntary spastic constriction of lower vaginal muscles, which may prevent intercourse

Causes: Physical factors such as hymenal abnormalities, genital herpes, obstetric trauma, or atrophic vaginitis; protective reflex to pain; psychological factors (such as guilty feelings about sex, fears resulting from traumatic sexual experiences, early traumatic experience with pelvic examination, or phobias of pregnancy, venereal disease, or cancer)

Treatment: Pelvic relaxation exercises, sex therapy, behavior therapy, psychoanalysis

VARICELLA
Common, acute, and highly contagious infection caused by herpesvirus varicella-zoster (also called chickenpox)

Cause: Direct contact (mainly with respiratory secretions or skin lesions); indirect contact (air waves); congenital varicella — acute maternal infection in first or second trimester of pregnancy

Treatment: Antipruritics, cool bicarbonate of soda baths, calamine lotion, antihistamine therapy; patient must be isolated until all vesicles and most scabs disappear

APPENDIX
3

Expected patient outcomes
for selected diseases

ACQUIRED IMMUNODEFICIENCY SYNDROME
• Patient remains free from chills, fever, and other signs or symptoms of illness or infection.
• Patient demonstrates use of protective measures, including conservation of energy, maintenance of balanced diet, and ability to get adequate rest.
• Patient demonstrates effective coping.
• Patient achieves diagnostic results indicating immune system improvement.

ACUTE RESPIRATORY FAILURE
• Patient maintains a respiratory rate within plus or minus 5 breaths per minute of baseline.
• Patient's arterial blood gas levels return to baseline.
• Patient reports feeling comfortable when breathing.
• Patient achieves maximum lung expansion with adequate ventilation.

ALZHEIMER'S DISEASE
• Patient remains safe and protected from injury.
• Caregiver identifies stressors that can and cannot be controlled.
• Caregiver identifies formal and informal sources of support.
• Family or significant other develops strategies to maintain patient's safety.

ASTHMA
• Patient remains free of adventitious breath sounds.
• Patient maintains a patent airway.

• Patient verbalizes an understanding of triggers for attacks.
• Patient reports signs and symptoms indicating the need for medical intervention.

BENIGN PROSTATIC HYPERPLASIA
• Patient maintains fluid balance, with intake equalling output.
• Patient verbalizes an understanding of treatment.
• Patient remains free of complications.
• Patient discusses impact of urologic disorder on self and family or significant other.

BREAST CANCER
• Patient acknowledges change in body image.
• Patient verbalizes feelings about change in body image.
• Patient verbalizes positive feelings about self.

CARDIAC ARRHYTHMIAS
• Patient maintains hemodynamic stability, as evidenced by stable vital signs.
• Patient's skin remains warm and dry.
• Patient remains free of complaints of chest pain.
• Patient maintains adequate cardiac output.

CARPAL TUNNEL SYNDROME
• Patient verbalizes relief of pain.
• Patient displays increased mobility.
• Patient demonstrates the ability to attain highest degree of mobility possible.
• Patient verbalizes feelings about limitations.

(continued)

Expected patient outcomes *(continued)*

CATARACT
• Patient discusses impact of vision loss on lifestyle.
• Patient expresses a feeling of safety, comfort, and security.
• Patient regains visual functioning.
• Patient states he plans to use appropriate resources.

CEREBROVASCULAR ACCIDENT
• Patient displays increased mobility.
• Patient maintains muscle strength and joint range of motion.
• Patient demonstrates ability to cope and adjust adequately.
• Patient and family or significant other display new coping strategies.

CHOLELITHIASIS
• Patient identifies specific characteristics of pain.
• Patient verbalizes relief of pain within a reasonable time after taking prescribed medication.
• Patient verbalizes possibility of physical pain being associated with dietary intake.
• Patient expresses a feeling of comfort.

CHRONIC FATIGUE AND IMMUNE DYSFUNCTION SYNDROME
• Patient identifies measures to prevent or modify fatigue.
• Patient explains relationship of fatigue to disease process and activity level.
• Patient verbalizes increased energy.
• Patient verbalizes plan to resolve feelings of fatigue.

CIRRHOSIS
• Patient shows no further evidence of weight loss.
• Patient tolerates oral, tube, or I.V. feedings without adverse effects.
• Patient maintains normal skin color and temperature.
• Patient maintains normal vital signs.

CORONARY ARTERY DISEASE
• Patient maintains hemodynamic stability
• Patient remains free of arrhythmias.
• Patient remains free from chest pain.
• Patient maintains adequate cardiac output.

CYSTIC FIBROSIS
• Patient maintains a patent airway.
• Patient remains free of adventitious breath sounds.
• Patient demonstrates the ability to breathe deeply and to cough to remove secretions.
• Patient shows no signs of pulmonary compromise.

DIABETES MELLITUS
• Patient and family members successfully incorporate components of therapeutic regimen into daily activities.
• Patient selects daily activities to meet the goals of treatment or prevention program.
• Patient and family members use available support services.
• Patient expresses intent to reduce risk factors for progression of illness.

DIVERTICULAR DISEASE
• Patient controls diarrhea with medication.
• Patient's elimination pattern returns to normal.
• Patient regains and maintains fluid and electrolyte balance.
• Patient practices stress-reduction techniques daily.

DYSMENORRHEA
• Patient verbalizes feelings about potential changes in sexual activity.
• Patient identifies specific characteristics of pain.
• Patient verbalizes possibility that physical pain is associated with emotional stress.
• Patient helps develop a plan for pain control.

Expected patient outcomes (continued)

ENCEPHALITIS
• Patient maintains body temperature within normal range.
• Patient exhibits no signs of compromised neurologic status.
• Patient's environment is modified to decrease stimulation.
• Patient maintains muscle strength and joint range of motion.

ENDOMETRIOSIS
• Patient reports freedom from pain.
• Patient verbalizes understanding of disorder.
• Patient acknowledges a problem or potential problem in sexual function.
• Patient expresses a willingness to obtain counseling.

EPIGLOTTITIS
• Patient maintains adequate ventilation.
• Patient maintains a respiratory rate within plus or minus 5 breaths per minute of baseline.
• Patient maintains arterial blood gas levels within the normal range.
• Patient reports ability to breathe normally.

GENITAL HERPES
• Patient verbalizes feelings about potential or actual changes in sexual activity.
• Patient expresses concern about self-concept, self-esteem, or body image.
• Patient states at least one effect of illness or treatment on sexual behavior.
• Patient and significant other state infection risk factors.

GLAUCOMA
• Patient discusses impact of potential vision loss on lifestyle.
• Patient expresses feelings of comfort, safety, and security.
• Patient regains visual functioning.
• Patient plans to use appropriate resources.

GLOMERULONEPHRITIS
• Patient maintains fluid balance, with intake equal to output.
• Patient remains free of complications.
• Patient discusses impact of urologic disorder on self and family or significant other.
• Patient maintains specific gravity within normal limits.

HEART FAILURE
• Patient reports feeling comfortable when breathing.
• Patient exhibits no pedal edema.
• Patient's cardiac workload diminishes.
• Patient and family or significant other state understanding of salt and fluid limits.

HEPATITIS, VIRAL
• Patient shows no further evidence of weight loss.
• Patient tolerates oral, tube, or I.V. feedings without adverse effects.
• Patient exhibits no evidence of skin breakdown.
• Patient shows normal skin turgor.

HERPES SIMPLEX
• Patient exhibits improved or healed lesions or wounds.
• Patient reports increased comfort.
• Patient expresses an understanding of skin care regimen.
• Patient verbalizes understanding of disease transmission.

HERPES ZOSTER
• Patient reports pain regimen success.
• Patient expresses feelings regarding changes in tactile perception.
• Patient exhibits improved or healed lesion or wounds.
• Patient remains free of skin breakdown.

(continued)

Expected patient outcomes (continued)

HIATAL HERNIA
• Patient reports no gastric reflux.
• Patient remains free of indigestion.
• Patient and family or significant other understand relationship of symptoms and dietary intake.
• Patient and family or significant other plan appropriate dietary modifications.

HYPERTENSION
• Patient's blood pressure remains within parameters established for him.
• Patient maintains fluid intake and output as recommended.
• Patient maintains blood urea nitrogen, creatinine, and sodium levels within acceptable limits.
• Patient demonstrates skill in selecting fluids and foods as permitted.

HYPOGLYCEMIA
• Patient expresses interest in learning new behaviors.
• Patient gradually sets realistic goals.
• Patient practices new health-related behaviors during hospitalization.
• Patient develops realistic plan for maintaining new skills at home.

LEUKEMIA
• Patient maintains adequate fluid and nutritional intake.
• Patient reports increased comfort.
• Patient remains free of complications.
• Patient verbalizes feelings about condition.

LYME DISEASE
• Patient expresses increased comfort.
• Patient remains free of complications.
• Patient, family, or significant other verbalize an understanding of disease prevention methods.
• Patient verbalizes an understanding of importance of taking medication.

MENINGITIS
• Patient maintains or attains an improved level of consciousness.
• Patient remains free of signs and symptoms of infection.
• Patient remains free of complications.
• Patient regains and maintains a normal body temperature.

MYOCARDIAL INFARCTION
• Patient remains free of further arrhythmias.
• Patient reports no chest pain.
• Patient identifies ability to cope and adjust adequately.
• Patient participates in health care regimen and plans care activities.

NEPHROTIC SYNDROME
• Patient maintains intake and output within prescribed limits.
• Patient maintains blood urea nitrogen, creatinine, sodium, and potassium levels within normal limits.
• Patient remains free of complications.
• Patient demonstrates ability to cope and adjust accordingly.

OSTEOARTHRITIS
• Patient reports no pain.
• Patient shows increased joint mobility.
• Patient tolerates medication regimen.
• Patient maintains daily exercise routine.

OSTEOPOROSIS
• Patient and family acknowledge presence of safety hazards in home.
• Patient acknowledges feelings and concerns about current situation.
• Patient makes decisions about course of treatment.

PANCREATITIS
• Patient maintains fluid intake and output within normal limits.

Expected patient outcomes *(continued)*

• Patient remains free of nausea and vomiting.
• Patient reports reduction in abdominal pain.
• Patient's laboratory values return to normal.

PEPTIC ULCER
• Patient experiences no further weight loss.
• Patient and family or significant other communicate understanding of special dietary needs.
• Patient's fluid intake and output remain within normal limits.
• Patient reports reduced abdominal pain.

PERICARDITIS
• Patient copes with current medical condition without demonstrating severe signs of anxiety.
• Patient reports feeing comfortable when breathing.
• Patient reports no pain.
• Patient's cardiac workload diminishes.

POLYCYSTIC KIDNEY DISEASE
• Patient maintains fluid balance.
• Patient maintains specific gravity within normal limits.
• Patient maintains nonfluctuating weight.
• Patient maintains hemodynamic stability.

PROSTATE CANCER
• Patient maintains fluid balance.
• Patient voices increased comfort.
• Patient expresses an understanding of treatment.
• Patient avoids bladder distention.

PULMONARY EDEMA
• Patient maintains blood pressure within prescribed parameters.
• Patient exhibits no pedal edema.
• Patient expresses comfort with breathing.

• Patient's urine output shows evidence of diuresis.

RENAL CALCULI
• Patient reports no pain.
• Patient verbalizes an understanding of the importance of straining all urine.
• Patient verbalizes an understanding of the importance of adequate fluid intake.
• Patient remains free of complications.

SALMONELLOSIS
• Patient controls diarrhea with medication.
• Patient's elimination pattern returns to normal.
• Patient regains and maintains fluid and electrolyte balance.
• Patient's skin remains intact.

THROMBOPHLEBITIS
• Patient expresses feeling of comfort or absence of pain at rest.
• Patient's peripheral pulses are present and strong.
• Patient's leg skin color and temperature remain normal.
• Patient demonstrates the ability to perform Allen exercises.

TUBERCULOSIS
• Patient expresses feelings associated with social isolation.
• Patient voices an understanding of disease transmission.
• Patient expresses an understanding of compliance with medication regimen.

ULCERATIVE COLITIS
• Patient controls diarrhea with medications.
• Patient's elimination pattern returns to normal.
• Patient regains and maintains fluid and electrolyte balance.
• Patient's skin remains intact.

(continued)

Expected patient outcomes *(continued)*

VALVULAR HEART DISEASE
• Patient maintains hemodynamic stability.
• Patient exhibits no arrhythmias.
• Patient is able to perform activities within limits of prescribed heart rate.
• Patient maintains adequate cardiac output.

Suggested readings

Corwin, E. *Handbook of Pathophysiology.* Philadelphia: Lippincott-Raven, 1996.

Cotran , R.S., et al. *Robbins Pathologic Basis of Disease,* 5th ed. Philadelphia: W.B. Saunders Co., 1994.

Everything You Need To Know About Diseases, Springhouse, Pa.: Springhouse Corp., 1995.

Huether, S., and McCance, K. *Understanding Pathophysiology.* Philadelphia: Mosby–Year Book Inc., 1996.

Isselbacher, K.J., et al., eds. *Harrison's Principles of Internal Medicine,* 13th ed. New York: McGraw-Hill Book Co., 1994.

Mulvihill, M. *Human Diseases: A Systematic Approach.* Norwalk, Conn.: Appleton & Lange, 1995.

Rakel, R.E., ed. *Conn's Current Therapy 1995.* Philadelphia: W.B. Saunders Co., 1995.

Thibodeau, G., and Patton, K. *The Human Body in Health and Disease.* Philadelphia: Mosby–Year Book, Inc., 1992.

Index

A

Abdominal aneurysm, 1
Acid loss, causes of, 204
Acquired hypogammaglobu-
    linemia, 68-69
Acquired immunodeficiency
    syndrome, 2-3
    drug treatment for, 3
    expected patient outcome
        for, 363
Acute angle-closure glauco-
    ma, 117-118. *See also*
    Glaucoma.
Acute febrile respiratory ill-
    ness, 7t. *See also*
    Adenoviral infec-
    tions.
Acute follicular conjunctivi-
    tis, 7t. *See also*
    Adenoviral infec-
    tions.
Acute glomerulonephritis,
    118-119
Acute herpetic stomatitis,
    302, 303
Acute leukemia, 182-184
    forms of, 183
Acute osteomyelitis, 219,
    220
Acute otitis externa, 222-223
Acute pharyngoconjunctival
    fever, 7t. *See also*
    Adenoviral infec-
    tions.
Acute poststreptococcal
    glomerulonephritis,
    118-119
Acute pyelonephritis. *See*
    Pyelonephritis,
    acute.
Acute renal failure. *See* Renal
    failure, acute.
Acute respiratory disease, 7t.
    See also Adenoviral
    infections.
Acute respiratory failure
    in COPD, 3-5
    expected patient out-
        comes for, 363
Acute transverse myelitis,
    209-210
    causes of, 210
Acute tubular necrosis, 5-6
Acyclovir, 114
Addisonian crisis, 8
Addison's disease, 8-9

Adenoviral infections, 6-8,
    7t
Adrenal crisis, 8
Adrenal hypofunction, 8-9
Adrenogenital syndrome,
    351
Adult respiratory distress
    syndrome, 9-10
Afro-Asian syndrome, 231
Agammaglobulinemia,
    68-69
Agranulocytosis. *See*
    Granulocytopenia.
AIDS. *See* Acquired immu-
    nodeficiency syn-
    drome.
Airway obstruction, prepar-
    ing for, 95
Alcoholism, 351
Allergic angiitis and granu-
    lomatosis, 341t. *See*
    also Vasculitis.
Allergic purpura, 10-11
    genitourinary features of,
        11
Allergic rhinitis, 11-12
ALS, 13
Alzheimer's disease, 12-13
    expected patient out-
        comes for, 363
    experimental drugs for, 12
Amyloidosis, 351
Amyotrophic lateral sclero-
    sis, 13
Anal fissure, 14
Anaphylactic reactions. *See*
    Anaphylaxis.
Anaphylactoid purpura, 10
Anaphylaxis, 14-16
    teaching patient how to
        use kit for, 15
Aneurysm
    abdominal, 1
    cerebral, 51-52
    femoral, 105-106
    popliteal, 105-106
    thoracic aortic, 313-314
    ventricular, 341-342
Angina, 71-72
Angioedema, 329-331
    triggers for, 330
Angioplasty, 72i, 73
Ankylosing spondylitis,
    16-17
    signs and symptoms of,
        17

Anorectal abscess and fistu-
    la, 17-18
Anorectal contracture, 18-19
Anorectal stenosis, 18-19
Anorectal stricture, 18-19
Antibody tests for HIV, 2
Antithyroid therapy, 159
Aortic arch syndrome, 341t.
    See also Vasculitis.
Aortic insufficiency, 337. *See*
    also Valvular heart
    disease.
Aortic stenosis, 337. *See also*
    Valvular heart dis-
    ease.
Aphthous stomatitis,
    302-303
Aplastic anemias, 19-20
Appendicitis, 20-21, 351
ARDS, 9-10
Argon laser trabeculoplasty,
    117
Arrhythmias, 46
Arterial occlusive disease,
    21, 23
    sites of, 21, 22i
Arthrodesis, 218
Arthroplasty, 218
Asbestosis, 23-24
Ascariasis, 351-352
Aspergilloma, 24
Aspergillosis, 24-25
    types of, 24
Asphyxia, 352
Asthma, 25-26
    expected patient out-
        comes for, 363
    forms of, 25
    treatments for, 26
Astrocytoma, 40. *See also*
    Brain tumors, malig-
    nant.
Atelectasis, 26-27
Atherosclerosis, 71
Atopic dermatitis, 27-28, 79
Autoimmune thrombocy-
    topenia, 165
Autoimmune thyroiditis,
    318
AZT, 3

B

Bacteremia, 283. *See also*
    Salmonellosis.
Bacterial conjunctivitis, 69,
    70

i refers to an illustration; t refers to a table.

i refers to an illustration; t refers to a table.

i refers to an illustration; t refers to a table.